A Companion Guide
for Wom...
Breast C...

De...

They

Sa...

...ancer

HOW...
A DIVISION...
NEW YORK LON...

...ompson

Author of the Woman to Woman Mentoring Series

Our purpose at Howard Books is to:
• Increase faith in the hearts of growing Christians
• Inspire holiness in the lives of believers
• Instill hope in the hearts of struggling people everywhere
Because He's coming again!

Published by Howard Books, a division of Simon & Schuster
1230 Avenue of the Americas, New York, NY 10020

Dear God, They Say It's Cancer © 2006 by Janet Thompson

ISBN-13: 978-1-58229-575-6
ISBN-10:   1-58229-575-1

10 9 8 7 6 5 4 3 2 1

HOWARD is a registered trademark of Simon & Schuster, Inc.

Manufactured in China

For information regarding special discounts for bulk purchases, please contact Simon & Schuster Special Sales at 1-800-456-6798 or business@simonandschuster.com.

Edited by Jennifer Stair
Interior design by Tennille Paden and Stephanie D. Walker
Cover design by John Lucas

To
Grace Marestaing, my "Grace Abounds,"
who mentored and loved me through my breast cancer journey and
continues to be my friend.

Leslie Furth and Nancy Tuttle,
who fought the good fight and finished the race.
Two breast cancer sisters who inspired and encouraged me
through their journals and their journeys.

Contents

Contents

Contents

Contents

Contents

Contents

Acknowledgments

I'M THANKING YOU, GOD, FROM A FULL HEART,
I'M WRITING THE BOOK ON YOUR WONDERS.

—*Psalm 9:1 MSG*

It takes a small village to write a book and an even bigger village to go to battle with breast cancer. My deepest love and gratitude go out to all who comprise my village.

My loving family. Dave, my godly hubby, helpmate, and lifeline through breast cancer, writing, and ministry. You make so many sacrifices for me in sickness and in health. I love you! Kim, "my baby." You are a loving daughter and my best friend. You and Toby so blessed me by efficiently taking over AHW Publishing. Shannon, Dan, and Joshua kept Grandpa company while I wrote at the cabin. Michelle, Giulio, Sean, and Janel encourage me; and my precious grandchildren bring healing, energizing joy, and fun into my life. I love you all so much.

My dearest Jane, cherished friend, speaking and traveling buddy, fellow ministry servant, and confidant. I pray I am half the friend to you that you are to me. I love you, my Enaj.

My "Grace Abounds," who mentored and prayed me through a new life journey.

Liz, who understood like no one else could because she had "been there, done that."

The Woman to Woman Mentoring team, who took the ministry beyond me. You rock!

Disciples of the Anne Ortlund group—Jeanette and Debbie for checking scriptures; Lorna for tracking down permission forms; Cathy, my "kitchen-packing angel," for all your faithful prayers for me to meet the goal.

The Woman to Woman Mentoring Ministry prayer chain, who cover me in prayer.

Linda and Sharron, my walking pals, who spurred me on with your encouragement and prayers.

My medical team, who used their expertise to prolong my life and care about me. Your names are certainly not in order of significance but how you sequenced into my life: Dr. James Carter; Dr. John West and the BreastCare Center & Oncology Center of Orange County; Donna Valentine PA-C; Barbara Ginesi, Patient Care Navigator, St. Joseph Hospital; Dr. Merry Tetif, Dr. Kenneth Tokita and the Irvine Cancer Center and Tokita Radiation Center; Mary Ann Green RT; and Frank De La Torre RT. You are all my Team Possible!

All the breast cancer sisters, plus Randy Niles and Bernard Wolfson, who openly and vulnerably share your stories and your hearts to help others on this journey. Health and peace.

Lesa Floyd and the women's ministry at Mobberly Baptist Church for giving me your ministry booklet *It's Breast Cancer*, which allowed me to meet new breast cancer sisters.

My pastor, Rick Warren, and Kay for pastoring my family and me and offering words of encouragement and inspiration from your own journey with breast cancer.

Jennifer Stair, for your careful editing and patience in teaching me what my computer and I are capable of and for always assuring me everything would be fine—this book is in God's hands!

Susan Wilson, my copy editor at Howard who continually reminded me that proofing should be fun, and the entire Howard Books team.

John and Chrys Howard; and Philis and Denny Boultinghouse, for embracing my vision.

My Lord and Savior, for using me and allowing me to live to write this book.

I thank God in remembrance of all of you.

INTRODUCTION

Sharing Sister to Sister

THE LORD WILL FULFILL HIS PURPOSE FOR ME; YOUR LOVE, O LORD, ENDURES FOREVER—DO NOT ABANDON THE WORKS OF YOUR HANDS.

—*Psalm 138:8*

IF ONLY MY WORDS WERE WRITTEN IN A BOOK—BETTER YET, CHISELED IN STONE!

—*Job 19:23–24 MSG*

I'LL WRITE THE BOOK ON YOUR RIGHTEOUSNESS, TALK UP YOUR SALVATION THE LIVE-LONG DAY, NEVER RUN OUT OF GOOD THINGS TO WRITE OR SAY.

—*Psalm 71:15 MSG*

1

Surviving for a Purpose

"Hi, my name is Janet Thompson. I am a breast cancer survivor."

Doesn't that sound like a recovery-meeting introduction? Many words associated with breast cancer trouble me. The worst offender is the word *survivor*. *Survivor* has become a household term from reality TV programs in which only the toughest, smartest, bravest, and most popular contestants survive the elements and win. To me, this is an unappealing concept. In heaven, the Lord says, the first will be last and the last will be first . . . and the sick will be well.

The branding *breast cancer survivor* created an internal struggle for me. My surviving insinuated others didn't—that made me sad. Having to survive in order to live—that made me mad. Maybe I wouldn't survive—that made me apprehensive. Stating I "survived" implies a hard struggle—that scared me. *Survivor* just didn't seem to fit me. I cringed every time someone used the word, especially when everyone felt the need to tell me stories of women who died from breast cancer, then ending with the *one* who survived. It was like fingernails on a chalkboard.

As I was settling in to write this book, the following press-release e-mail flashed across my computer screen:

> HOWARD SIGNS SADDLEBACK LEADER. Howard Publishing signed Saddleback Church (Lake Forest, CA) women's leader Janet Thompson for a book that encourages women battling breast cancer. Thompson, a breast cancer survivor, has an extensive national speaking ministry.

There it was for the entire world to see—I am a "breast cancer survivor." Like it or not, it is a fact; so I had better get used to it. I would love to tell you that happened and I now freely use the word *survivor*. Not the case. I continuously seek a new term to describe the ordeal because I'm more than just a "survivor"; I'm also a "winner"! You see, there is a spiritual battle going on around us—a battle for our souls, our hearts, and our minds—and God does not want us merely to survive this battle. He assures us that with His help we will be victorious. Wounded but not defeated. Not just surviving, implying we barely made it, but energized by running the race, staying the course, and fighting the good fight. Somehow, some way, we will be better women because of this experience.

I don't feel I just survived; rather, I believe God had a purpose and a plan in my breast cancer. He wanted my heart to break for every woman going through this. He intended for me to write this book and speak freely so others also might find purpose in their breast cancer.

It took me months to write the first words of this book. I wanted so badly for you to have it in your hands, but every time I thought about putting my journey into words, it seemed too painful. Finally, I cried out to God to release what was holding me back and discovered that freeing power came when I wrote through the pain and despite the pain.

Tears and sadness consumed me as I penned the first pages to you. But I broke through the wall as I poured out my thoughts and heart to the Lord and to you, and before long I wasn't crying anymore . . . well, most of the time.

This book is for you, my breast cancer sister. While I may not know you by name, I know you by heart. I understand your feelings and pain, and I want to walk beside you as only a friend who has been there can. *Dear God, They Say It's Cancer* is the book I longed for during my own breast cancer journey. Its purpose is to be a mentoring tool, a comfort, a companion, a journal, a record keeper, a devotional, and a source of information for you. It provides a place for you to take notes and store some of the pieces of paper you receive at doctors appointments along with treasured keepsakes. I trust it also will be an oasis of solace and comfort from the Lord's Word. My prayer is to mentor you from others' and my experiences and to wrap you in God's love.

Writing to you today, in early November, I have not yet reached my one-year surgery anniversary. This time last year, I was in limbo between finding out the biopsy was positive and waiting for the surgery date. There is no way to know in those countdown days how your life is about to change. You live in a continual state of shock. The world keeps going around, but yours has stopped. You desperately want to relive the day before you felt the lump or had the mammogram or the doctor said he thought he felt something in your breast. You pray, "Lord, could You just turn back the clock so I can replay those days and have them turn out differently?"

However, the minutes and days keep ticking by, the surgery date looms on your calendar, and you wonder what to do. *Do I live life as normal? How do I prepare? It doesn't really hurt or look that bad. Do I really need to do this? Maybe it will just go away. I'll wake up relieved that it was just a bad dream.*

Awakened from your thoughts by calls from the doctor's office, you are not sure which way to turn. Should you check out more information on the Web? Read more books? Talk to people? Who should you tell? How will they react? How and when do you tell your children? What about your job? What about your hair? What about your husband? You feel your life spinning out of control, filled with overwhelming decisions and public conversations about parts of your body you thought good girls kept private. Now everyone wants to take pictures, poke, and look at your breasts. Overnight, you have gone from modest to what feels like an exhibitionist!

My purpose in writing *Dear God, They Say It's Cancer* is to help you and me be more than women who do or do not "survive" breast cancer, but, instead, women who seek and find God's purpose in it. God never wastes a hurt. Nothing happens by accident in a believer's life. For each of us, God's plan and purpose will be different. I know my purpose is to share my God-given passion to raise the awareness of prevention and early detection of breast cancer, as well as help those on the breast cancer journey live a quality life in the secure arms of the Lord.

Where to Begin?

Dear God, They Say It's Cancer will be relevant wherever you are in your breast cancer or faith journey. This is your book to use in whatever way serves you best. There is no right or wrong way. The book starts at the beginning of your breast cancer journey and progresses through decisions, treatments, emotions, things to remember, things to forget, and tools to assist. Along the way it explores a gambit of feelings and circumstances we all share on this journey.

If newly diagnosed, you can start right from the beginning and journal as you go along, or you might choose to go to the topic touching your life that day. For those of you in the middle or maybe even several years past your breast cancer treatment, let this book be the means to work through any lingering feelings of grief, sorrow, hurt, and brokenness, as well as to remember joys and blessing. Each chapter has the following subsections:

The Topic Title—A quote from the Lord and/or a breast cancer sister.

 Dear God—My letter to God. A window into my breast cancer story.

 A Sister Shares—A fellow breast cancer sister shares her story.

 Mentoring Moment—Lessons learned, helpful tips, encouragement.

 God's Love Letter to You—Paraphrased scriptures to personalize.

 Let's Pray—Praying through a scripture or praying with me.

 Your Letter to God—Each chapter ends with encouraging prompts to help you journal your own breast cancer story.

Journaling

The journal section, "Your Letter to God," is one of my favorite parts of this book. It is an opportunity to record a major event in your life. If this is your first experience journaling, what a great time to start! Healing often happens when we talk about it—or write about it. Please don't be afraid or apprehensive. Journaling is simply writing down and documenting your feelings. Think of it as writing a letter to God. Not everyone understands how you feel, but God always understands, and He is eager to hear from you. No matter what faith you are or are not, you matter to God. God will fill the pages, nudging you toward helpful things to put down on paper. Maybe He will help you remember a good time to laugh about or a different way of looking at a person who said something hurtful without even knowing it. I suggest you pray before journaling and then let your pen flow freely. Some days you will write pages; other days you won't feel like writing more than a sentence. Here's what three breast cancer sisters said about journaling:

Once you start writing, it all comes back to you. I could go on and on! This book is exactly what all of us survivors need to document this miserable journey and to remember God's faithfulness and lessons learned. —Darlene Gee

I kept a journal of my feelings and the things for which I was grateful. —Nancy Tuttle[1]

Every day I wrote something—how I was feeling, things family and friends helped with, especially God's special blessings. It is important to journal because you can go back and read how faithful God was and still is! —Linda Taylor

One of my visions for *Dear God, They Say It's Cancer* is that it be a safe place to document an epic time in your life. Take this book with you to doctor appointments, tests, scans, mammograms, radiation, chemotherapy, the hospital, and wherever the twists and turns of your cancer journey take you. With your book in hand, you can . . .

- Take notes

- Journal

- Read

- Write questions to ask the doctors or technicians, and record their answers

- Read an encouraging story from a breast cancer sister

- Note something to remember about a fellow patient you meet

- Receive God's comfort from His "Love Letter" to you

You may need more than the space provided for journaling. If you feel up to a shopping trip, visit a stationery store and pick out a journal that reflects your personality. You may want it to be quite feminine and pink, which is the breast cancer color, or perhaps you prefer something more utilitarian. A spiral-bound notebook works fine too. If a trip to the store is not possible, ask someone to pick up a journal for you. Often, people want to get you something, and I have found you can never have too many journals.

Your journal will be personal. Don't feel you have to share it with anyone; however, as God did with me, He might give you the opportunity to mentor others with the wisdom and encouragement that comes from putting your thoughts into words. I am going to let you read my journal. I wish there had been a book like this to journal in while I was going through my breast cancer treatment. I grabbed whatever was available at the time. Unfortunately, my journey is scattered between Realtor notepads, scraps of paper in my purse, or whatever was handy by my bedside. I longed for a book to record everything in one place. For an organized person, breast cancer definitely caught me unprepared to make sense out of a confusing period.

My "Dear God" letters in this book are a compilation of reflections from those scattered notes, as well as current feelings. If you acquired this book after treatment, you may wish to follow my format in looking back at experiences combined with what you are currently encountering. I think you will agree that even after the intense treatment slows down, breast cancer always will be a part of your life. Hearing women speak in terms of how long they have been cancer free assures me breast cancer is now a permanent component of my persona.

Breast cancer sisters have confided in me that if they didn't journal during their journey, they now regret it. They long for a record of this life-impacting event to leave a legacy for future generations. During the heat of the battle with the daily barrage of decisions and assaults to your body, you often don't feel like doing or thinking anything. However, when the crisis subsides, you will wish you had written things down.

If you are in the group of women now looking back at the breast cancer journey, it's not too late. This book is for you too. While often writing my "Dear God" in the present, I am actually reflecting back from notes made along the way and from memory. You may be saying to yourself, "Memory? What memory? Between radiation, chemotherapy, Tamoxifen, or some other drug, my memory is shot." I thought the same thing, but when I took pen to paper or fingers to keyboard, God brought it all back to me, and I'm confident He will for you too!

If you are just beginning the journey and don't feel like journaling right now, just make notes in the lines provided in the margins and come back to it later.

If you are in the midst of your journey, some of your entries will be in the present, and other times you will write in the past tense.

Don't worry about grammar or spelling or sounding articulate. Remember, this is *your* book, and there is no right or wrong way to use it. By the way, the note-taking area in the margins is for you to use however you choose. You may want to write down what you are feeling as you read that page or note something you want to remember. This area gives you an opportunity to interact with the material you are reading.

I share parts of Nancy Tuttle's story in this book. Nancy's son, Randall Niles, who accepted Christ during his mom's breast cancer, found all her journals after she went to be with the Lord, and it changed his life. He says:

> One of the last messages Mom received from God was "to write." Although she never fully understood God's purpose for this calling, she accepted the challenge with a servant's heart. As her health declined, she was increasingly frustrated with her inability to focus. She was discouraged that her lack of physical strength prevented her from accomplishing God's work.

About one month after her death, God revealed to me that His calling for my mother was not yet complete. Through a series of visits and letters from Christian friends who knew and loved her, God hit my heart with the fact that I was part of this calling! As a prodigal son, I was integral to God's purpose for Mom's life!

Filled with conviction, I returned to her desk, computer, files, and bookshelves in order to discover the full impact of God's mission for us—as a Christian mother and prodigal son. I was stunned to find a wealth of material she had been inspired to write over the years. Letters, journals, testimonies, essays, church devotionals, Bible study notes—they were fantastic, rich with insight and heart. In tears, I collected my mother's works and spent that weekend reading. In prayer, I humbly realized that I was a prodigal son saved by God's patient grace. Through my mother's words, I saw that my relationship with Jesus was the ultimate hope and purpose for her life of fervent prayer.[2]

Maybe you are thinking, *I don't want anyone reading what I write.* That's OK too. No one has to read it but you. Make that clear to your family and friends and even put it in writing! Whether you have journaled regularly for years or this is your first time, let me assure you there is freedom and healing in expressing your thoughts and feelings in writing.

The best part about journaling is that God is ready to receive our words with a faithful, listening ear. He can take it all: the good, the bad, and the ugly. He beckons, "Come to me, all you who are weary and burdened, and I will give you rest. Take my yoke upon you and learn from me, for I am gentle and humble in heart, and you will find rest for your souls. For my yoke is easy and my burden is light" (Matthew 11:28–30). We can't refuse that offer.

Annually, I disciple a small group of women. Journaling prayers to the Lord is the first spiritual habit I introduce to them. You should hear the rumble around the table: "That doesn't seem natural." "I don't like to write. I just want to talk to God." "This is going to be hard." "Why do we have to do this when He can read our mind?" "I won't have the time!" Maybe these are some of your thoughts too.

After the protests fizzle down, I ask, "Does your mind ever wander when praying?" The unanimous answer is, "Always." Wandering minds are corralled when we journal. Then I probe deeper. "How often do you mean to pray, but the time just slips away?" Knowing looks and nodding heads around the table. Ah, that won't happen when we stop, sit down, and write out our prayers. Next, I ask, "Do you always remember everything you pray for? Do you go back and thank God for every answer?" The answer: "Of course not." So I encourage them, "Make journaling a habit and a spiritual discipline in your life, and I promise it will be a blessing!"

The group always struggles through the first few weeks, and then the breakthrough comes. The grumbles turn to, "I can't believe I have not done this my whole life!" "I really miss it when I don't take the time." "It has kept me faithful and focused during my quiet time with the Lord." Soon their journals are full, and they are buying new ones.

Let me give some tips to help journaling become a blessing for you too:

- Pray before you start.

- Select a journal that reflects your personality and style.

- Write your heart. Don't worry about grammar or sounding spiritual. Let your pen flow with your thoughts and feelings.

- Think of journaling as simply writing a letter.

- Date your journal entries.

- Experience journaling as a conversation. Freely write all that is on your heart and mind. By the way, prayer is simply talking or writing to God.

- You might want to reflect on my "Dear God" letters or comment on one of the "Sister Shares" stories or "Mentoring Moments" and how it applies to you.

- Just in case your mind goes blank, there are thought-provoking questions to get you going at the end of each chapter under "Your Letter to God." Don't feel confined to answering them. Write whatever you desire.

- If you want to write confidential things and worry someone might read your journal, come up with abbreviations and symbols only you understand.

- Don't feel you must be positive all the time. When it hurts, talk about it. When you are sad, cry out. When you are mad, God can take it.

- Express the good things that happen, too, and the days where everything does seem better.

- Journal in doctor or treatment waiting rooms, while receiving chemotherapy treatments, sitting in the car while your ride runs into the store for you, nights when you can't sleep, lying down to rest but your mind is racing, long hospital days and nights . . . let this book be your constant companion.

- Keep this book and your journal with your purse, and regard both with equal value. Your words to God, and His back to you, are treasures.

- If you aren't up to journaling and the pen seems too heavy, don't worry—it shouldn't make you feel guilty. When the time is right, you will get at it again. Maybe reading "God's Love Letter to You" will provide more comfort that day than writing.

- Use the "Prayer-and-Praise Journal" in appendix B (page 378) to record your prayer requests and God's answers.

Personalizing and Praying the Scriptures

Another purpose of this book is to be a devotional—a study of how God's Word, the Bible, applies to your life and specifically your breast cancer. No other book can give us the guidance, direction, peace, and answers we seek. The Bible is "a manual for living, for learning what's right and just and fair; to teach the inexperienced the ropes and give our young people a grasp on reality. There's something here also for seasoned men and women, still a thing or two for the experienced to learn—fresh wisdom to probe and penetrate, the rhymes and reasons of wise men and women. Start with God" (Proverbs 1:3–7 MSG).

I invite you to pray Psalm 32 with David, who wrote many of the psalms while running for his life and under great siege, so they apply to your and my life right now too. The Bible is your personal guide for life. There is no other like it. *Nothing else* will fill the deep need and hole in your heart except God and His words in the Bible.

Therefore, throughout this book we will be learning to pray through the Scriptures. That means we personalize them by putting our names in place of all the pronouns and/or adding personal pronouns . . . another name for this is paraphrasing. *The Message* (MSG) affords itself well to this because it is actually a paraphrase of the Bible rather than a literal translation in modern-day language like the *New International Version* (NIV) or the *New Living Translation* (NLT).

We will prayerfully personalize the Scriptures many times in the "Let's Pray" sections, and often I will join you in this prayer by adding my name. Since we are paraphrasing, these sections will not be the *exact* original text. Let's try it here to give you some practice:

Let's Pray

Prayerfully personalize Psalm 32:1–11 MSG by inserting your name in the blanks:

Count yourself lucky, how happy you, _____, must be—you, _____, get a fresh start, your slate's wiped clean. Count yourself lucky—God holds nothing against you, _____, and you're holding nothing back from him. When I kept it all inside, my bones turned to powder; my words became daylong groans. The pressure never let up; all the juices of my life dried up. Then I let it all out; I said, "I'll make a clean breast of my failures to God." Suddenly the pressure was gone—my guilt dissolved, my sin disappeared. These things add up. Every one of us needs to pray; when all hell breaks loose and the dam bursts we'll be on high ground, untouched. God's _____'s island hideaway, keeps danger far from the shore, throws garlands of hosannas around _____'s neck . . . Celebrate God. Amen.

The Lord and I want to walk with you through your breast cancer journey. I hope the "Mentoring Moments" give you some new ideas and helpful hints. In addition, many breast cancer sisters graciously contributed their stories to help encourage, inform, and mentor you. We pray it will give you inspiration to write *your own* story.

Things never seem as scary when you have a friend next to you. Ecclesiastes 4:9 says, "Two are better than one," but verse 12 adds, "a cord of three strands is not quickly broken"—the Lord, you, and me.

Your Victorious Breast Cancer Sister,

Janet

CHAPTER ONE

Making the Annual Appointments

I HAVE HEARD ALL ABOUT YOU, LORD, AND I AM FILLED WITH AWE BY THE AMAZING THINGS YOU HAVE DONE. IN THIS TIME OF OUR DEEP NEED, BEGIN AGAIN TO HELP US, AS YOU DID IN YEARS GONE BY. SHOW US YOUR POWER TO SAVE US.

—Habakkuk 3:2 NLT

It's That Time of Year Again

During my routine annual exam my doctor detected a small lump in my breast. He wasn't that concerned about it, but I was due for a mammogram anyway, since I was then forty. —Lisha

I squeezed a mammogram appointment into my busy travel schedule. —Heather

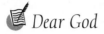 Dear God

Dear God,

Thank You for the reminder that I didn't receive the appointment letter for my annual October mammogram. When I called in September and told the receptionist of the oversight, she said, "Oh, I've been getting a lot of calls saying the same thing. We've had changes back there, and I guess they got behind." Behind? I never received a letter. All the emphasis on being diligent with annual mammograms, and she just shrugged this off like I was making a nail appointment. Oh, and now they can't see me until November 18. No worry though. It's just routine anyway. Father, please protect me, and don't let this delay be a problem. I also want to pray for all the other ladies who did not get their annual mammogram reminder letter. I hope they are diligent and remember to call anyway.

Thank You things went better setting the appointment for my annual physical with my gynecologist. It's in early October. What a relief! With these appointments set, I now can focus on the traveling and speaking engagements remaining this year.

Diligently Yours, Janet

A Sister Shares

For my fortieth birthday in April, at the recommendation of my gynecologist, I added a mammogram to my yearly workup. I went willingly as a firm believer in preventative healthcare. A week after my *first* mammogram, I was called back by the surgeon's office. There was a "thickening." Probably nothing, but a repeat mammogram was in order. The repeat mammogram indicated the thickening was not an illusion. A sonogram, or ultrasound, was done. As the surgeon closely examined my internal tissue, she explained that very often malignancies appear on sonograms as a starburst-type mass with a shadowy tail. "Let's do a core biopsy." She explained that she would insert a relatively large-gauge needle to extract a core of tissue, much like the bulb planter used by gardeners to remove a plug of dirt, though on a much smaller scale. She cautioned me that small tumors, she estimated mine at 5 mm, are sometimes hard to pinpoint in a core biopsy. A negative result was not necessarily a confident analysis. An excision biopsy would follow. —Bonnie[1]

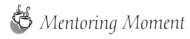 *Mentoring Moment*

Annual mammograms, breast self-examinations, and gynecological checkups, including clinical breast exams, are a must for every woman. Breast cancer is occurring at higher rates among younger women. I fervently encourage every woman, even in her twenties or thirties, if she has breast cancer in her family or feels something suspicious, to schedule an immediate appointment with her doctor. It doesn't mean she won't get breast cancer, but early detection increases the chances for complete recovery. At the age of thirty-five, I was a dietitian at a hospital that purchased its first mammogram machine, and they gave all the female staff free mammograms. That baseline mammogram started me on an annual schedule.

The American Cancer Society posts recommendations for all women on their Web site (www.cancer.org.) It reads:

> Women age 40 and older should have a screening mammo-gram every year, and should continue to do so for as long as they are in good health. Women in their 20s and 30s should have a clinical breast examination (CBE) as part of a periodic (regular) health exam by a health professional, preferably every 3 years. After age 40, women should have a breast exam by a health professional every year.
>
> Women at increased risk should talk with their doctor about the benefits and limitations of starting mammograms when they are younger, having additional tests, or having more frequent exams. Women should discuss with their doctor what approaches are best for them. Although the evidence currently available does not justify recommending ultrasound or MRI for screening, women at increased risk might benefit from the results.[2]

I will never forget an overnight hospital stay in my early twenties. All night I listened to the muffled crying of the woman in the other bed. She was having a mastectomy the next day. Repeatedly, she warned me *never* to put off annual checkups and mammograms, as she had done. I heeded her advice; it saved my life.

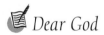 God's Love Letter to You

Dear_____, (fill in your name)

Do you not know that your body is a temple of the Holy Spirit, who is in you, whom you have received from me? You are not your own; you were bought at a price. Therefore honor Me with your body (1 Corinthians 6:19–20 paraphrased).
Your Creator, God

Let's Pray

Father, You made us women, crafting our bodies with breasts. We want to honor You with our bodies, and we understand that means avoiding sinful activities with our bodies, as well as taking excellent care of them. Life is Your gift to us in the form of breathing, functioning bodies. Our responsibility is to cherish this gift and do everything we can to keep our bodies in good, running order.

Lord, help us to encourage others to be diligent in scheduling regular examinations and tests. If we have been negligent in the past, we ask Your forgiveness and help in avoiding procrastination in the future. Thank You, Lord, for our bodies and breasts. Let us use and maintain them to Your glory. Amen.

The Suspicious Alarm

IN MY ALARM I SAID, "I AM CUT OFF FROM YOUR SIGHT!" YET YOU HEARD MY CRY FOR
MERCY WHEN I CALLED TO YOU FOR HELP. —PSALM 31:22

Dear God

Dear God,

Oh no! I had my annual October physical with my gynecologist, and he feels "something" in my right breast and wants me to have my mammogram at a breast care center out of the area. I told him I already had an appointment in November at my regular mammogram center, but he stressed I could get in right away at this new one. "They will do everything all in one place. The ladies appreciate that," he added. I assume "everything" means the mammogram and ultrasound he ordered as well as seeing the breast specialist while I'm there. I guess that would be convenient. I'm not worried though . . . it's just the "right-breast alarm" again.

I remember in my midforties receiving a call back for an ultrasound on my right breast after a routine mammogram. I really was nervous that time, because it had never happened before. Boy, did I praise You when it turned out there was no problem and the doctor only commented on my dense breasts full of great milk ducts! I cried. My husband, Dave, didn't understand why I was crying. Men just don't get it. It was such a release from the fear of not knowing. Dave and I celebrated with going out to dinner.

Then just five years ago during my annual physical, another doctor thought he felt a mass in my right breast. So, off to the specialist, only to find this, too, was just a false alarm. Lord, I am sure this is another right-breast false alarm, and my doctor wants me to drive such a distance to have the mammogram and see a new specialist. There is no breast cancer in my family. No reason to worry.

Cautiously Yours, Janet

 ## *A Sister Shares*

Back in 1975, I suffered for months with pain in my back and left arm. My doctor thought it was just a cyst. As the pain became more intense, I decided to consult a dear friend of our family, a doctor in San Antonio who had delivered my children. He told me to get on a plane and come to San Antonio for some tests. The first test was a mammogram, which showed I had advanced breast cancer. I was in a state of shock! Surgery was scheduled, and I had a radical mastectomy. The doctor came out of the operating room and told my husband, Tom, he believed all of the lymph nodes were cancerous and that I had only a short time to live.

When my husband and children came in to see me following the surgery, I knew they were very sad. I was unaware of the prognosis the doctor had given them. When the pathology report came back, it showed none of the lymph nodes were malignant! The nodes were hard and inflamed, but not cancerous. Praise God! I felt it was a miracle. Perhaps they detected the four-inch malignant tumor just before it could spread throughout my entire body! —Grace Bell

 ## *Mentoring Moment*

Grace Bell flew to another city, yet I complained about going twenty minutes out of my way to one of the best breast cancer centers and specialists in our area. When the alarm sounds, we need to diligently follow through, no matter how sure we are it is "nothing" or how far we have to travel. Maybe your alarm was a lump, soreness, or drainage, but whatever form it took, if you are reading this book, the alarm probably was something.

I know of one grandma who felt a suspicious lump in her breast and waited eighteen months to get it checked out. It was cancer. She seemed to know that all along but either didn't want to face it or didn't want to disrupt the family flow. I think it is natural for all of us to go into a period of denial. Worrying in advance does not help anything, but where there is a reasonable suspicion, we need to get it checked out ASAP.

God's Love Letter to You

Dear_____, (fill in your name)

Dear friend, guard clear thinking and common sense with your life; don't for a minute lose sight of them. They'll keep your soul alive and well; they'll keep you fit and attractive. You'll travel safely; you'll neither tire nor trip. You'll take afternoon naps without a worry; you'll enjoy a good night's sleep. No need to panic over alarms or surprises, or predictions that doomsday's just around the corner, because I will be right there with you; I'll keep you safe and sound (Proverbs 3:21–26 MSG paraphrased).
Your Protector, God

Let's Pray

Father, You know what a difficult time this is for us. We fear something is not right, and it is so hard not to worry as we go through the process of determining if there really is a problem. Lord, we come asking You to remove our worries, fears, and doubts. Let us put our energy and efforts into pursuing more information, and help us remember that worry does not come from You. Give us a calm spirit, and let this not be a distraction to the other things You are doing in our lives. We trust You and put our confidence in You alone. Amen.

Setting the Follow-Up Appointment

One evening in August 2001 when I was showering, I discovered a small lump on my right breast. I quickly told my husband what I'd found and not to worry. Nevertheless, I made an appointment with my family doctor, and he ordered a mammogram. —Gloria

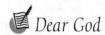 Dear God

Dear God,

Reluctantly, I set the appointment at the breast care center my gynecologist recommended. I had an immediate check in my spirit when they answered, "BreastCare and

Oncology Center." I didn't like hearing the word *oncology*. After all, I am only going for a mammogram. I don't have cancer for goodness' sake, and the term *oncology* makes me so uncomfortable. However, what a contrast to calling my regular mammogram center. Here they were apologetic of a two-week wait for the mammogram, ultrasound, and surgeon's appointment all in the same day! "Is that too late?" the receptionist asked. "Are you worried?" Before I could answer, she began telling me how worried she was about waiting two weeks for her own appointment with a doctor. Lord, there I was, comforting and assuring her two weeks was fine. There was no definite problem and this was a month earlier than the one I previously scheduled.

Reluctantly Yours, Janet

 ## A Sister Shares

With the results of the mammogram in hand, the doctor said, "It's just a cyst." At his suggestion, I saw a surgeon on November 1, 2001. The surgeon also verified the lump was just a cyst and told me to return for another checkup in six months. In the meantime, the lump was getting bigger, but I thought, *It's just a cyst*, so I didn't think any more about it.

When I returned to the surgeon in July 2002, he was surprised at how much the "cyst" had grown. Twice he attempted to drain it but was not successful. At this point I thought, *a cyst drains. Cancer doesn't.* The surgeon looked at me and said, "It needs to come out." I knew then it was cancer.

I had surgery on July 25, and it went well. Afterward, as the surgeon walked toward my husband and me, I sensed something was wrong by the look on his face. I was right. He told us, "It's cancer."
—Gloria

 ## Mentoring Moment

Still confident there was no problem, I put the appointment date on my calendar and continued with my schedule. Looking back, I see God protecting me from the anguish of worry. He says in the Bible, "Do not worry about tomorrow, for tomorrow will worry about itself. Each day has enough trouble of its own" (Matthew 6:34). These verses comforted my family and me through the days to come.

The difference between making an appointment for a "routine" and a "diagnostic" mammogram is quite significant, both to the mammogram center and to you. While arranging for a diagnostic mammogram means you will probably get an appointment sooner, it also moves you out of the ho-hum "It's that time of year again" attitude and into every woman's worst fear. It does not matter how rich or famous you are, this is stressful. Last night I heard Nicole Kidman interviewed after receiving an award for promoting women's health issues. On national TV, Nicole commented that she recently had a mammogram and was called back to take more x-rays. She explained that since her mother is a breast cancer survivor, it was an agonizing two-day wait to discover all was fine with Nicole.

Don't ever let the fear of finding out prevent you from making all the necessary appointments and following through with them. Fortunately, we live in an age of technology with incredible diagnostic tools to avert, treat, and often cure potential problems at early stages.

God's Love Letter to You

Dear_____, (fill in your name)
Shout for joy, O heavens; rejoice, O earth; burst into song, O mountains! For I, the LORD, comfort my people, and I have compassion for my afflicted ones (Isaiah 49:13 paraphrased).
Your Comforter, God

Let's Pray

Lord, You are our source of comfort, our shelter from the storm. We come to You with our worries and concerns and ask You to give us peace. Restore our faith where doubt prevails. Assure us with Your love that You always are near and will never leave or forsake us. Don't let us be overcome by apprehension and fear. Keep us diligent in our pursuit of good health. We love You, Lord. Amen.

It's Mammogram Day

I found the lump myself. The day I went for the mammogram and sonogram, God gave me Deuteronomy 31:8: "The LORD himself goes before you and will be with you; he will never leave you nor forsake you. Do not be afraid; do not be discouraged." God did indeed go ahead of me in many ways. —Linda Taylor

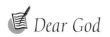 Dear God

Dear God,

Driving up to the BreastCare Center, the big letters on the next building sent a shiver down my spine: ONCOLOGY. *There is that word again,* I said to myself. *Only sick people with cancer need oncology. I don't have cancer—I'm not sick—I don't need oncology! I'm just here for a mammogram.* Parking a distance from *that* building, I averted my eyes from the sign as I prayerfully entered the building with a more assuring sign—the BreastCare Center.

When it was finally my turn, I noticed they had digital mammography. That's cool—high-tech! It was also comforting to see my neighbor Patty. She raves about working here. We exchanged pleasantries, and then another technician did my mammogram. Next, the breath-holding, nervous wait while the radiologist checks it. Uh oh, the technician called me back for more pictures. This time, she practically shoved my entire upper body into the viselike machine, grumbling all the while about the radiologist's wanting these difficult views. More waiting. Back for additional pictures. Finally, she said, "Your right breast looks fine, but since your doctor ordered an ultrasound, we have to do it." The ultrasound looked good. "Go get dressed." Relief!

Running into Patty on my way back to the dressing room, we chatted about her new kitchen remodel. Abruptly, my technician interrupted to say the radiologist wanted to talk to me. Patty suddenly looked serious and quickly ended our conversation. While dressing in that tiny cubicle, I heard Patty's voice outside the curtain saying to me: "Good-bye. Good luck! These are really great doctors." I assured her everything was just fine. "The technician told me the ultrasound looked great!" Buttoning my shirt, I felt an uneasy check in my spirit. Why had she come back to tell me this? Did she know something was wrong?

Emerging from the dressing room, I felt the first waves of apprehension. It almost felt like stepping out of real life into a movie—more as an observer than a participator. The technician ushered me into a dark room only slightly illuminated by several large, glaring computer screens. One screen had a baby picture on it, and a female radiologist sat working in front of another one. In typical grandma style, I babbled on about the baby. The radiologist asked me to sit next to her. She was all business—no baby talk. I sat down, awkwardly juggling my belongings in my lap. Right on top sat my Bible.

The radiologist didn't mince words. "Your problem is not on the right." Ah, a split second of relief as I let out my breath, only to quickly take it in again as she pointed to the screen and continued, "It's on the left. See these white spots? They are clustered calcifications. See how this large one has a ragged edge?" She kept talking, as busy doctors often do. "I am 99 percent sure they are cancer. You have two options—one is a needle biopsy to see if I am right, and that is about a thousand dollars—or the other is to go ahead with my opinion and schedule surgery to remove it. Either way, the choice is yours."

Surreal! Those white spots looked perfectly innocent. One minute I was chatting about a baby picture, now cancer . . . options . . . decisions. *I have cancer?!* The words resounded in my mind. My immediate thought was, *I am "one of them"! How should I react? What should I say? What questions should I ask? Don't I need more information to make this kind of decision?* I held on to the shred of possibility she was wrong. Surely, the surgeon would assure me this is just a false alarm like all the previous times.

The radiologist continued, not missing a beat. She would do the needle biopsy, and the surgeon I was to see next would do the surgery. "Do you have any questions? What do you want to do?" What should I ask?

I prayed, *Lord, help me respond intelligently. These are all new terms—calcium deposits that were always no problem before. Needle biopsy—is that painful? Where do they do it? Am I awake? What will it show them?* Eventually finding my voice, I asked these questions along with, "Did these show up in the previous films sent to you?" "No," she said. "This is the first time they increased in size for us to clearly see them. They can lay dormant for years. You probably didn't do anything to cause them. They are a mutation of cells."

She continued explaining that if I chose the needle biopsy, the procedure would be at this office. It would be painful, although they would numb the area, and I would lie on my stomach with my breast hanging through a hole in the table without moving for perhaps an hour. Did I want to see the room and table where they would perform it?

All I wanted to do was run! Awkwardly gathering my things and heading for the door, I heard over my shoulder, "By the way, if this helps in your decision, I don't get paid more whether you have the needle biopsy or not." I think she meant that to reassure me she was not trying to sell me on this. She really did think it was cancer and wanted me to take action. At least, that is how I received it. But it didn't make me feel better . . .

Nervously Yours, Janet

A Sister Shares

In the movie *Erin Brockovich*, Erin is helping a family when the wife learns she has breast cancer after already enduring uterine cancer. She sobs to Erin, "Whew, well, I'd got so used to having them come up benign. Guess I just didn't expect it. Oh, I sure wish I had longer to get used to the idea." Then she asks Erin, "Do you think if you've got no uterus and no breasts, you're still technically a woman?"

☕ *Mentoring Moment*

From our very first mammogram, we each develop our own coping style. Some go in with a certain amount of confidence that the card coming in the mail or the phone call will tell us, "All is well. We'll see you next year." Others sit on pins and needles. I don't think we ever prepare for bad news. Then one day it happens. Just like in the movie, the results are not normal. I don't know how I thought it would happen or how I would feel.

I went to this mammogram in complete denial. For whatever reason, I was so sure all would be fine. I had an extensive covering of prayer; it seemed inconceivable breast cancer could happen to me. My stance always has been that I would read up on breast cancer when and if it ever came up close and personal. If I didn't think about it, maybe it wouldn't happen to me.

Willing it not to happen does not work. We can't outrun breast cancer, but we can nip it in the bud, so to speak. Annual mammograms are a start, but women must do monthly breast self-exams so they know the feel of their breasts and can detect anything abnormal. Our role as breast cancer sisters is to help other women learn from our experience.

📖 *God's Love Letter to You*

Dear_____, (fill in your name)

Whoever obeys My command will come to no harm, and the wise heart will know the proper time and procedure. For there is a proper time and procedure for every matter, though your misery weighs heavily upon you (Ecclesiastes 8:5–6 paraphrased).
Wisely yours, God

🙌 *Let's Pray*

Prayerfully personalize Linda Taylor's verse, Deuteronomy 31:8:

The Lord himself goes before _____ and will be

with _____; he will never leave _____ nor forsake _____. Do not be afraid; do not be discouraged.

Thank You, Lord, for going before us in every step of the journey unfolding in our lives. It is so comforting to know You will never leave our side, no matter what the circumstances. We admit to being fearful and ask forgiveness for our doubts. We worship You and want to honor You in everything we do and say. Amen.

This Is Surreal!

I knew the nurses in the office, and they were very quiet when I arrived, but the sad look in their eyes gave them away. I could have left the office and known my results without seeing the doctor. —Martha[3]

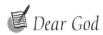 ## *Dear God*

Dear God,

I barely remember walking downstairs from the radiologist's office to the surgeon's waiting room and receiving a vibrating pager to await my appointment. My legs felt like Jell-O. I am sure a glazed look revealed my recent shocking news to all who looked my way. Sitting down and trying to absorb my surroundings, my eyes darted blankly around the room, filled with women obviously in cancer treatment. My heart sank. There were so many of them. *Lord, what is going on? This room is full, and it is only one of many such waiting rooms in Orange County alone!* Was I going to become one of them? Was this now my fate? A mere half-hour ago I lightheartedly chatted with my neighbor. Suddenly, without warning, my serene life was tumbling into an abyss. I felt alone. I didn't want to be here. Why hadn't I brought someone?

Lord, I prayed, *please be with me. I am scared.* It seemed I sat speechless for hours, staring into space, avoiding eye contact with anyone in the room. One regretful glance to the right took my breath away—a gift shop displaying wigs and head bandanas. The vibrating pager jumping on my leg mercifully jolted me from my racing, gloomy thoughts.

Lonely Yours, Janet

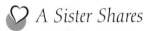 ## *A Sister Shares*

I was setting up my classroom for the fall in August, and I was actually annoyed at having to take time for a mammogram. I had to do it; I had cancelled a few months earlier. I rushed in, had the mammogram, and hurried back to my classroom. When I went home for lunch, a phone message said I needed to return for an ultrasound. This wasn't too earth shattering, since it had happened before. I had fibrocystic breasts and expected this was the reason for the callback. I had the ultrasound and drove home, suspecting nothing.

About 4:00 p.m. a nurse called and asked me to come back in with my husband, if possible. He met me there, and I felt rather numb, not upset. The doctor told us there was something suspicious about the ultrasound. We could schedule a biopsy, or he could try a fine needle aspiration now. I don't like waiting, so I told him to do the needle aspiration. He proceeded, and it really was a needle in my breast, through the side of my nipple to be exact. I don't really like pain, and this was excruciating! The doctor told me he might not have enough to tell anything but volunteered to wait around while the lab tested it.

It was about 6:30 now. The test came back positive and showed very aggressive cancer. I still felt no emotion. He wanted to schedule surgery as soon as possible, but I needed time to think this out and declined to schedule anything. —Lynn

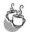 Mentoring Moment

If you are going for your diagnostic mammogram or surgeon's appointment, I suggest you take someone with you. Often we women don't want to bother others, but this is the time to call in favors from our best friend or ask a favorite relative to tag along for moral support. I felt so alone in the surgeon's waiting room. If all is OK, you have someone to celebrate with; and if it is unnerving news, someone is near for comfort while you cry, talk, shout, hug, pray, and maybe just to hold your hand while you wait.

God's Love Letter to You

Dear_____, *(fill in your name)*
    If you fall down, a friend can help you up (Ecclesiastes 4:10 paraphrased).
I will be with you, God

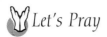 ## Let's Pray

Prayerfully personalize Psalm 42:5–8 NLT.

Magnificent Lord, boldly . . .

I, _____, will put my hope in God! I, _____, will praise him again—my Savior and my God! Now I, _____, am deeply discouraged, but I, _____, will remember your kindness. . . . I, _____, hear the tumult of the raging seas as your waves and surging tides sweep over me. Through each day the LORD pours his unfailing love upon me, _____, and through each night I, _____, sing his songs, praying to God who gives me life. Amen.

Meeting the Breast Specialist

In July 2002, I had my annual mammogram, followed by a spot compression mammogram. A few days later my doctor's nurse phoned to say I needed to consult a surgeon concerning the results. When I heard that, my heart sank immediately. —Anita

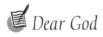 ## Dear God

Dear God,

I was so nervous. Everything happened so fast, yet part of me did want to get it over with quickly and behind us. As I was ushered into the exam room, we passed a man in greens talking to a workman about problems with the wood floor. From their conversation, I learned that this was a new building. Once in the exam room, the nurse took the usual information and then told me to undress from the top up and the doctor would be in to see me.

Boy, was I surprised when the door opened and the "man in greens talking to the workman" walked in and introduced himself as Dr. West! He apologized for keeping me waiting and then explained his concern over the Sunday grand opening for this new facility and the wood floor buckling. He seemed very nice, and I was trying to be sympathetic about the floor, but I was thinking, *I might have cancer. Please focus on me. I need your full attention. Get to know me. I need to know who you are. I have heard great things about you, but I don't know you.*

Instead of saying all that, I mumbled something about the floor and then went into a full explanation of what the radiologist had just told me. He was all business now . . . no lumps felt. I wasn't reassured; the problem was not a lump; it was calcium deposits. *I will never take another calcium supplement again,* I told myself.

"A high percentage of calcifications are benign," he assured me, pulling up my mammogram pictures and report on the computer screen. As if reading my mind, he added, "We call these calcifications, but they have nothing to do with your dietary intake of calcium." I reminded him of the radiologist's report. "She does seem pretty concerned about this," he noted, his voice subtly changing toward concern and a frown appearing between his eyebrows. "Let's get you scheduled for that needle biopsy."

Back upstairs to make the appointment. They insisted I take a tour of the biopsy room. Yes, it would be good for someone to drive me. Was I claustrophobic? Yes. Could I lie on my stomach for that long? I didn't know. I have a bad back, but I would try.

Appointment made, I headed for the car, carefully avoiding even a glance at the blatant ONCOLOGY sign on the building next-door. I was hanging on to the "high percentage of calcifications are benign" comment from the surgeon. That was a better statistic than the radiologist's. I prayed nonstop and sent an e-mail asking everyone I knew to pray this was just a scare and that I could lie still on my stomach for as long as they needed. And so we prayed.

Prayerfully Yours, Janet

A Sister Shares

I had seen the doctor, but Sue [her daughter] was in for her judgment. . . . He walked in with his cowboy boots on—after all, we were in Cowtown. . . . He sat down in his big, overstuffed chair—propped his elbow on his knee and fist under his chin, and said, "Your mother needs a mastectomy, and I recommend we remove both breasts."

You think it is quiet in the Carlsbad Caverns when they turn the lights out—we weren't even breathing or batting our eyes. . . . Finally, we came up for air and blurted out some silly question, and he gave us several answers we never heard—our ears were still dead. Color came back to our faces, and we looked at each other, and then we became human and could talk with a little knowledge and got down to serious business, and he was a right nice doctor . . . but he was as serious about me being double flat-chested as the day I was born.

"Mother, I don't like him. I sure wouldn't want to go to him with

a sore foot; he would cut off both feet." We both laughed out loud—now we could get down to serious talk. I agreed with her. If it ain't broke, don't fix it . . . but what if we liked the other doctor less? We could really choose as we had all the details taken care of, and I could cancel if need be. We both knew more about a mastectomy now than we had ever known in our life and would become more of an authority before this case was finished.
—Martha[4]

Mentoring Moment

My ministry is to women. Having gone through menopause myself already, I knew how scary that can be, so I started a file titled Menopause and saved helpful articles and information. My diagnosis was in October, which is National Breast Cancer Awareness Month. During this month, our local newspaper provides an entire special section devoted to breast cancer awareness. It includes many articles, as well as listing breast care facilities in the area. I had tucked the current one in my Menopause file.

Arriving home from my mammogram experience, I quickly tore upstairs and pulled out the Menopause file. I needed education fast. Browsing through the recent newspaper section on breast cancer, my eyes abruptly landed on a picture of two people I recognized. There was Dr. West, the surgeon who had just examined me, looking over the shoulder of the radiologist who had given me the dreaded suspected diagnosis. The article was about the new Orange County BreastCare Center & Oncology Center opening this month—the same place I had just left! It touted digital mammography, allowing the surgeon to immediately see the pictures and receive a quick report of the findings. What a major confirmation I was at the right place . . . buckling floors and all.

It is important to realize doctors are only human. They are very skilled, intelligent, brave people through whom God works and to whom He allots all their gifts and talents. Some doctors acknowledge that; others don't.

My breast specialist and surgeon, Dr. West, is a very capable and humble man whom I grew to appreciate. As we became acquainted, I could feel his care and concern for my recovery, and he always cheered me on with a reassuring hug. Realizing that a big focus in my life at the time was our home remodel helped me understand my doctor's concern with his facility's floor. It did not reflect his putting the floors as a priority over me. I had to extend grace and mercy to him, and you may need to do the same to your doctors.

Being comfortable with your doctor is so very important. I felt confirmed that I was where the Lord wanted me and saw His hand in getting me there. Remember, you have a choice in all this. You will spend hours with this doctor, so if you aren't clicking with him or her, you might want to try another one.

- Ask around to see if family or friends recommend a good breast specialist.

- Ask your gynecologist or family doctor for referrals.

- Check the Internet.

- Go to a support group, and talk to women there about their doctors.

- Pray.

I appreciate these words on the BreastCare Center brochure, which advise: "Select a health professional who is committed to quality breast care . . . a health practitioner who responds appropriately to your symptoms." I'll add, "Look for God's confirming hand in your final decision."

God's Love Letter to You

Dear_____, (fill in your name)
    Have no fear of sudden disaster. . . . I will be your confidence (Proverbs 3:25–26 paraphrased).
Your Confidence, God

Let's Pray

Father, You know us better than we know ourselves. You understand how badly we don't want even to have a breast cancer specialist in our lives—not to mention having to select one. Help us with our choices. Guide us and give us wisdom. We are tired and confused, and decisions don't come easily right now. Keep us sensitive to Your gentle nudging, and give us clear vision to recognize the signs of You at work in our lives. We praise You as the Great Physician. Amen.

Your Letter to God

How did your journey begin? When the doctor told you he was suspicious, what were your thoughts? Did something comfort you, or did you experience pure anguish? Describe awaiting the test results. Journal your thoughts and feelings when there was just suspicion but nothing definite. Share it with the Lord. Pour it out to Him. It helps, even through the tears. How might you help other women take proactive measures?

Dear God, _____ Date: _____

_____

_____

_____

_____

_____

_____

_____

_____

_____

_____

_____

_____

_____

_____

_____

_____

_____

_____

_____

_____

_____

_____

_____

_____

CHAPTER TWO

Facing the Dreaded Diagnosis

TELL ME, WHAT'S GOING ON, GOD? HOW LONG DO I HAVE TO LIVE?
GIVE ME THE BAD NEWS! . . . WHAT AM I DOING IN THE MEANTIME, LORD?
HOPING, THAT'S WHAT I'M DOING—HOPING. . . .
AH, GOD, LISTEN TO MY PRAYER, MY CRY—OPEN YOUR EARS.
DON'T BE CALLOUS; JUST LOOK AT THESE TEARS OF MINE.
I'M A STRANGER HERE. I DON'T KNOW MY WAY.

—*Psalm 39:4, 7, 12 MSG*

Life Is Messy Right Now

AND ME? I'M A MESS. I'M NOTHING AND HAVE NOTHING: MAKE SOMETHING OF ME.
YOU CAN DO IT; YOU'VE GOT WHAT IT TAKES—BUT GOD, DON'T PUT IT OFF.
—PSALM 40:17 MSG

I RUN FOR DEAR LIFE TO GOD, I'LL NEVER LIVE TO REGRET IT. DO WHAT YOU DO SO WELL:
GET ME OUT OF THIS MESS AND UP ON MY FEET. PUT YOUR EAR TO THE GROUND AND LISTEN,
GIVE ME SPACE FOR SALVATION. BE A GUEST ROOM WHERE I CAN RETREAT; YOU SAID YOUR
DOOR WAS ALWAYS OPEN! YOU'RE MY SALVATION—MY VAST, GRANITE FORTRESS.
—PSALM 71:1–3 MSG

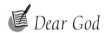 ## Dear God

Dear God,

Ironically, just like the BreastCare Center, we, too, were having work done at our home. We were remodeling the living room, dining room, and kitchen. So You helped me empathize with Dr. West and his floors. We were at the demolition stage where cement mixers and my kitchen stove sat in the middle of the living room—of course, You saw it all. Everything torn up, dust filled the air, and workers invaded my space each morning ready to make more of a mess. All of a sudden, life seemed messy.

Messily Yours, Janet

 ## A Sister Shares

On September 1, 2002, I felt a lump in my breast. I knew immediately in my heart it was cancer. Of course, I went through the usual thoughts of denial. I had just had a mammogram in May. My husband had died the previous September. This could *not* be happening! I had a daughter in college. I had to work! Then I began to pray, and it was as if I heard the Lord say, "I will take care of this." I immediately had a peace that continues through today. —Cheryl

 ## Mentoring Moment

Our life was in chaos. I longed for the comfort and security of a calm and peaceful home, while all around me destruction reigned with strangers traipsing in and out from morning until night. Maybe this was the Lord's way of taking my focus off myself and giving me something else to think about. However, all the plans for our home now took a backseat in light of the possibility of breast cancer.

More than likely you have something happening in your life, too, that makes this potential cancer crisis very inconvenient. Maybe . . .

- You are facing a deadline at work

- You're selling or buying a house

- You or one of your kids is planning a wedding or just got engaged

- You just started back to school or a new career

- You just met Mr. Right

- You just had a baby or, worse yet, are pregnant

- You have the trip of a lifetime planned

- It's the holidays, and company is coming to visit

- Like me, you are redecorating the house, *plus* it is the holidays and company's coming

- You have a major project planned

- You have a thesis or manuscript due

- You are preparing for a mission trip

- You just started a new ministry

- Or fill in the blank: _____

How did I know something was going on in your life? Because none of us wakes up one morning with the premonition we should plan breast cancer into our calendar. However, suspected breast cancer does put many things of this world into perspective, doesn't it? If we don't survive, who cares about our house or any of the plans we had? Someday it will all be gone, but our relationship with God endures forever.

God's Love Letter to You

Dear_____, (fill in your name)
Pile your troubles on my shoulders—I'll carry your load and help you out (Psalm 55:22 MSG paraphrased).
Your Burden Carrier and Caretaker, God

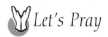 Let's Pray

Prayerfully personalize Philippians 3:7–9:

Lord, I am humbly coming before You to admit that . . .

I, _____, once thought all these things were so very important, but now I, _____, consider them worthless because of what Christ has done. Yes, everything else is worthless when compared with the priceless gain of knowing Christ Jesus, my Lord. I, _____, have discarded everything else, counting it all as garbage, so I, _____, may have Christ and become one with him. I, _____, no longer count on my own goodness or my ability to obey God's law, but I, _____, trust Christ to save me. For God's way of making us right with himself depends on faith. Amen.

It's Diagnostic-Test Day

As I moved through the biopsy, lumpectomy, MUGA Scan, CT scan, and bone scan, I knew God would take care of this in His way. —Cheryl

> Don't look the other way; your servant can't take it. I'm in trouble. Answer right now! Come close, God; get me out of here. Rescue me from this deathtrap.
> —Psalm 69:17–18 MSG

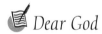 Dear God

Dear God,

You know how much I dreaded biopsy day. What an array of mixed feelings—thoughts of wanting it over, wrestling with apprehension about the needle-biopsy procedure, colliding with the nagging fear it was cancer. I am so glad Dave went along for moral support and to pray for me. Climbing on the table and positioning myself facedown with my breast hanging through a hole confirmed my fears. Boy, that was awkward. Trying to calm myself, I jokingly said they needed a head hole like a massage table so your neck doesn't crank to the side. As the words left my mouth, I realized the foolishness of that comment. I would be looking directly at everything they did. The technicians didn't think it was funny either. They were all business, covering me in a warm blanket with instructions to "get comfortable." Right! They cautioned that the radiologist didn't want patients talking, so I should lie perfectly still and be quiet. *Oh Lord, I need You now. You know neither of those things comes naturally.*

The technicians went right to work numbing the suspicious area and several times referred to "drilling" the needle into my breast and the "hook" they use to get the biopsy specimens. *Lord, You made me such a visual person—sometimes that's detrimental.* Immediately, Dave's power drill with a hook at the end came to mind. I felt faint. In walked the same radiologist who only days before had sent my world swirling with her "I'm 99 percent sure they are cancer" bombshell. Acknowledging my presence, she sat down on a stool and elevated the table where I lay with my breast suspended through the strategic hole with a vice tightly clamping it. "Hi," I mumbled, heeding the technician's warning not to talk. After a brief explanation of the procedure, the whirring drill fired up and my vivid imagination went wild. Heat filled my body. Using as few words as possible, I blurted out, "Take off the blanket!" They did.

"OK," the doctor said. "I'll go look at this and be back. You lie still." How could I do anything else? I wasn't going anywhere. Lord, how I prayed the feelings of panic and claustrophobia would subside. Deep breaths and many prayers to You kept me calm until the doctor returned, announcing she needed four more biopsies. FOUR MORE! The drill started whirring, and I started counting. That made it worse. Number three, I felt faint. I knew sometimes your fainting body jerks. What would happen to my clamped breast with a drill in it? Panicking, I spoke, "I think I am going to pass out." "Are you feeling it?" they asked. "No, I am *hearing* it," I cried. "Hold on." Then the infamous words, "We're almost done." But they meant done with the four drills. Again, the radiologist left the room to look at the samples. Mercifully, she returned quickly. She had enough. I couldn't get off that table fast enough.

Stumbling out to the waiting room, I saw such compassion in my husband's eyes. I knew he had been praying. Words could not convey to him what just happened, so I blurted out, "That was a torture chamber." He got the picture. Returning to my torn-up house, I laid down to reflect on the recent happenings. I must have slept from the sedation. I awoke to hearing the workers leaving. Walking out to check their progress, to my surprise, I saw a bouquet of flowers with a balloon and a bag of snacks. They were from my two dear friends, Jane and Cathy, who had been praying at the exact time of the biopsy. Those snacks, prayers, and friends were the beginning of a lifeline through my cancer battle and the chaos in both my life and house.

Painfully Yours, Janet

♡ A Sister Shares

At age thirty-nine, Margaret Kelly underwent her first mammogram. When the doctor's office called her back to redo the test, Margaret thought the follow-up was routine. When the office called a second time to schedule an ultrasound, she still saw no reason to be concerned. Fear didn't set in until she heard the word *biopsy*. A day later her doctor called to deliver news no woman wants to hear: *breast cancer*, and her survival depended on a double mastectomy.[1]

☕ Mentoring Moment

"What a wimp!" you might be saying about me. One woman I talked to had no problem with this biopsy. She even liked being tucked under the warm blanket—the same blanket I threw off. Again, we each are so unique and individual. This test was hard for me. If you had this or some other equally painful, awkward test, I hope your experience was less traumatic.

If you still have tests to endure, take someone with you. Even to a blood test. You have no idea how you will react. You are under a lot of stress. Knowing that someone is in the waiting room praying and will be there to give you a hug and drive you home brings such solace and comfort. When I became claustrophobic in the MRI tube, my friend Jane was with me and quickly started reading the Bible to me. I went from panic to peace.

📖 God's Love Letter to You

Dear_____, (fill in your name)
    As a mother comforts her child, so will I comfort you (Isaiah 66:13).
Your Comforter, God

🐰 Let's Pray

Oh Lord, hear our cry. We are scared—frightened. How did we come to this place in our lives? We will never make it through this without You, Lord. Please slow our rapid hearts, remove the sinking feeling in our stomachs, and soothe our aching heads and troubled minds. Let us feel Your presence during the tests. Give the doctors wisdom and clear vision to see and diagnose any problems. If it be Your will, we ask for good results. If the tests confirm our worst fears, give us grace and courage to take the next step to wellness. We depend on You. Wrap us in Your loving arms, and let us crawl up into Your lap. Today we need the comfort of our Abba, Daddy. Amen.

The Agonizing Wait for Test Results

I quietly talked with God and said, "Here I am again." To know you have a loving God and it will work out according to His plan is a great comfort. —Martha[2]

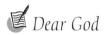 ## Dear God

Dear God,

Now we wait. The results will determine whether or not my life continues on as normal. For now I am just going to carry on business as usual. With so many speaking engagements coming up between now and the end of the year, at least there is work to keep my mind preoccupied. The radiologist said to call in three days.

We aren't talking about it much at home. In some ways it's like tiptoeing around an elephant in the living room, hoping if we don't acknowledge it, we won't have to admit its presence. For me, I am not going to spend my time worrying until I know positively there is something to worry about. Plus, here we are in the middle of this house remodel. Like Cathy e-mailed after delivering the balloons on biopsy day, "Honey, your house is a disaster!"

Praise You for so many distractions to help me focus on daily life. It normalizes this difficult time for all of us.

Impatiently Yours, Janet

 ## A Sister Shares

A few days after my annual mammogram in July, my doctor's office phoned me to say I needed to consult a surgeon concerning the results. When I heard that, my heart sank immediately. From that moment, I began to pray it was not cancer. Then I prayed, *Lord, if it is cancer, give me the grace to face it.* My husband and I had a trip to Europe planned for the first three weeks in August, and I was unable to consult with a surgeon until after our return. For a few days I let this news weigh on my mind. Then I thought, *This is silly. There's nothing I can do about it now. I'm going to enjoy my trip, and I will deal with this when I return. Besides, it may be nothing.* Thankfully, I was able to turn this over to the Lord, and we had a great time on our vacation. —Anita

☕ *Mentoring Moment*

My statement in the above prayer, "Praise You for so many distractions to help me focus on daily life," might seem like an oxymoron. Usually distractions take us off focus, but during the waiting period it is best to continue with life as planned before the threat of cancer entered the picture. My previously planned tasks, obligations, and to-dos helped distract me from worrying. Instead of my focus going to what might be, I kept my mind and energy on what was currently before me, as did Anita. I made a conscious decision not to speculate on pointless what-ifs. There would be plenty of time for that later if, indeed, the diagnosis was positive. Until then, there was work to do, trips to take, life to live.

If you are currently in this waiting period, try to keep your mind occupied with daily tasks, plans, and activities. Can you cherish these transition days and not jump ahead of yourself? If your diagnosis is positive, you will expend future time and energy on cancer; but until you know for sure, pray and ask others to pray you would have freedom from time and energy wasted on tormenting fears and anxiety.

📖 *God's Love Letter to You*

Dear_____, (fill in your name)
    Wait passionately for Me; don't leave the path (Psalm 37:34 MSG paraphrased).
Waiting with you, God

🙏 *Let's Pray*

Prayerfully personalize Psalm 130:5–7 MSG.

Coming before Your throne, O Lord . . .

I, _____, pray to GOD—my life a prayer—and wait for what he'll say and do. My life's on the line before God, my Lord, waiting and watching till morning, waiting and watching till morning,_____ waits and watches, for with GOD's arrival comes love, with GOD's arrival comes generous redemption. Amen.

They Say It's Cancer!

"It's cancer." My heart sank, and I held my breath with disbelief. My husband's eyes filled with tears and so did mine. I asked God to give me strength, and He did. —Gloria

PILE YOUR TROUBLES ON GOD'S SHOULDERS—HE'LL CARRY YOUR LOAD,
HE'LL HELP YOU OUT. —PSALM 55:22 MSG

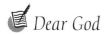 Dear God

Dear God,

"Call on Wednesday morning," the biopsy technician said. Impatient me called first thing. "No results yet. Try in the afternoon, or it might be a day or two more." The initial two-day wait was doable, but waiting another day . . . Why? What's wrong? Grabbing my cell phone, I headed out the door to run errands. There were tile samples to pick out—I was a woman with a house remodel going on.

That is how I happened to be sitting in my car in front of a tile store when I received the news. At 3:00 p.m., I called again. They were anxious to talk to me this time. "Hold just a minute . . . the radiologist wants to talk to you." Waiting for her to come to the phone, my eyes landed on a National Breast Cancer Awareness Month poster in the front window of the tile store. It touted a group of smiling women under a heading asking for breast cancer support. The women were bald or wearing bandanas. In those brief moments I pleaded my oft repeated, "Lord, please don't let me be one of those women. I don't want to have breast cancer. Please protect me from this!"

Even as I cried out to You, I knew doctors seldom come to the phone for good news. If she wanted to talk to me, it probably was to confirm her speculation. I don't remember her saying "Hello." In her quick, to-the-point manner, she said, "I was right; you have DCIS, ductal cancer in situ, which needs to be removed. You are going to be fine. You should have 100 percent recovery. Call the surgeon and set it up. Any questions?"

The cell-phone line crackled. Here I am staring at the breast cancer poster as she tells me I *am* one of them. I mumbled back, "Does this mean it's noninvasive?" Now she was getting a little perturbed. "Yes, I just told you it was in situ. Your prognosis is the best you can have." She didn't understand that *in situ* is a phrase she uses freely, but until a couple of days ago I never heard that term before. I needed reassurance I understood what it meant. Sometimes doctors forget they are talking a new language to their patients. "Good luck!" and she was off the phone. That was the same thing my neighbor Patty said after my mammogram. Luck was not what I needed now. What I needed was You, Lord, and lots and lots of prayer. That was the only sure thing I could count on—that was my only hope.

Still in shock, on-task me got out of the car and walked into the tile store, past the smiling faces on the breast cancer poster. I was on the verge of tears, and those breast cancer ladies had the audacity to smile back at me. How had they found something to smile about? I hope You keep a smile on my face. Holding back the tears, I waited as the store clerk helped another customer. Standing at the counter, my eyes fell on Breast Cancer Month brochures. I wanted to yell, "Help me so I can get out of here. I am one of these women. I just found out I have breast cancer. Help!" Finally, I left with tile samples in hand. I didn't take any of the Breast Cancer Month brochures. I wasn't ready yet to be one of them.

Hopefully Yours, Janet

 ## A Sister Shares

On November 1, 2001, I had an appointment for a mammogram and ultrasound in the morning, followed by an appointment with Dr. West, the surgeon who gave such excellent care to my mother. He did a fine-needle aspiration that afternoon. At 6:00 p.m. he called my office with the positive cancer diagnosis and set up a meeting for the next morning at 7:45 to discuss options. I had about a half-hour drive home that night, and I truly don't know how I made it. Even with my intuition confirmed, the reality of the word *cancer* was a shock. A year later, as I reflect on that day, I don't remember anything after my phone conversation—not even driving home. —Grace Marestaing

 ## Mentoring Moment

I let my impatience get the best of me. About to receive some of the most important information of my life, I took it on a cell phone in the car while running errands! What was I thinking? No one around to comfort and cry with me or share the call on another extension, making sure I got the facts straight. Like Grace, I also had to drive home alone. I would not recommend doing as we did. Instead . . .

- Receive news from doctors in a safe, comfortable place, preferably with someone you love and trust.

- Ask the doctor to wait while the other person gets on an extension phone.

- Give a pen and this book turned to the "Phone Notes" (page 359) to the other person, and instruct the person to write down what the doctor says. If it is just you, try to write down everything the doctor tells you.

- Ask another person to go with you to provide arms for hugging, a shoulder to cry on, and a prayer partner to pray with; or if the news is good, to celebrate with you.

📖 *God's Love Letter to You*

Dear_____, (fill in your name)

I am a good GOD, a hiding place in tough times. I recognize and welcome anyone looking for help, no matter how desperate your trouble (Nahum 1:7–8 MSG paraphrased).
Your Hiding Place, God

🙏 *Let's Pray*

Prayerfully personalize Psalm 39:2–7 NLT.

Father, You are our one and only hope . . .

As I, _____, stood there in silence—not even speaking of good things—the turmoil within me grew to the bursting point. My thoughts grew hot within me and began to burn, igniting a fire of words: "LORD, remind me, _____, how brief my time on earth will be. Remind me, _____, that my days are numbered, and that my life is fleeing away. My life is no longer than the width of my hand. An entire lifetime is just a moment to you; human existence is but a breath." We are merely moving shadows, and all our busy rushing ends in nothing. We heap up wealth for someone else to spend. And so, Lord, where do I, _____, put my hope? My, _____'s, only hope is in you. Amen.

Telling the Family

I don't remember when or how I told my parents, my sisters, my best friend—it is just a kind of blank. —Grace Marestaing

ALL HIS SONS AND DAUGHTERS CAME TO COMFORT HIM.
—GENESIS 37:35

FAMILIES STICK TOGETHER IN ALL KINDS OF TROUBLE.
—PROVERBS 17:17 MSG

📝 *Dear God*

Dear God,

That was the hardest drive home. Needing to tell someone, I called Dave and blurted it out. Then I called my anxiously waiting best friend, Jane. I don't remember her exact words, but what I do remember is an e-mail later that night: "So does 'malignant' mean you have cancer? It doesn't, does it?" Why was I doing all this in the car? Driving? On the cell phone? Lord, You know I wasn't thinking clearly. If I had it to do over again, I would come home and spend time with You before making those phone calls . . . but I didn't.

At least I waited to get home before calling my daughter, Kim. She was at work but expecting the call. As she started crying, my tears unleashed. We were both unable to talk. After attempting to explain what I knew, we hung up. Five minutes later she called back, saying she couldn't keep working and was coming over. I welcomed her company. We are kindred mother-daughter souls, and You know the many things we have been through together. She would understand how I felt without my even explaining, just as I knew she was thinking about her high-school friend's mother who died several months ago of breast cancer. Oh, God, it is so hard to tell my daughter I have breast cancer, because I may be passing on that possibility to her too. I want to leave my daughter an inheritance—a legacy—but not this. I introduced breast cancer into our lineage. Lord, please don't make it "our disease."

Fearfully Yours, Janet

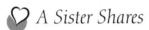 A Sister Shares

Sue [her daughter] and I discussed the recommendations of the two doctors. We decided I should have only the cancerous breast removed and have the surgery in Longview. Surgery was scheduled. . . . I closed my eyes, saw each of my children's faces, and thought, *How can I tell them?* . . . Sue phoned my other daughter, and I called my two sons to notify them of my upcoming surgery. Then it was time for me to tell David [her then fiancé], and I knew that wouldn't be easy. —Martha[3]

Mentoring Moment

Our immediate family is the hardest to tell. They are dealing with their own feelings and may not react the way we want. Don't be surprised if at first they draw into themselves or are not as supportive as you hoped. Setting your expectations too high could lead to disappointment, depression, and anger. Breast cancer is a shock to them as much as it is to us. Instinctively, I knew my husband would be OK, but many husbands aren't. Give them time to adjust. Fiancés quickly learn the meaning of "in sickness and in health" and whether they are truly ready to make that commitment.

I think daughters are the hardest to tell because never again can they check No on a health application asking if there is breast cancer in their family. Some breast cancer is genetic—passed down through generations—and with that comes a certain amount of guilt for mothers and fear for daughters, often leading to an initial strain on the relationship. It is important to remember that not all breast cancer is genetic. There is no breast cancer in my immediate family. My oncology radiologist assured me there is no reason to fear that Kim will get breast cancer. Mine was a mutation of cells that really had no determined cause. However, I have since read there is speculation that the numerous diagnostic x-rays I had during treatment for scoliosis as a young girl could have been a contributing factor.

For both you and your daughters' peace of mind, invite them to attend doctors appointments so they can hear the doctor and ask their own questions. If your breast cancer is genetic, your daughters can start taking precautionary steps and having regular early screening tests.

Still, it seems no matter how old our daughters are when they hear Mom has breast cancer, later they say it was all just a blur. During the initial stages when my daughter thought I might die, I was amazed at the research she did and how many of the details she remembered. After the initial shock and realization I would survive, I think she went into a survival mode of her own, trying to balance fear with the adjustment that Mom, who had always been the pillar of strength and independence, was vulnerable. One single mom said she was concerned about her youngest adult daughter taking her on as a "project."

One woman said her daughter refused to discuss her mom's breast cancer. Mom understood her daughter's fears but insisted that she and her daughter receive genetic testing. Perhaps this pressure caused the daughter's distancing. If your daughter doesn't want to know if it is genetic, don't push. It could push her away. There are breast cancer support groups for us and maybe even our husbands, but what about our daughters? Maybe when you feel better, God will prompt *you* to look into starting one in your area.

It can also be quite difficult telling our *own* mothers. My mother is deceased, but when fifty-nine-year-old Carol was diagnosed with breast cancer, she found it difficult to tell her ninety-four-year-old mother. She discussed with her sister not even telling their mom, but they eventually decided she was "a pretty tough old gal" and could take it. As it turned out, Carol's mom did just fine. On the other hand, Jamie, whose mom had a lumpectomy in her seventies, still has not told her mom about her own breast cancer and lumpectomy two years ago. She says, "My mom is ninety-three years old, and she would get too upset and nervous."

Telling young children also has its heartbreaking challenges. Household routines change during treatment, so we can't hide this from the kids. It could be very scary and traumatic if they see us sick and don't know why or hear from someone else that we have breast cancer. Check the Web sites under "National Contacts" (page 345) for help in finding the appropriate words and support resources available for your children's ages.

📖 *God's Love Letter to You*

Dear_____, (fill in your name)
Then I, the LORD, reached out my hand and touched your mouth saying, "Now, I have put my words in your mouth" (Jeremiah 1:9 paraphrased).
Your Courage, God

🙌 Let's Pray

Lord, we feel inadequate for the task of telling our loved ones. We can barely grapple with it ourselves, not to mention trying to help them with their shock and fear. They take their cue from us; we set the pace for the family's emotions. Help us get through this. Heal any rifts; bind up wounds. We so badly need our families to be strong right now. Draw us *all*

Talking to Children

When a woman with young children is diagnosed with breast cancer, she faces a delicate balancing act. How do you talk to your children honestly without scaring them too much? Psychologist Sandy Finestone, a twenty-year survivor and coordinator of cancer-patient services at Hoag Memorial Hospital Presbyterian in Newport Beach, California, recommends the following:

- Talk to children at their comprehension level and be honest. "The bad thing is to keep them out of the loop," she said. "Tell them my treatment is going to take this amount of time; I may be tired. If my hair falls out, it is good because that means the chemicals are working."

- Get them involved in positive events, like the Race for the Cure.

- Demystify cancer. "I've had children draw on their mother's head," Finestone said.

- Look for good resources, and get children in touch with other kids who understand. Finestone recommends Kids Konnected, an online community for children whose parents are battling any type of cancer (www.kidskonnected.org). There are also books and other links recommended on the Susan G. Komen Breast Cancer Foundation Web site (www.komen.org).[4]

closer to one another and closer to You. Let them see us praise Your name and love You more than ever as we put our trust and hope in You working through our doctors. Amen.

Who Else to Tell and Who Should Do the Telling?

I know when I was going through this walk, I was careful whom I shared with. I didn't want to hear anyone's horror stories. I needed encouragement and a listening ear. —Darlene M.

I am indebted to the ladies who made telephone calls and sent e-mails to tell everyone for me. It was very hard to call the people I needed to tell, and I so appreciated not having to verbalize these words more often than I did. —Sue

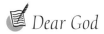 *Dear God*

Dear God,

You tell us we have not, because we ask not. The prayers of others are so important at this time, but that means telling them. Eventually, everyone will know, but who first? I was so grateful for e-mail. I composed the first group letter to close friends and family, asking prayer for the biopsy. When the results were positive for cancer, I informed by e-mail those who had been praying. Then Dave took over giving updates to friends and family, and my dear friend Jane ran interference in the ministry. I did not have the energy emotionally or physically. Often, not knowing how to respond to the news, people would tell stories that actually made me feel worse!

As surgery approached, Dave gradually expanded the e-mail list. It was the best we could do, but all seemed encouraged by it. I hope You don't think that was impersonal, Lord, but it allowed us to reveal things at our own pace. Dave could also screen responses. Such a relief . . . I was so fragile those first few weeks. When the many medical bills overflowed our mailbox, Dave offered to negotiate payment plans and write the checks. Again, he seemed to know the monthly reminder would not help me heal and move on.

Gratefully Yours, Janet

Two Sisters Share

I remember when first diagnosed, all my friends were calling with names and phone numbers of people to call whom they knew had experienced breast cancer. Not a good idea. After talking to three or four people, I came downstairs and told my husband I couldn't take one more sad story. I told him those were *their stories*, and I was going to have *my own*; and as it turns out, mine is a story filled with hope, joy, and love! —Darlene Gee

In this e-mail, and this e-mail only, I will talk BRIEFLY about the "How long does she have" question I know people ask. This is normal; however, it won't be a subject past this e-mail for me. It will be something for discussion among yourselves as the ones who sit on the outside of the disease and watch. I encourage you to talk to each other and find comfort I can't afford to get involved in. For me it will be to live one day at a time, not dreary but positively. And last, please feel free to share any e-mails I pass along. I know I don't have everyone on the list who will ask how I am, so please share if someone inquires. —Linda M.

Mentoring Moment

I recommend not doing the communicating yourself. It is physically, mentally, and emotionally exhausting. Repeatedly explaining your situation and listening to comments, reactions, stories, and shock wears you down. Many know someone with breast cancer and feel compelled to tell you the story. It doesn't help. Those of us who have "been there, done that" often lament that we were doing pretty well until our friends tried "cheering us up." Stunned and unable to interrupt or stop them, I would listen to tales of women who had not survived, occasionally hearing a happy ending. Others told their own stories. Nothing prepared me for the dreary responses. It opened my eyes to how ill prepared many are to interact appropriately with someone going through a crisis. In hindsight, I was much too polite.

Don't get me wrong. Many people had loving, kind responses, and likely you have received those too; but few people really know what to say. Maybe shock or feeling uncomfortable causes them to say things you both regret. Right now all we can handle is *our story*.

My best friend, Jane, took over the leadership and communication responsibilities for the Woman to Woman Mentoring Ministry and *About His Work* Ministries, my speaking and writing ministry. My husband found e-mail the quickest and easiest way to disseminate information, developing a group e-mail of friends and family and sending periodic updates. What a relief to them and me. I was fortunate my husband and best friend took on these roles, but maybe for you the filtering spokesperson will be a sister, adult child, best friend, your mom, coworker, or church representative. They can relate to you all the *appropriate* thoughts and prayers people are conveying.

Set boundaries. If you don't want informed people telling others right now, make that clear. It is your right, and they should honor it. However, people have a difficult time keeping secrets, so it is better not to put them in that awkward position. If you truly don't want others to know yet, only tell a select few. Conversely, if you are fine with people sharing, let them know that too.

Providing answers to the following questions helps prepare the spokesperson:

- Who to tell?

- What to tell? Give basic information . . . nothing speculative, just the facts. If you start talking of *possible* outcomes, that's where the stories grow.

- Who should tell?

- What words to convey? No more and no less.

- Can those receiving the news tell others?

- Can they forward e-mails?

- Do you want doctor referrals? If you don't, let them know you have picked excellent doctors.

- How can they pray for you?

- Where do you need immediate help?

God's Love Letter to You

Dear_____, (fill in your name)
A reliable messenger brings healing (Proverbs 13:17 NLT).
Your Voice in the Storm, God

Let's Pray

Lord, we come exhausted. This has been a difficult few weeks and days—wow, has it only been that? We know our friends and families love us, but we are so sensitive, and sometimes their words hurt and sting. Help us be loving and forgiving. We still are adjusting to this bombshell, and we don't even like the way we ourselves react sometimes. Please give extra discernment and compassion to those around us. We praise You for our families, friends, and most of all for being the Great Communicator in our lives. In Jesus's name, we pray. Amen.

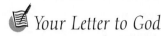 *Your Letter to God*

Breast cancer is a surprise that throws our world out of kilter or helps us put everything in perspective. Which happened in your life? What was (or is) the waiting like? It may be painful to revisit, but comfort comes from writing it down. If you are awaiting tests, ask God to remove anxious thoughts. How did you tell family, and how did that go? If you have not told your family or friends, ask for wisdom, courage, and words. Have you identified a spokesperson? If not, ask the Lord to bring one or two forward quickly.

Dear God,   *Date:*

CHAPTER THREE

Paralyzing Shock

TAKE A GOOD LOOK AT ME. AREN'T YOU APPALLED BY WHAT'S HAPPENED? NO!
DON'T SAY ANYTHING. I CAN DO WITHOUT YOUR COMMENTS. WHEN I LOOK BACK,
I GO INTO SHOCK, MY BODY IS RACKED WITH SPASMS.

—*Job 21:5–6 MSG*

A State of Shock

I have been in my own world since the diagnosis, and although many have offered their expertise or willingness to talk with me about their own experiences, I have been reluctant to do so. I can't explain why—it just hasn't felt like a pressing need. That may all change afterward—I may still just be in shock. —Kay Warren

I left the office in shock. I was there a total of seven hours as they diligently tried to assess my situation. How was I going to cope with waiting over the weekend for a report? —Bonnie[1]

The first test was a mammogram, which showed that I had advanced breast cancer. I was in a state of shock! —Grace Bell

 ## Dear God

Dear God,

I go through the motions each day, but I am numb. A little tape keeps playing in my head: "You have breast cancer." It seems surreal. Impossible. This is something that happens to other women, not me. Right now, little has changed in our life and yet everything has changed. I feel like this must be happening to someone else. If we just don't follow up on the biopsy results, maybe it will all go away. My mind seems frozen. I am in a state of shock. I can't even think of words to write.

Numbly Yours, Janet

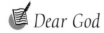 ## A Sister Shares

After the initial shock of learning I had cancer, came the overwhelming task of choosing doctors and treatment options. . . . I would like to say I turned to the Lord, but I didn't. Instead, I read everything I could get my hands on about breast cancer. I felt like I was cramming for the most important exam of my life. —Nancy Tuttle[2]

 ## Mentoring Moment

The dreaded diagnosis sends us all into shock. Every woman's testimony about her breast cancer story includes the word *shock*:

- "When I heard the word *cancer*, I was in shock."

- "When I got the diagnosis, my heart stopped."

- "I went into my own little world."

- "When I got over the shock . . ."

- "You are never prepared for such shocking news."

- "My whole family was shocked that I had cancer."

- "We were so shocked to get the news that you have breast cancer."

- "I was shocked when they said, 'Breast cancer.'"

- "You just never think it will happen to you."

You get the idea. I said it. You said it. Others said it to you. It is natural.

A cancer diagnosis affects the whole family, and their world starts to whirl with yours. My own adult children responded to the positive diagnosis with alarm. Kim was sure I was going to die. Shannon was "shocked by the news." Michelle wrote from Italy, where she lives, "The word *cancer* is so scary. We are so sad." Sean and his family were living in Spain at the time, and his in-laws were visiting. When he told his father-in-law, who had fought his own battle with cancer, they were all sad, knowing what lay ahead for me.

Most of us don't spend our days wondering if we are going to get breast cancer. Bad news is shocking. *Webster's* defines *shock* as "a sudden or violent disturbance of the mind, emotions, or sensibilities." The synonym, *startle*, implies "the sharp surprise of sudden fright." Our body reacts with dry mouth, racing heart, sinking stomach, sweaty palms, numbness, flushed face, maybe fainting or sickness—it is a terrible feeling. We can't live in a state of shock for long without our body completely shutting down, so mercifully, the shock phase passes and myriad reactions follow, including denial, frantic research, anger, depression, and eventually, acceptance.

📖 God's Love Letter to You

Dear_____, (fill in your name)
I am holding you by your right hand—I, the LORD *your God. And I say to you, "Do not be afraid. I am here to help you" (Isaiah 41:13 NLT).*
Your Shock Absorber, God

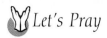 Let's Pray

Oh, Father, no one but You and another breast cancer sister can fully appreciate how this news has devastated our families and us. Help us go forward. Remove any paralysis in our spirits from this dreaded diagnosis, and replace it with a purpose and a plan. We cannot live in shock. Please replace the numbness and long, sleepless nights with conviction to do whatever we must to get well. Comfort our loved ones and friends. Help them overcome their initial reaction so they can be there for us like we have never needed them before. We are women with heartache, longing to be hopeful. Only You, precious Lord, can break down the wall that has dropped around us. We ask for an infusion of courage to go on. Amen.

It's All So Confusing!

IT IS A LAND AS DARK AS MIDNIGHT, A LAND OF UTTER GLOOM WHERE CONFUSION REIGNS AND THE LIGHT IS AS DARK AS MIDNIGHT. —JOB 10:22 NLT

PEOPLE CAN NEVER PREDICT WHEN HARD TIMES MIGHT COME. LIKE FISH IN A NET OR BIRDS IN A SNARE, PEOPLE ARE OFTEN CAUGHT BY SUDDEN TRAGEDY. —ECCLESIASTES 9:12 NLT

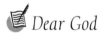 *Dear God*

Dear God,

Confusion almost engulfed me in the beginning. I remember when I called the surgeon's office to tell them the biopsy was positive and I needed to set an appointment. The response surprised me: "No, you must be wrong; we haven't had any positive reports or faxes today." Even after explaining my talk with the radiologist, they still insisted it was not possible. It wasn't the procedure. "The surgeon likes to call and give you the news. Patients like that better. They expect to hear it from their doctor. The radiologist never does that."

So what to do now? Procedure seems to have been broken. The radiologist told me the biopsy results were positive; I needed to know what to do next. Why were they making this hard situation even harder for me? So there I was, trying to convince the surgeon's office I really did have cancer—that I was, if you will, "a positive report." But wasn't it really a negative report? It seemed that way to me anyway. Wow, that was bizarre.

Then, early the next morning, Dr. West himself called to apologize for the way I found out. I said that was quite all right, and I actually appreciated the radiologist caring enough to relieve my anxiety. Besides, I didn't know the procedure. Her telling me seemed normal.

Again, the surgeon explained this was a new office and they hadn't worked out all the procedures. I thanked him for his personal call and concern. Then he put someone on the phone to set my appointment, and she proceeded to scare me to death by saying we needed a family conference appointment where we would decide if I was going to have a lumpectomy, partial, radical, or bilateral mastectomy, reconstruction . . . she lost me there. *Wait a minute; I am just having a lumpectomy, that's what the radiologist said. No one said anything about a mastectomy.* She explained that some women want the option of eliminating any potential chance of future cancer by removing both breasts. This was way too much information for first thing in the morning . . . in fact, it was too much, period. Not on the phone. Not from this person. We are talking about my breasts, not changing the tires on a car.

Lord, I decided to ignore what she said and set the appointment for my family and me to meet with Dr. West. Let him explain it all to us. I was not jumping to conclusions worse than anyone had told me so far. That would be the first of many times I consciously chose not to react to someone's insensitivity or mistakes. We set the appointment for Dave, Kim, and me to meet with the breast specialist and surgeon, Dr. West, and let him explain our options. "The doctor sees 'positives' on Tuesday morning." There it was again—was this my new label? This must be a pretty regular and common thing if they schedule "positives" every week. Oh Lord, that many positives? How negative.

Positively Yours, Janet

A Sister Shares

When first diagnosed with breast cancer, I initially thought I was going to die soon. After talking with the other women in the Reach for Recovery program, we discovered that all of us felt the same way! How about you? —Jamie

A Doctor Shares

In December 2000, I met a patient named Barbara Wilson. . . . Some three years earlier Barbara had found a lump in her breast that was shown to be cancer. She had a lumpectomy and six months of chemotherapy. Now the cancer was found to be growing in her bones and liver.

It was a typically frigid January day in New England. Barbara was seated in the waiting room, wearing a heavy woolen sweater, flanked by two women from her church. She was tall and slim, with angular features and serious blue eyes. I asked whether she wanted her friends to sit in on our discussion. "Do I need bodyguards?" Barbara asked with a laugh. "I suspect what I am going to hear will unnerve them more than me." —Dr. Jerome Groopman[3]

Mentoring Moment

Early on, it was apparent that cancer is not a spectator sport. Often we double as the participants in the race or fight as well as the assistant coaches and trainers with our doctors. No watching from a distant position and letting everyone else direct the plays and moves. We must take an active role in our treatment. God is God; doctors and their staffs are human. Just like the rest of us, they make mistakes, forget, and say the wrong thing. As much as we would like to put ourselves at their mercy, close our eyes, and wake up with it all over, we must actively engage in this journey. Always have a pen and paper in your hand the minute one of them starts talking. I still have the notes from that early-morning phone conversation with the surgeon and nurse. Not expecting the call, I grabbed a notepad near the phone.

Let me advise you to expect the unexpected. Whenever you are talking with anyone involved in your treatment, use the "Phone Notes" (page 359) or "Appointment Notes" (page 353) and write down everything they say. Then if you need to make a decision, go to the "Peacekeeping Worksheet" (page 349). If the doctor's office calls and there is someone else with you, ask that person to get on an extension phone to hear the conversation too.

Be prepared. Some things you hear may throw you into shocked confusion, and you just can't take it all in at once. Have someone go with you to all doctor appointments, and let him or her take notes in this book while you converse with the doctor. Your mind will be in a swirl, and there is no way you can think to write everything down, much less remember it. If the doctor or doctor's office does something that's unnerving or you are confused, tell them. You may be helping the next patient. I did, and they were grateful.

God's Love Letter to You

Dear_____, (fill in your name)
I will guide you along the best pathway for your life. I will advise you and watch over you (Psalm 32:8 NLT).
Your Guide, God

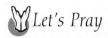 Let's Pray

Prayerfully personalize Job 37:20–24 NLT.

My Lord, in wonderment I pray . . .

Should God be told that I, _____, want to speak? Can we speak when we are confused? We cannot look at the sun, for it shines brightly in the sky when the wind clears away the clouds. Golden splendor comes from the mountain of God. He is clothed in dazzling splendor. We cannot imagine the power of the Almighty, yet he is so just and merciful that he does not oppress us. No wonder people everywhere fear him. People who are truly wise show him reverence. Amen.

Becoming "One of Them"

It was unbelievable. There I was in the same waiting room, the same medical offices where I had brought my mom for some of her appointments and chemotherapy. I was now a part of that community—a breast cancer patient. Never in a million years would I have imagined it! —Grace Marestaing

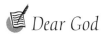 ## Dear God

Dear God,

You know how I prayed over the years not to be "one of them." The statistics leaped out at me: "One in every eight women will get breast cancer." Even worse, in Orange County where we live, I have heard one in four! Worldwide, every three minutes a woman is diagnosed with breast cancer. *Oh Lord*, I pleaded each time my eyes fell on a new statistic, *Please don't let me be one of them.* The thought haunted me at speaking engagements or while leading women's Bible studies or meeting with groups of women. Scanning the room, I mentally took in the number gathered and said to myself, "Lord, if we can believe the statistics, several poor women in this group are going to get breast cancer. Please, Lord, I have so much work to do for You. There is no history of breast cancer in my family. Give me peace that it will not be me!"

Lord, You were preparing me; I see that now. Just the weekend before my now infamous "routine" annual gynecologist's appointment, which ended up anything but routine, I was in North Carolina speaking at a women's retreat. Saturday night the emcee wore a robe to announce their slumber party and made the comment she had received it as a gift when she was in the hospital. My eyes darted to her very short hair. The ladies at our table filled us in—the emcee had just gone through breast cancer treatment. "Oh Lord, don't let it be me."

Actually, it was a relief from my tormented thinking when, indeed, it was me! It had to be me. Why not me? Of course, me. I could never relate to all those hurting women in my audiences if it had not been me. I get it now and can truly say, "Thank You, Lord, that it was me."

Acceptingly Yours, Janet

 ## A Sister Shares

I had leapt through the looking glass. I was to become one of those people in the chemo room whom I had always been afraid of, those whose cancer had spread, deviously robbing them, sometimes again and again, of sustained life without cancer treatment. But one cannot be afraid of oneself. One can simply inhabit one's situation, with or without grace, and astoundingly, find comfort and normalcy, even in circumstances that, looked at from afar, couldn't support that. —Leslie Furth[4]

 ## Mentoring Moment

It may take you awhile to comprehend this new identity, and that's all right. If you are not yet ready to be "one of them," don't worry about it. You might not want to wear a pink ribbon; I couldn't for almost a year. People gave them to me, and I saw them in the doctor's office, but they stayed in my jewelry box or purse as a gentle reminder. Somewhere around the end of the first year—a milestone anniversary—I started embracing the sisterhood of courage and commitment to life we all share and that binds us together. Today I actually am proud to be "one of them."

After the initial shock I truly can say there was comfort in realizing the Lord was in this from the beginning. God planted those questioning thoughts in my mind. I was arguing with the Holy Spirit's whispers. Prior to God's nudging, I heard other women's breast cancer stories from a remote, detached distance. Poor things. So grateful it was not me. Were you like that too? Now overnight—we are *one of them*. We have joined a sisterhood you and I never wanted or anticipated. Our worst nightmare has come true.

God had to show me it was not about me. It was about the work He needed to do *in* and *through* me. This was the way He chose to do it. When that light dawned, I immediately knew this experience would not be wasted. Hard to believe, I know, but I had a sense of anticipation of how God was going to use it. Of course, this book is one of the ways, but I will share many others as we journey together. With the Lord in your life you know that the plans He has for you are for good and not for evil, to give you hope and a future.

📖 God's Love Letter to You

Dear_____, (fill in your name)

    Even to your old age and gray hairs, I am God who will sustain you. I have made you and I will carry you; I will sustain you and I will rescue you (Isaiah 46:4 paraphrased).
Your Rescuer, God

🙏 Let's Pray

Lord, You are so holy and awesome, but how did You let this happen to us? We are numb, overwhelmed, sad, resentful, mad . . . That feels better to let it out.

    Now, Lord, help us move to the next step—acceptance. Remove any desire to isolate ourselves from other breast cancer sisters or the world in general. That would be such a waste of our hurt. There is a new group of women coming into our lives, and because of this common bond of breast cancer, we will embrace one another. Give us courage to reach out to those needing a hug and to let others know when we need that hug ourselves. Help us be compassionate and understanding and lean on each other when our paths cross. Amen.

Single and Sick!

Since I'm a single mom to three boys, my diagnosis made me feel extra vulnerable and helpless. —S. K. Whang[5]

✒️ Dear God

[Written by Grace Marestaing]
Dear God,

    Help, Lord, I'm single, a family of one—discovering, one more time, the lessons of radical reliance and trust in You. Lord, I'm single and I am so grateful for the family that is surrounding me and for the friends who have become dearer than I could have imagined. But Lord, why is it that I feel alone in this journey? The tests, the procedures, the surgeries—those ultimately are just You and me, and I cling to the comfort of Your promised presence. Lord, how I need to feel You close.

How I need to know You as Provider, Father, in those moments when panic sets in about my finances and my mind says, *If you don't work, there is no income.* But Your Word says, "The Father knows what you need."

How I need the mind of Christ as I catapult into the decision-making process with my doctors, and as I work at absorbing the seeming mountains of information. Lord, I need Your holy guidance to help me through the maze. All along, Your sustaining hand is there. "My grace is sufficient . . ." Your Spirit brings those amazing words to mind when my body feels so worn down that I don't have the strength to read them. "My strength is made perfect in your weakness." Bring on the perfection, Lord . . . or I don't think I'll make it.

Lord, I'm single. You are my intimate Friend. You know precisely how You made me. You know my thoughts before I speak them. You knew exactly when the cancer cells began to divide in my body. It was not a surprise to You. And You know the number of my days. Loving and gracious Lord, I'm single . . . but I am not alone. I put my trust in You.

Singly trusting You, Grace

 ## Three Sisters Share

I just wanted to remove my illness and get on with my life . . . I had just met the most precious man, and I wanted nothing to interfere with our relationship as we had planned to be married. I would have cried had he left; that would have been the greatest loss I could have suffered in a long time. . . .

Then our discussion began. . . . He needed to feel free to leave with no guilt attached. He was a healthy man that needed a healthy wife who could go fishing, golfing, dancing, to football games, and on and on for a full life. After he listened to me until he was sick of what I was saying, he began reading me the "Ramsey Act," and when he finished, I felt pretty important after all . . . no matter what I removed. I had his full consent to lose a breast, I had my children's love and special strengths, my church was praying day and night with the twenty-four-hour prayer room, and I had an open line to God . . . so how could I lose or sit here and moan about something that could be removed and I could be with my family, and David [Ramsey] and I have a continued wonderful life that I loved so much.
—Martha[6]

Here are some thoughts on going through cancer as a single person. For me, the hardest part is not having a husband and/or children as caregivers. My mother has been here for six months, and she's been wonderful. I couldn't have gone through it without her. At eighty-three, this really has been hard on her. I also have wonderful friends at work, at church, and in my neighborhood who have done everything from clean my home to grocery shop, take me to appointments, bring meals, do pharmacy runs, even take me to the ER at 10:30 at night!

A strong support system of friends is a must for a single person. I also had to get over my hesitation to ask for help. I've always been so independent, not wanting to ask others for help too often. I've had to get over that! I've discovered giving others a chance to help is as much a blessing to them as it is to me. I struggle with the fear of the cancer returning and wondering if the strong support system will be there if that happens. I also struggle with wondering if I'll ever be attractive to a man again. It's hard to feel attractive now with a bald head and one breast! It's really a faith walk that I struggle with. I hope I have developed a stronger faith in God through this experience, but I have to admit, I really struggle with it some days. —Cindy

I went through the whole process living by myself. My older sister was my physical support; she went with me to visits with the surgeon, drove me to the hospital, picked me up, and took me for the first visit to radiation only because she used to take my mom to the same place. —Jamie

 ## *Mentoring Moment*

Having been a single parent for seventeen years, I have a window into your experience as a single woman. During my single-parenting years I contracted an illness that had me down for two months. I remember the same look of terror in Kim's eyes then that I saw when I told her I had breast cancer. She was a little girl depending on her single mom for everything, and I was helpless. It was a scary time for both of us, wondering if I would regain my energy to work and be a mom and provider again. Not living near family, I hired someone to care for both of us during my convalescence. So having walked in your shoes a bit, I know the engulfing panic and fear—especially in the middle of the night.

Now married, I could not write this section's "Dear God," but knowing many of you reading this book are single, I wanted specifically to address issues you face. Grace Marestaing was my volunteer patient representative at the BreastCare Center, who went on to become a dear mentoring friend. Discussing this book at dinner one night with Grace, the Lord put on my heart the special challenges of going through breast cancer as a single woman—the decision process, treatment, recuperating, how it might affect any future plans for marriage. I asked Grace if she would write this "Dear God," and she eagerly agreed. She later e-mailed, "Writing that 'Dear

God' piece has continued to bless me and minister to me. It's a wonderful thing when that happens." I trust you are finding the same thing as you journal *your* "Dear God's."

The breast cancer sisters who shared their stories above have completely different experiences, and yours will be unique and specific to you. We can't measure our lives by someone else's, but we can ask God for guidance and direction with our particular situation.

God's Love Letter to You

Dear_____, *(fill in your name)*

Sing to me, sing praises to my name and extol me—my name is the LORD *and rejoice before me. I am a father to you who are fatherless, a defender of widows and in me you find a holy dwelling place. I set the lonely in families (Psalm 68:4–6 paraphrased).*
Your Heavenly Husband, God

Let's Pray

Father, we call out as women experiencing the loneliness of going through illness without a husband or the loss of a husband because of our illness. You tell us singleness is a way of life—some will choose or have it chosen for them. But when we are sick, we desire for someone to shoulder the burden. Thank You for family and friends who rally around, but most of all thank You for Your never-ending presence. We know the emptiness that comes from going through trials—especially illness—on our own. Help us remember You are always near, and draw us closer when others let us down. This is a growing experience for sure . . . growing closer to You every day, in every way. Amen.

Your Letter to God

If you are currently in the "shock phase," you may be able to write little more than acknowledging that is where you are right now. You don't have to say much. God knows your heart, and He hurts with you. Maybe you just want to write down a list of words that describe how you feel, or felt, in those first few days after diagnosis. Then ask God to give you a clear mind and inner peace, free of any confusion.

Dear God, _____ *Date:* _____

_____

_____

_____

CHAPTER FOUR

Asking What If? What About? Why?

I REMEMBER GOD—AND SHAKE MY HEAD.
I BOW MY HEAD—THEN WRING MY HANDS.
I'M AWAKE ALL NIGHT—NOT A WINK OF SLEEP;
I CAN'T EVEN SAY WHAT'S BOTHERING ME.
I GO OVER THE DAYS ONE BY ONE, I PONDER THE YEARS GONE BY.

—*Psalm 77:3–5 MSG*

What If?

I questioned what I had done to get cancer—maybe too much coffee, or wine, or stress, or the estrogen therapy I had been on for five years since my hysterectomy. —Nancy Tuttle[1]

I know there's always room for self-doubt and "what-ifs," and I reassure myself with the thought that in the midst of such fear and uncertainty, we had to do what felt right. —Bernard Wolfson, Leslie Furth's husband[2]

When I start what-ifing or worrying about tomorrow, I lose my peace. —Darlene M.

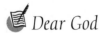 ## Dear God

Dear God,

I can't help asking myself if there is something I did to bring this on. Did I miss something along the way? While going through menopause in my early fifties, I felt Your nudge to change gynecologists. That doctor routinely put all his patients on hormones with the caveat, "Unless you are afraid of breast cancer." Of course I am! No woman wants to take that chance. He kept talking about "quality of life"; I just wanted a life to worry about the quality of. He wouldn't talk about anything else but hormones.

Then I switched to Dr. Carter, who prescribed a light, natural hormone cream. Rubbing it on each night felt so safe, but was it growing this cancer in my breast? Was that You, Lord, giving me a nagging doubt? I weaned myself off even before the cancer diagnosis, but was it too late? What if I had gone off sooner? What if I never went on hormones at all—just toughed it out? It really was tolerable; I could have done without it. Why didn't I, Lord? There was just so much confusion at the time. Everything I read gave both sides and then pretty much said, "You have to make the choice." It was so undefined, as if we were guinea pigs in one big human experiment that went bad. Now the pendulum has swung the other way, and they say hormones have too high a risk even to continue the studies. What if I had been born ten years later, allowing more time for research and breakthroughs? Would I still have gotten breast cancer?

What if I had not used two microwaves—or not even one? What if I had learned more about the dangers of pesticides and preservatives? Would I have listened? Probably not. What if I hadn't consumed so much coffee since childhood? What if I hadn't had scoliosis and all those x-rays as a young girl? What if I hadn't worn underwire bras? I read something that said they might cut off the circulation to your breasts. What if I had nursed Kim longer? What if I'd had more children and nursed all of them? Would that have helped? What if I'd had digital mammography earlier? What if I had gone to the BreastCare Center years ago instead of the one that didn't even send me a reminder letter? Did a radiologist miss something in my previous exams?

What-ifingly Yours, Janet

♡ A Sister Shares

I journal spasmodically, and looking back, I see my initial reaction was to put down a lot of "what-ifs." Maybe I could have been diagnosed earlier? Should I have taken Prempro when I really didn't think it was necessary? Was that the beginning of a cancer seen way back in 1992? Dr. Bodai [the promoter of the breast cancer stamp] said, "We are in the *present* and worrying about the *past* wasn't going to change things."—Shirley

Mentoring Moment

I hit a hot button here, didn't I! I hope you found a way to quiet those what-ifs in your mind, but if not, you have that opportunity now. As if reading my mind before I could even ask the questions, the diagnostic radiologist assured me, "You didn't do anything to cause this. You would have had to be on hormones much longer than you were for it to be a contributing factor. This has probably been going on in your body for maybe ten years and has just now become big enough for us to detect on the screen. It was not evident in any of the previous films you had sent to us. It's in early stages, so let's just take care of it. You are going to be fine."

I appreciated her assurance and tried to find refuge in it. Still, I had to work hard at casting out the arrows that pierced my mind and heart with doubt, unrest, guilt, worry, shame, and sorrow for what might have been. I constantly had to remind myself that doubt and faith cannot coexist in the same heart. If I doubted, then my shield of faith had slipped.

One way that helps me cast out doubt and what-ifs and face each day with renewed courage and faith is daily to put on the armor of God found in Ephesians 6:11–18. This has been a morning practice of mine for many years, even before I brush my teeth. God provides us this protection; we just need to remind ourselves how to claim it. You will see these verses in today's "God's Love Letter to You."

There is no turning back. There is nothing we can do about the *past*—only the *present* has an outcome on our *future*. Worry about the past or the future is pointless, another one of those things we cannot change. However, what we do *now* will influence the future. My pastor, Rick Warren, compares worrying about the past or future to driving a car, looking in the rearview mirror or way out in the distance. Either way, we crash. The only safe way to drive and live our life's course is:

- An occasional, quick glance at what's behind us

- A quick, long-range glance ahead to see if we want to proceed

- An alert, steady focus on our current surroundings

I won't tell you to do the impossible and not play what-if. So, like my letter to God, get it all out. Think of every what-if that comes to mind—even the inapplicable ones that still hound you. Write them all down on the next page. Then once they are out of your mind and onto paper, mark a huge X through your list, and clear them out of your mind. Move on to what we can do in the present—now—enjoy life. OK!

God's Love Letter to You

Dear_____, (fill in your name)
Put on the full armor of God so that you can take your stand against the devil's schemes. For your struggle is not against flesh and blood, but against the rulers, against the authorities, against the powers of this dark world and against the spiritual forces of evil in the heavenly realms. Therefore put on the full armor of God, so that when the day of evil comes, you may be able to stand your ground, and after you have done everything, to stand. Stand firm then, with the belt of truth buckled around your waist, with the breastplate of righteousness in place, and with your feet fitted with the readiness that comes from the gospel of peace. In addition to all this, take up the shield of faith, with which you can extinguish all the flaming arrows of the evil one. Take the helmet of salvation and the sword of the Spirit, which is My Word. And pray in the Spirit on all occasions with all kinds of prayers and requests (Ephesians 6:11–18 paraphrased).
Your Commander in Chief, God

Let's Pray

Lord, You gifted us with incredible minds, which can be our friends or enemies. Satan loves to put doubting, fearful what-ifs in our heads—nagging, worrisome thoughts we replay over and over in our minds like an old bad movie. One we don't want to watch and yet feel compelled and drawn to like a magnetic force drawing us into the eye of a tornado that tosses us around and then cruelly spits us out battered, bruised, and emotionally devastated.

Lord, those destructive what-if thoughts are not from You. We know that. Please take hold of our minds and help us heed Paul's reminder in Philippians 4:8 to "Fix your thoughts on what is true and honorable and right. Think about things that are pure and lovely and admirable. Think about things that are excellent and worthy of praise" (NLT). Fill our minds with the hope, endurance, and love of Jesus Christ. Protected by You, we rest. Amen.

Every "What-If" I Have Heard or Can Think of

_____

_____

_____

_____

_____

_____

_____

_____

_____

_____

_____

_____

_____

_____

_____

_____

_____

When you have them all written down—can't think of any more what-ifs—ceremoniously mark a huge X through them. Now move on to getting well!

Maybe It's All a Mistake

If I didn't have the scars, I might have thought it was all just a dream. —Lisha

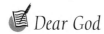 ## Dear God

Dear God,

Is it possible I could wake up and this would all have been a bad dream? You know, those first few days I honestly expected to receive an apology call. They made a mistake. "So sorry! Everything is fine—see you next year." Maybe they mixed up my test results or put the wrong name on a slide. Right up until surgery, I still hoped.

It all seemed so surreal. Only three days after the positive diagnosis, I was onstage speaking at a conference. While my mouth gave the familiar talk, my thoughts raced: *I have breast cancer! Here I am going about life as usual. None of these people in the audience know that in a few short weeks I am having surgery! My life may never feel this normal again. I have breast cancer . . . How could this be? No history in my family. I exercise regularly, watch my diet, have mammograms religiously—I've done it all, and yet it still happened.*

Oh Lord, it wasn't a mistake at all. You knew from the time I was born, this would happen. Every day You were preparing me to take it, grow through it, and come out the other side ready to help whomever I can in whatever way I can. There are no mistakes in a believer's life. Help me to spread that encouraging message.

Unmistakably Yours, Janet

 ## A Sister Shares

The doctor gave me a booklet to read about the possible side effects from chemo. I put off reading it until the day before I was to have my first treatment because I really didn't want to know all the terrible things that were going to happen from putting a poison in my body.

I had to take my daughter and her friend to dance class that evening and decided to go to Starbucks to read it while I waited for their lesson to be over. Bad idea! It hit me full force what I was in for, and I couldn't imagine assaulting my body that way. I started to cry, and then I started to sob and had to leave quickly. I really lost it. I sat in the parking lot waiting to pick up the girls, trying to get control because I didn't want them to see me that way. They came out, and as soon as I looked at them, I started bawling again and cried all the way home. What a meltdown!

The next morning I had my treatment, and although I did get sick that evening, almost none of the other side effects occurred during the full course of chemo. Sometimes ignorance is bliss. —Darlene Gee

Mentoring Moment

Each of us has that "it's all a mistake" feeling sometime during this ordeal. Or we fantasize that this crisis will go away if we put off dealing with it. These are natural thoughts that help us get through those first difficult days after diagnosis. Even if just for a moment we can cling to the notion it might possibly be a terrible mistake or a really bad dream, we have hope. Soon, however, we must come to grips with painful reality and accept our situation.

Often, like Darlene, we find what we worried about doesn't turn out as bad as we thought. Many of us discover that the only thing we can count on for sure to provide true lasting hope and alleviate our worse fears is knowing that Jesus Christ loves us and wants the very best for us. Somehow—some way—He will turn it all into good. That's no mistake!

God's Love Letter to You

Dear_____, (fill in your name)

This is My, God's, Word on the subject: I know what I'm doing. I have it all planned out—plans to take care of you, not abandon you, plans to give you the future you hope for. When you call on Me, when you come and pray to Me, I'll listen. When you come looking for Me, you'll find Me. Yes, when you get serious about finding Me and want it more than anything else, I'll make sure you won't be disappointed (Jeremiah 29:10–14 MSG paraphrased).

Your Sure Thing, God

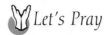 Let's Pray

Our Father in heaven, as little girls, we spent many childhood hours playing make-believe. Now we regress a bit to those sweet, carefree days when with a little improvising and a lot of imagination, the world was at our command. If we didn't like the rules of the game, we left or picked a different make-believe game where the rules fit us. Now we want to play a different pretend game, where we win and are well and the bad guy, cancer, loses. Help us absorb or accept reality. Let us crawl up into Your lap until the nightmare is over. You are the Truth, the Light, and the Way. Amen.

What About My Schedule and My Plans?

My oldest daughter left the day after Christmas for New Orleans to perform with her cheerleading squad in the halftime show of the Sugar Bowl. I had planned on accompanying her as a chaperone but was too debilitated by the radiation treatments. It was very disappointing to me not to be able to share one of the most exciting moments of her life. I had been there for everything my children did. —Bonnie[3]

> JOB ANSWERED GOD: "I'M CONVINCED: YOU CAN DO ANYTHING AND EVERYTHING. NOTHING AND NO ONE CAN UPSET YOUR PLANS." —JOB 42:1–2 MSG

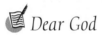 Dear God

Dear God,

Boy, You sure used breast cancer to help me slow down and focus. You know I plan my calendar several years in advance, so my first thought was, *What about all my speaking commitments?* Thank You for boldness to share this part of my life with the surgeon and his team and get them involved in determining what to keep on the calendar and what to reschedule. My speaking between the diagnosis and surgery was probably some of the best ever. I even got back on the road again before radiation ended!

I am glad we went on the planned Thanksgiving trip with Kim and Toby and Toby's parents, Pat and Cheryl, even though it was only one week after surgery! Crazy as it seemed, it did alter my focus. I cherish the memory of those early-morning coffee chats when Cheryl, an early riser, found me on the couch after a sleepless night. Cheryl planned the whole trip, cooked, and then insisted Dave and I take the biggest and best room. I felt so loved and cared for.

Cancer happens while doing life. It brought home the brevity of my earthly existence. My time really is Your time; Your plans become my plans. Thank You for helping me clearly see which commitments to keep and release a perfectionist attitude toward the ones I could not.

In Your time, Janet

♡ A Sister Shares

During my routine annual exam, my doctor detected a small lump in my breast. He wasn't that concerned about it, but being forty, I was due for a mammogram anyway. The day after the mammogram, I got a call to have a second mammogram. As I was sitting, waiting for the results, my brother-in-law walks in [he is a general surgeon] and tells me I have a spot that looks suspicious and I need a biopsy. I asked if he would be comfortable performing the procedure, and he said, "Absolutely!"

He performed the biopsy immediately and told me the results— it was malignant! I was stunned. Everything was happening so fast. The one thing I did know was that I didn't have time for anything to be wrong with me. After all, I had a one-year-old daughter with Down's syndrome, and *she* had her own health problems. The next day I had a lumpectomy and, because the margins were not clear, had a second surgery the following day. This time the margins were clear. Within two weeks I went on a trip to New Mexico and still had in that surgical drain! It was so sore and uncomfortable. But alas, all in good time, the fluid subsided and I was drain free. —Lisha

Mentoring Moment

Cancer seldom gives us warning. It rudely intrudes into our lives. A legitimate question is, "What happens to all my plans?" Ask your doctor that question right up-front. Don't feel that your plans are unimportant. Your life just took a significant sidetrack. You need to discuss how cancer will impact your future.

The fall of 2003, our pastor, Rick Warren, announced that his wife, Kay, had breast cancer and would be undergoing surgery, chemotherapy, and radiation. He also mentioned this meant canceling their plans and speaking engagements through April 2004. The month of Kay's surgery, Pastor Rick and Kay unveiled their Global PEACE Plan to launch our church into changing the world. Then Kay started difficult chemotherapy treatments requiring hospitalization. Pastor Rick only gave one sermon of a five-part Global PEACE Plan series when he realized Kay needed him by her side. They rescheduled the launch of the plan.

That Christmas, Pastor Rick sent the following e-mail to the congregation:

I want to thank you for allowing me the freedom personally to take care of Kay during her cancer. My wife is the love of my life, and this is what God intended families to do. I'd want every husband in our church to do the same if the situation arose in their family. God blesses us when we keep our commitments. So this year will be the first Christmas Services that Kay and I have missed in Saddleback's 23 years. I've prepared a message entitled, "When God Messes Up Your Plans." (How appropriate!) I've always been struck by the fact that EVERYONE at the first Christmas had their plans messed up by God—because God had a bigger and better plan. When life doesn't work out the way we intended, God wants us to trust Him.[4]

Our church launched the Global PEACE Plan God put on Pastor Rick's heart—just a little later than planned—well, maybe right on God's time plan.

I had plans, too, and so do you. As an author and speaker, I had publicized speaking engagements on the calendar. Money was paid; plans were made. If possible, I wanted to honor those commitments. I was very specific with the surgeon and his staff. As we planned surgery dates and treatment, I brought my calendar, told them the commitments I preferred to work around, and asked their realistic opinion of what needed altering. We found a surgery date that allowed me to finish my remaining 2002 commitments. The last speaking engagement was on a Saturday, with surgery the following Wednesday. This meant surgery and treatment during the Thanksgiving and Christmas holidays—a concession willingly made. The first speaking engagement scheduled for January 2003 was in Alaska. With surgery now on the calendar for November 20, 2002, we all agreed that was pushing it. So Alaska moved to September 2003; but, hey, Alaska in January is pretty cold anyway.

I also told the doctor we had planned a family Thanksgiving trip to Sun Valley, Idaho. His smiling response was, "I don't think you will be able to ski!" He was saying, though, that I could go. Surgery was a week before we were to leave. Tickets were purchased; plans were made. I was hesitant; my daughter hopeful. Daily I saw her watching me for progress. The first time she saw me dressed was when they picked us up to drive to the airport. I had a pillow protecting my chest, and Fleece (my new stuffed sheep) tucked under my arm, and lots of prayer. The stitches just removed that morning, we had to be nuts! It was tiring for sure. I slept through much of the festivities, but it was a great opportunity to get away and relax with family. I have no regrets. It is a fond memory for us all.

The Bible tells us "plans fail for lack of counsel, but with many advisers they succeed" (Proverbs 15:22). Ask your doctors' advice for the smallest detail. It's all part of your life. Let them advise:

- When should you take an absence from work, and when should you start back?

- If you have small children, what can you do, and where will you need help?

- What is a realistic time frame to resume current obligations, knowing everyone's recovery is different?

- When can you drive?

- How will you feel after surgery? During radiation? Chemo? Reconstruction? Ask for openness and honesty as to average recuperating times, and then allow for delays or complications. If they don't happen, you have extra time. If they do, you have some planned-in margin.

Don't add to your plate during this time, and don't feel guilty about postponing or canceling your plans. Your life is on the line. Nothing is more important. People will graciously understand. If they don't, it's probably not something you should participate in anyway. The important thing is to grant yourself understanding and grace. Be realistic, not heroic.

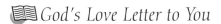 God's Love Letter to You

Dear_____, (fill in your name)
Listen to advice and accept instruction, and in the end you will be wise. Many are the plans in your heart, but it is my purpose and plans that will prevail (Proverbs 19:20–21 paraphrased).
Your Life Planner, God

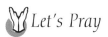 Let's Pray

Lord, we are busy women with schedules and plans. Many people depend on us; we don't want to disappoint them. Help us release expectations of others and ourselves. Presented with this life-threatening situation, everything else pales in comparison. We ask for eternal perspective to remember that what we miss or reschedule in this life is insignificant. We pray for anyone inconvenienced by our absence or inability to perform our usual duties. Shower with grace and mercy those who replace us or do the tasks themselves. Thank You in advance for rearranging our schedules and our lives. Help us rest in Your assurance it will all turn out for good with our plans in Your capable hands. We stand in awe that You, the Creator of the universe, care about our schedules. Amen.

Why?

I have cancer. I knew it in her office a month ago but had hoped my intuition would prove false. This is the sort of thing that happened to other people. Why me? The question everyone asks. The one without any answers. —Bonnie[5]

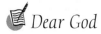 Dear God

Dear God,

Continually I search for answers to the whys . . . Why now? Why breast cancer? Why radiation? Why Tamoxifen? Why an oncologist? Why go through any of this? Why was my life spared? Why did You let this happen? Why a frozen shoulder? Why constant pain? Why more suffering after a life with scoliosis? Why not peace in my middle years? Why the struggle? Why the financial strain? So many whys . . .

Questioningly Yours, Janet

A Sister Shares

I questioned why God allowed this to happen, now that my new husband and I were so happy. Hadn't God just promised He had a wonderful plan for my life and Bob's? I felt terrible that I was going to put Bob through another battle with cancer. He had just lost his daughter to the disease. —Nancy Tuttle[6]

Mentoring Moment

Are you letting out a big sigh of relief that it is OK to ask why? Not only is it OK, I would wonder if you didn't. Our humanness makes us search for answers. Initially, we stoically go through the motions, but in the quiet of the night we ask, *Why?* We ask our doctors, "Why did this happen to me?" If a recurrence, we want to know why didn't they heal us permanently the first time? If complications, like my frozen shoulder, we want to know how and why it happened, and who's at fault? When I tell people about my frozen shoulder, they often ask, "Why did that happen?" My only frustrated answer, "I don't know, and neither do the doctors." In the world of quick, ready information at our fingertips on the Internet—we expect an instant answer. When we don't get it, we aren't satisfied until we do.

I do understand why it had to be me, but on days when my arm is killing me, or I cry all day, or am just plain down, I ask the questions. The answer I hear so often is, "Why *not* you? Will you still serve and honor Me, even if I never reveal the answer to you?" I know my answer to that tough question—"Yes, of course I will." I have.

This morning I woke up with all your faces on my heart. In my quiet time with the Lord, I read the opening chapters of 1 Chronicles with the many lists of names skipped over in past readings. Suddenly, the Lord reminded me that the Bible is a book about people! Not nameless, faceless people, but hundreds of real people, and God put all their names in the Bible for us to know them.

I may never know all your names or see your faces, but I do have the long-sought-after answer to my question, "Why me, Lord?" *You* are the reason I had breast cancer, and I love you for that. My heart breaks that you need this book, but I am grateful and hopeful it brings you closer to the One who has all the answers and the Book that records them. "For God sometimes uses sorrow in our lives to help us turn away from sin and seek eternal life. We should never regret his sending it" (2 Corinthians 7:10 TLB).

Every time someone asks about Dave and my new organic diet and I share the life changes we made since cancer—there is an obvious "why?" answer. Friends and acquaintances now faithfully getting mammograms—another answer. Are you seeing that in your life too? I hope so. At the end of this chapter I've provided you an opportunity to record those "whys" and the "what-for" answers. We may never have all our *earthly* whys answered, but for now take comfort in knowing the Bible is an *eternal* Answer Book. Read it, study it, have it read to you, and pray for God to relieve your worried whys and fill you with the peaceful what-fors.

God's Love Letter to You

Dear_____, *(fill in your name)*
I tell you, don't worry about everyday life—whether you have enough food, drink, and clothes. Doesn't life consist of more than food and clothing? Look at the birds. They don't need to plant or harvest or put food in barns because I feed them. And you are far more valuable to me than they are. Can all your worries add a single moment to your life? Of course not (Matthew 6:25–27 NLT paraphrased).
I AM the Answer to All Your Questions, God

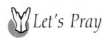 Let's Pray

Lord, we believe and pray together Hebrews 11:1–3 MSG:

The fundamental fact of existence is that this trust in God, this faith, is the firm foundation under everything that makes life worth living. It's our handle on what we can't see. The act of faith is what distinguished our ancestors, set them above the crowd. By faith we see the world called into existence by God's word, what we see created by what we don't see.

Help us be women of faith, trusting in Your divine providence, moving forward even when we don't have all the answers, remembering that You do! Impossible on our own, but with You as our Strength and Guide, we will flourish. Thank You for the example of Your Son, Jesus Christ, who did not ask why but only that Your will be done on earth as it is in heaven. This is our plea . . . this is our prayer. We are trusting You more and more each day. Amen.

Your Letter to God

Have the nagging, stomach-churning what-ifs, maybes, might-have-beens, if-onlys, what-abouts, and whys invaded your peace and sleep? Ask God for release to spend energy on the present. Ask for discernment and wisdom of where to delegate or ask for help. Pray that your doctors and their teams have patience and expertise in advising how to alter your life for this season, and pray for your willingness to listen and heed their answers. Can you find hope in knowing God's plan for your life is for good, not evil? Journal asking for the everlasting hope you can count on forever, and make a journal entry when you receive it.

Whys?	What-Fors?
_____	_____
_____	_____
_____	_____
_____	_____
_____	_____
_____	_____
_____	_____

CHAPTER FIVE

Dealing with People's Reactions

MY HEART BEATS WILDLY, MY STRENGTH FAILS, . . .
MY LOVED ONES AND FRIENDS STAY AWAY, FEARING MY DISEASE.
EVEN MY OWN FAMILY STANDS AT A DISTANCE. . . .
DO NOT ABANDON ME, LORD.
DO NOT STAND AT A DISTANCE, MY GOD.
COME QUICKLY TO HELP ME, O LORD MY SAVIOR.

—Psalm 38:10–11, 21–22 NLT

People Say the Darnedest Things

I FOUND MYSELF IN TROUBLE AND WENT LOOKING FOR MY LORD; MY LIFE WAS AN OPEN WOUND THAT WOULDN'T HEAL. WHEN FRIENDS SAID, "EVERYTHING WILL TURN OUT ALL RIGHT," I DIDN'T BELIEVE A WORD THEY SAID. —PSALM 77:2 MSG

KIND WORDS HEAL AND HELP; CUTTING WORDS WOUND AND MAIM.
—PROVERBS 15:4 MSG

WELL-SPOKEN WORDS BRING SATISFACTION. —PROVERBS 12:14 MSG

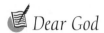 ## Dear God

Dear God,

Forgive me for all the hurtful things I callously say to others. Breast cancer impressed upon me how ill equipped we often are to say the right thing at the right time. So often our careless words inflict pain and heartache. For example, questions often asked when someone finds out I have breast cancer are, "In both?" "Are you losing both of them?" "Did they take them both off?" In my case they didn't, but what if they did? It sounds so sterile. So cold. So harsh. So personal. So impersonal. Not wanting to say the word *breasts,* they reduce this body part to inanimate objects—"them." Do they realize "taking them off" means cutting my breasts from my body? I recoil at these questions often asked with the casualness of, "Do you want one scoop or two?" I hurt deeply for all those women who did lose their breasts, and it casts the shadow of a doubt as to whether I should have kept mine. It is simply the wrong thing to say to any of us.

I've also noticed everyone seems compelled to comment on how I look. They either say with great shock, "You look so good! Doesn't she look good?" with the unspoken insinuation, " . . . for a person with cancer!" Or they comment on how great I look when I know I really do look bad. I asked Dave, "Why is everyone saying this to me? Did I really look that bad?" Dave's answer was that with the changes we made in our diet, I actually look better than before cancer. I think that is a compliment!

Lord, how can I graciously let people know the inappropriateness of their questions and comments and help them take my cue as to what is comfortable discussion? Please give me words that build up and do not tear down.

Frustratingly Yours, Janet

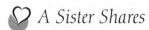 ## A Sister Shares

While grocery shopping, I literally ran into our former tax consultant, Linda Ferrigno, and her husband, Vince. Linda is recovering from lung cancer. We spent most of our time telling stories

of the darnedest things people say. Linda had one lung removed and becomes winded easily, so they have a handicapped sticker on their car. Vince told me that once he and Linda attended an event with a busy parking lot, and someone actually came up and told him how *lucky* they were to park in handicapped! He could not believe his ears! Linda would rather be healthy and walk from the farthest corner of the parking lot than have close parking because she is handicapped. People often have things all out of perspective. —Janet

 Mentoring Moment

Maybe my discomfort comes from not having had a mastectomy. Answering those intrusive questions creates a collision of emotions— gratitude, unease, guilt, sadness, and doubt. I lose my peace. There is a check in my spirit and a sinking in my stomach. What difference does it make? Why would they need to know? Are they asking out of compassion or curiosity? If you had a mastectomy, I can only imagine the affront of callous and careless questions and comments you are enduring.

Some people are very gentle and kind, but so many others are abrupt, curious, and clueless. Linda Ferrigno and I also compared notes on our frozen shoulders we each incurred after surgery and radiation. Vince said people often got the strangest look on their faces when he said his wife had a frozen shoulder—almost like, *So what?* Yet Martha Ramsey wrote an entire book about the pain she suffered with her frozen shoulder. I found that the same people *repeatedly* asked the same question, "What caused that? Why do you have that?" Were they not listening or unable to accept the only answer I had? "No one knows for sure which part of the treatment caused it, but it is there." Renewed pain and sadness floods my heart each time I have to say that.

My solution is to stop talking about it. This might help you too. If *we* bring up a topic, then it sends a message that it is fair game as a discussion subject. Therefore, consciously choose not to discuss parts of your treatment or physical condition that are particularly uncomfortable or known to bring hurtful responses. We all struggle with speaking the truth in love. I find a good response to a painful question is, "You know, I am really not comfortable talking about that right now, but I could use your prayers for my recovery." Then change the subject. It is honest—you didn't embarrass them but lovingly conveyed that a more appropriate question for them to ask is, "How can I pray for you?"

If we feel compelled to answer their inappropriate questions, we run the risk of plummeting into a sea of breast cancer stories we don't want or need to hear. Most people think we want suggestions, or they have to come up with something oh so spiritual to say, or someone else's story will make us feel better about ours. What clearly needs expressing is that we just want their love, help, and prayers.

A friend told me that without thinking, she commented to a breast cancer survivor, "I sure am glad I have *my* breasts." To which the survivor responded, "I sure am glad I don't." I advise all women speaking to a breast cancer woman, *if you have not had breast cancer, don't say anything about your breasts or hers. There is no way you can understand how she feels, and there is no way she is going to be comforted about how you feel about your breasts. Either way, you have inflicted pain.*

I talk about my breast cancer from the speaking platform. Fellow breast cancer sisters or their relatives come up at breaks to share their stories, and I let them tell as much or little as they want. I respond the same way. The particulars are not as important as learning we are meeting a sister with a similar experience. We don't have to know all the gory details to share a common bond revealed in our eyes. Words aren't necessary to give a hug and a prayer.

Through my own discomfort, God revealed how innocently hurtful words come out of our mouths. My daughter, Kim, struggled with infertility. She and I were talking with an acquaintance married fifteen years with no children. I asked if this woman had considered adoption, because Kim was leaning that way, and I thought she might have some information for her. The woman said, "No, we did not pursue that." Later Kim gently said to me, "Mom, that was one of 'those questions' you are always talking about. If they don't have children after fifteen years, they probably chose not to adopt and that was a very personal question. If she wanted to talk about it, she would have brought it up on her own." I thanked Kim for bringing this to my attention and sought out the woman to apologize for being insensitive since I, of all people, should know better.

So don't be too judgmental or condemning. Just help others learn how to be more considerate and loving in their conversation, and learn from it yourself.

God's Love Letter to You

Dear_____, (fill in your name)

My dear sisters, be quick to listen, slow to speak, and slow to get angry because your anger can never make things right in my sight (James 1:19–20 NLT paraphrased). Forgive others from your heart (Matthew 18:35 paraphrased). Above all else, guard your heart, for it is the wellspring of life (Proverbs 4:23).
Your Forgiver, God

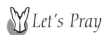 Let's Pray

Lord, please give us "tough skin" so the callous, unthinking remarks of others don't puncture our courage or daunt our fight for life. Provide us with loving, forthright words. Let us be instruments You use to help others know how to respond to someone going through a crisis. Help us be sensitive to our words spoken to others. Guard our tongues and hearts. Use us as instruments of Your love. Amen.

Top Thirteen Dos and Don'ts

When my mother was diagnosed with breast cancer in 1995, I automatically dropped into my natural state. I provided energy, positivism, and intellectual counsel. I focused on the inevitable victory of recovery, rather than the daily drudgery of treatment. As she probably expected, I removed myself from the emotional and concentrated on my role as the strong-willed only child with the unyielding positive attitude.
—*Randall Niles*[2]

IF SOMEONE COMES TO SEE ME, HE MOUTHS EMPTY PLATITUDES.
—PSALM 41:6 MSG

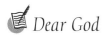 Dear God

Dear God,

You know how badly I needed "The Top Ten Things Not to Say or Do to Someone with Breast Cancer," which I jokingly talked about but never took time to write and use. Consequently, I struggled through a painful time. Some people, even those I love dearly, had a look in their eyes I have never seen before—it conveys "death." I was still trying to process that I had cancer, and they seemed already to have me buried!

It was eerie . . . I had dreaded this all my life, praying it would not be me and I wouldn't be part of an ever-growing group of women with the "big C," as some refer to it. Finally, I couldn't take another phone call, read any more e-mails, or see another mournful face. I knew they loved me, and like Jesus said on the cross, "They know not what they do." They needed education, but I didn't feel like being the teacher yet. Eventually, but not now. Lord, I prayed You would forgive them and

Book Pick

Simple Acts of Kindness: Practical Ways to Help People in Need by Terri Green is a sweet book you might find helpful to hand to people. Terri also attends my church, Saddleback. The caption on the outside cover reads: "Whether you have a friend struggling through a trial or simply want to learn how to reach out, *Simple Acts of Kindness* will show you how to become a vehicle for Jesus's love in practical and meaningful ways."[1]

forgive me for some of the thoughts that went through my mind. I fought the urge to scream, "Just tell me you love me! You are praying for me. You will be there for me. I don't want to hear one more horror story or self-righteous 'God is in control,' or 'You know, it could have been worse' comment! I can't take it!"

I prayed for the right heart and healing of each wound from careless comments. What saved me during that time was my constant prayer, "Lord, what is the purpose of all this? What do You want me to learn? What difference do You want me to make?" Graciously, You answered me. Many go through this. Maybe I had been one of those people who said the wrong thing at the wrong time. How many times had I hurt someone? So *first*, I needed to pray for forgiveness and wisdom never to do that again. *Second*, I needed to acknowledge gratefulness for those who gave a comforting response, sent a card, or helped. Like Jane, who made a quick recovery from the shock of my diagnosis and just said to me, "I have never known anyone with breast cancer before. This is all new to me." Then putting her hand on my knee, she said, "I will be there for you." *Third*, I needed to be in the shoes of someone experiencing this onslaught, so I could eventually help others know how to respond. Use me, Lord. Help me be strong. My prayer continues to be, "Give me courage throughout the breast cancer experience."

Wounded and Yours, Janet

A Sister Shares

The one thing I felt somewhat uncomfortable about was that my sister never once asked me how I felt: What did it feel like when I was told I had breast cancer? What does it feel like having to go to radiation therapy every day for eight to nine weeks? How does it feel now? I got the feeling if she didn't talk about it, then she didn't have to deal with it. However, maybe my sister was thinking she might someday get breast cancer, too, since my mother and I both were diagnosed with it, so she should go to the doctor with me to see what happens—which she did. My sister is five years older and in the insurance business. She has quite a few clients with breast cancer. —Jamie

Mentoring Moment

Just today at the grocery store I ran into a woman from church. Within seconds of our mutual greeting, she launched into two stories of people with cancer—one who died. Neither of these people had breast cancer, but she seemed compelled to share about everyone she knew with *any kind* of cancer—even though mine was now over a year ago. She never asked how I was doing. It doesn't bother me as much now as it did in the thick of it. Yet still I wonder, *What makes people do that*?

I jokingly told doctors and friends, "I am going to come up with a list of the Top Ten

Things Not to Say to Someone with Breast Cancer!" The doctors and staff all responded, "That's a great idea!" I asked, "You mean you don't already have that to hand out to patients?" They said, "No, but if you write one, we'll use it. It is so badly needed." When I mentioned this top ten list to friends and family, almost unanimously they would ask, "What are you going to put on it? We need to know." I discovered they sincerely wanted to know, because no one has ever taught them. They seriously need and desire help. So I did write that list, but it turned into the Top Thirteen Dos and Don'ts! Maybe you can help educate your friends and family. Most people will be quite grateful if you do it in love.

Try not to let yourself dwell on reactions that disappoint you. It is difficult to tell how certain family members or friends will react. Don't set your expectations too high. It will only make you mad, angry, or depressed, and that won't help. Focus on those who show their love and concern, and make every effort to surround yourself with them. It takes a person who understands giving selflessly and loving unconditionally to really meet your needs at this time. This is new territory for everyone, and honestly, most people receive no guidance or instruction in how to respond to someone in crisis. God may be at work changing their hearts—that calls for a praise reaction!

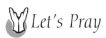 *God's Love Letter to You*

*Dear*_____*, (fill in your name)*

You must make allowance for each other's faults and forgive the person who offends you. Remember, I forgave you, so you must forgive others. And the most important piece of clothing you must wear is love. Love is what binds you all together in perfect harmony. And let the peace that comes from my Son, Jesus Christ, rule in your hearts. For as members of one body you are all called to live in peace. And always be thankful (Colossians 3:13–15 NLT paraphrased).
I love you, God

Let's Pray

Prayerfully personalize with me Psalm 19:12–14.

Our Father in heaven, we know we have said and done hurtful things ourselves, and so we pray . . .

Forgive _____ and Janet's hidden faults. Keep your servants, _____ and Janet, also from willful sins; may they not rule over _____ and Janet. Then will we, _____ and Janet, be blameless, innocent of great transgression. May the words of _____'s and Janet's mouths and the meditation of _____ and Janet's hearts be pleasing in your sight, O LORD, _____'s and Janet's Rock and _____'s and Janet's Redeemer. Amen.

The Top Thirteen Things to Do or Say
and Not to Say or Do to Someone with Breast Cancer

WORRY WEIGHS A PERSON DOWN; AN ENCOURAGING WORD CHEERS A PERSON UP.
—PROVERBS 12:25 NLT

After I joked about coming up with a list of the Top Ten Things Not to Say to Someone with Breast Cancer, I read an article from a wife who lost her husband in the 9/11 tragedy She had put together a similar list for those who have encountered the loss of a loved one for the same reason I finally did: people are clueless.

Here is my version specific for breast cancer, and hopefully the Lord gives you courage to share it with those well-meaning people who really don't know what to say or do. They will be grateful. Some people actually avoid us just because they are afraid they will put their foot in their mouth or because words escape them. In their desire to prevent hurt, they create it. We feel alone and abandoned because others are uncomfortable around us. Try using this list. (I expanded the list to the Top Thirteen, then added thirteen do's, as well.)

DON'T . . .

1. Talk about people you know with breast cancer. Good or bad stories are not helpful.

2. Tell me God is in control, has a plan, or knew it was going to happen.

3. Say "I'll pray for you" unless you mean it. I will be counting on those prayers.

4. Say, "Call me if you need anything." I don't know what you are willing to do and might be too sick or sad to pick up the phone.

DO . . .

1. Let me talk about mine and listen.

2. Just show me the love of God.

3. Pray for and with me.

4. Offer to do something specific; then do it.

5. Look at me like I am dying. I can read your body language and eyes, and it scares me.

5. Show genuine compassion and concern.

6. Avoid me. It makes me feel rejected, different.

6. Keep normal contact with me.

7. Act like nothing is happening, minimize my situation, or compare me with someone else.

7. Take your cue from me as to how comfortable I am talking about it.

8. Tell others, unless you have asked if it is OK.

8. Ask me if it is OK to tell others, and honor my wishes.

9. Feel bad if I can't return phone calls or cards.

9. Keep calling and leave a message. I love to hear your voice and look forward to the mail.

10. Be resentful of how my illness affects you.

10. Help me learn to live with my "new normal" that might also change my life.

11. Forget about me after the initial flurry of the diagnosis. This will be a long haul, and I need you.

11. Let me grieve, and understand that takes time. Stick with me.

12. Feel you have to say you "understand" how I feel. If you have not had breast cancer yourself, you don't understand.

12. Let me talk without trying to fix it or feel you have to comment. I might just need a listening ear.

13. Ask me questions like, Are you having them both taken off? Or on both sides? In fact, don't ask me any personal questions about my condition.

13. Let me tell you what I am comfortable saying. Keep your curiosity curtailed. I will tell you what I want you to know right now.

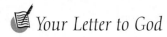 *Your Letter to God*

Can you forgive those who said and did hurtful things? If God brings to mind someone you need to ask forgiveness of or to forgive, write his or her name in your journal entry and pray for the right time and place. Forgiveness frees you from the burden of bitterness that can get a foothold on your mind and heart. Give praise for those who are encouragers.

Dear God,   *Date:* _____

_____

_____

_____

_____

_____

_____

_____

_____

_____

_____

_____

_____

_____

_____

_____

_____

_____

_____

Chapter Six

Preparing for What Comes Next

With your very own hands you formed me;
now breathe your wisdom over me so I can understand you.
When they see me waiting, expecting your Word,
those who fear you will take heart and be glad.
I can see now, God, that your decisions are right;
your testing has taught me what's true and right.
Oh, love me—and right now!—hold me tight!
just the way you promised.
Now comfort me so I can live, really live;
your revelation is the tune I dance to.

—Psalm 119:73–77 MSG

Putting Together Your Treatment Team

Now to choose the doctor. . . . I'll make the decision now that I think is right—if it proves wrong, I thought it was right at the time. . . . I realize some decisions can't be changed once they are made and . . . so, we just trust and trust and trust. —Martha[1]

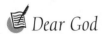 Dear God

Dear God,

I always said, "If ever I have cancer, I want the very best doctors. I'll go anywhere to find them. Get the cancer out right away." That's incongruous, since finding the best doctors could take time, which might not allow the "right away" part. I pray You picked my doctors even before I had cancer. When my gynecologist, Dr. Carter, sent me to a breast care center and breast specialist and surgeon out of my immediate area, a place I never would have known to select on my own, it seemed a sign from You. There were so many other signs—meeting my friend Grace at the BreastCare Center, discovering they would connect me with the other treatment doctors, seeing the surgeon's and radiologist's picture in the newspaper—all gave me a sense of peace that Dr. West was the right surgeon and that the Orange County BreastCare Center & Oncology Center was the right place.

I can talk to Dr. West. I always take a list of questions, and he actually seems appreciative of that. When he starts talking fast, I ask him to slow down so I can write the answers. I feel when it comes to skill, heart, and knowledge, he is the one. And it really is a short travel compared to where others might have to go to find their surgeons.

Lord, I also feel comfortable with the suggested radiation oncologist and oncologist, who both have offices near our home. Your hand is visible every step of the way. That gives me solace.

Trustingly Yours, Janet

A Sister Shares

In late August my husband and I had a consultation with a surgeon in Longview, Texas. The following week the surgeon performed a stereo tactic breast biopsy. Two days later, he phoned with the news: "You have ductal carcinoma in situ, the earliest detectable form of breast cancer. It's noninvasive." The news shook me, but I focused on what the doctor said: "earliest detectable form, noninvasive." I thought, *That's positive. That's good news. This can be cured!*

The next week my husband and I met with the surgeon again. He went over the diagnosis and options for treatment. My options were lumpectomy or mastectomy. I felt very blessed to have the cancer detected at such an early stage. My prognosis was excellent! I sought a second opinion from a surgical oncologist in Dallas, and he gave me the same diagnosis and options for treatment. I felt confident I had the correct diagnosis, so I scheduled a lumpectomy in Longview. Since I had an excellent prognosis with either lumpectomy or mastectomy, I chose lumpectomy because it was the less radical procedure. —Anita

 ## *Mentoring Moment*

Breast cancer suddenly brings a multitude of new doctors and decisions into your life. The treatment decisions we make influence the types of doctors we need. Some of us will need a bigger team than others. Maybe you were someone who seldom went to a doctor; now your calendar is full of doctor and treatment appointments. New faces, new relationships, new personalities, men and women all working together to save your life. That is their call and life mission; however, some are a better fit for you than others.

The important thing is to feel peace and confidence in your medical team. I hope you have that. If you can't talk to them, or if you don't feel they take you seriously, or if you question their expertise, then get a second opinion. Do research and make an appointment with another doctor to see if your personalities fit better or he has a strategy you prefer. Obtaining a second opinion will not threaten a confident doctor. Actually, some insurance companies require it. What works for one person might not for another. Maybe someone loves a certain doctor, but you aren't comfortable with him. This is your body and your treatment. It is extremely important that you feel at ease with your medical team.

Just be cautious not to use this search as an excuse to postpone necessary treatment. If your situation is urgent, research these doctors immediately. Use the "Peacekeeping Worksheet" on page 349, and prayerfully arrive at a decision. Once you make your *peaceful decision*, don't look back. You are going to meet other patients during this journey and exchange names of doctors, and each one thinks her doctor is the best. That can start you second-guessing; there is no point in that. Nor should you try to convince another patient you have the best doctors, because that will make her feel insecure. Just like there are many good pastors, there are many good doctors. Be grateful you each found the right one for you.

I felt it important to establish a personal and medical relationship with each of my doctors and their teams. I wanted them to know more about me than just my diagnosis and treatment, so I gave each one a brochure about the Woman to Woman Mentoring Ministry and a flier with my picture and a brief biography. It is always comforting at appointments when they open my medical file and there is my flyer reminding them of who I am and what I do. Ask someone to help you put together a simple flier on the computer with a picture of you or you and your family and a brief personal biography. Or paste a picture on a piece of paper and write a few words about yourself. Hand your flier to each of your doctors during your introductory meeting. We go to see doctors armed with medical records, copies of x-rays, and reports, but we often forget the human element. You can take the lead in establishing personal rapport from the very first appointment.

God's Love Letter to You

Dear_____, (fill in your name)

Trust in me, GOD, with all your heart and lean not on your own understanding; in all your ways acknowledge me, and I will make your paths straight. Do not be wise in your own eyes; fear me and shun evil. This will bring health to your body and nourishment to your bones (Proverbs 3:5–8 paraphrased).
The Great Physician, God

Let's Pray

God, You are the Great Physician working mightily on our behalf and using mere mortals to do Your earthly work. The medical teams watching over our health hold our lives in their hands. Help us make peaceful decisions. Give us confidence and courage to ask questions. We never wanted these doctors in the first place; part of us is resentful for even having to search them out. Yet we should be grateful there are men and women who dedicate their lives to saving ours. You can make good out of any decision we make, so let us rest in that comforting thought. Thank You for your presence during this process. In Your Son's precious name we pray. Amen.

The Planning Conference

My faith was tested when Earl, my husband, and I went to see my doctor for the conference to schedule surgery. —Linda Taylor

I looked at my surgeon and asked, "What do we do next?" —Gloria

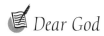 *Dear God*

Dear God,

Your presence filled the conference room as Dave, Kim, Dr. West—my chosen surgeon—his assistant Donna, and I sat around a table as Dr. West drew pictures and diagrams explaining my options—all of them. Yes, just like the nurse on the phone had said, I could choose a complete mastectomy, although he added it was not his recommendation for me. In my early stage of detection, his recommendation was partial mastectomy, also called a lumpectomy, followed by radiation, and Tamoxifen. Since my cancer was noninvasive, I would not need chemotherapy. Did I want my lymph nodes checked? The doctor expected them to be clear. That is what statistics said about my calcium deposits too. Things weren't turning out like expected. He said I could sleep on that decision. Dave and Kim looked at me as we said in unison "and pray on it." Amazingly, after all the drawings, arrows, scribbling, and detailed discussion, the only question I had was, "Am I going to lose my hair?" He was talking about losing my breast or breasts, and I asked about my hair. I am sure he hears it all. No, he assured me, I would not lose my hair.

Vainly Yours, Janet

 A Sister Shares

My doctor called to say I needed a mastectomy. When my husband and I talked with him in his office, he told us he had spoken with another doctor who specialized in breast surgery. This doctor said, if possible, they try to save the breast by doing a lumpectomy. I was fearful of having just the lumpectomy, but Earl spoke up and said, "I prayed asking God for you to have the cancer removed and keep your breast." I honored his prayer. —Linda Taylor

 Mentoring Moment

If you have not had the planning conference, pray about who should attend with you and what questions to ask and write them down on the "Appointment Notes" (page 353). My surgeon actually called it a

family conference, so I knew my family would attend. You may only want members of your immediate family or a close relative or friend to attend. I wish I had invited my best friend, Jane. It would have helped as she walked beside me every step of the way. A close friend will consider the invitation an honor.

I knew my daughter, Kim, needed to be present because this was now her heritage. It wasn't just happening to me; it was affecting *all* our lives. It would be great if your teenage and adult children attend, but especially try to have your daughters go with you. Since my other two daughters are stepdaughters, my diagnosis did not impact their health directly, but we kept them informed of all the details. If you are married, be sure your husband attends, even if he has to take off work—especially if he is having difficulty dealing with the reality of your breast cancer.

If possible, also have someone else present who is not as emotionally involved. Asking a representative from your church staff to attend is quite appropriate. He or she can be an objective person asking questions you can't formulate and taking notes while you and your family interact with the doctor. You receive a tremendous amount of overwhelming new information at this treatment launching point. It is very difficult to absorb everything in one sitting. You need freedom to talk, cry, and question, without trying to remember everything.

God's Love Letter to You

Dear_____, (fill in your name)
The heartfelt counsel of a friend is as sweet as perfume and incense. Never abandon a friend—either yours or your father's. Then in your time of need, you won't have to ask your relatives for assistance. It is better to go to a neighbor than to a relative who lives far away (Proverbs 27:9–10 NLT).
Your Great Counselor, God

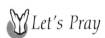 Let's Pray

Oh God, this is one of the hardest things our families have encountered. We need their support so badly, but they are afraid too. Some don't really want to hear about what is going on, not to mention attend this planning conference. Lord, help us bravely listen to the options and choices presented. Give us ears to hear and eyes to see. Help us not to become overwhelmed but to peacefully and carefully sort through the options and arrive at the course of treatment best for us. Thank You in advance for going with us. Amen.

Time to Make a Decision

Fortunately, where emotions shut down, my brain took over, and I went into a very practical, calm cognitive state: What were the steps? What did I need to do next? I gathered as much information as possible in a very short span of time. —Grace Marestaing

My greatest difficulty was actually deciding which avenue to take: lumpectomy or mastectomy? My answer came when a bouquet arrived at the door delivered by a former pastor-friend who's now a florist. On the doorstep we prayed together for guidance, and I got such a peace, a real physical rush, followed by total calmness and knowledge of what I should do. —Shirley

 ## Dear God

Dear God,

After the family conference, Grace Marestaing, the patient representative volunteer, gave us a tour of the BreastCare Center, showing us their extensive library and available computers, but the last thing I wanted right then was more information. I had just received more than I wanted to hear.

Lunchtime was emotional. I cried. Kim tried to be strong. Dave had listened carefully and arrived at a decision. We tried to eat and talk over the options. All three of us agreed we wanted something done soon. We reviewed our notes and concluded I should have the lumpectomy and radiation. We did want the lymph nodes checked just to be sure. Things hadn't been going as we thought or hoped, so we'd better cover our bases. Of course, there was always the possibility I could get the complications in my arm the doctor mentioned. We would deal with that when and if it happened. For now we would just focus on keeping me alive to feel the pain.

Decidedly Yours, Janet

 ## A Sister Shares

The decision to have a bilateral mastectomy with reconstruction was the result of experiences with my mother's mastectomy a year and a half before my diagnosis and the process of decision making with my doctors. I had read about breast cancer, was familiar with what a mastectomy looked like, and had helped my mother shop for her prosthesis. As my surgeon presented the options, I first decided not to do radiation, which was a must with a lumpectomy. Besides, my cancer was invasive. So my decision was mastectomy. I asked about the other noncancerous breast, and he was neutral. If I decided to go that route, he would do a simple mastectomy on the other side. The reconstructive surgeon helped me process through the next steps with his expertise and experience.

I must point out this is a very personal decision-making process for each woman. Breast cancer varies from person to person in type, severity, and options for treatment—as well as the personal preferences and dynamics of one's life. Three years, five surgeries, and chemotherapy later, I am very happy my process of decision making took me down this path. —Grace Marestaing

 Mentoring Moment

During the decision-making process I made a conscious decision to:

- Wait and hear my options from the doctor at the planning session

- Listen to his recommendations

- Ask questions

- Then determine how much research I needed or wanted to do

This method has served its purpose in my life to avoid unnecessary worry until I know what, or if, there is something to worry about. I wish we had the Peacekeeping Worksheet (page 349) to use with our decisions. We didn't. I hadn't designed it yet. I was in no condition to design a rational form, and you probably won't be either. That's why the Peacekeeping Worksheet is ready when you need it. Here's how to use it in decision making:

- Write down all your options, noting the pros and cons of each.

- Record all the doctors' comments, information, and recommendations.

- List results of research.

- Consider information from other breast cancer patients.

- Consult with your family.

- Pray over the completed worksheet.

- When you have peace with a decision, go with it, and don't look back.

Have the planning conference with the surgeon, and hear what he or she has to say *before* doing extensive research. You don't have to make any hard decisions at that conference. The doctor gives you pictures, explanations, and recommendations preparing you for what to investigate. Then set up another meeting or phone conference to ask questions after you research your specific type of breast cancer and surgery. It is pointless to research *all* the different kinds of breast cancer. Many women search the Internet relentlessly and come to the planning conference with their eyes glazed over and a thick folder that has them more confused then ever. I am not saying don't do research; however, when you reach a point of information overload and nothing seems clear . . .

- Stop and pray over what you have compiled.

- Remove information that contradicts each other.

- Hone in solely on what applies to you.

- Stay in the moment.

If you are not a research person, don't worry about it. Your doctor has done tons of research, and hopefully, you feel comfortable enough to respect his or her recommendation. Get a second opinion if you want; this is a huge decision. However, eventually you need to move on with your treatment. Don't torment yourself second-guessing every decision. God can and will grant you discernment and peace. It won't necessarily be a choice you like. Nothing about this is something we like or want.

Many of us have the fleeting thought that if we stall making a decision, we can crawl under the covers and wake up one day with our old life back. Others just want it over with as fast as possible so they can put it behind them and move on. Do not feel guilty about any of your reactions. You have a diagnosis all women dread. You never wanted to make any of these decisions . . . not to mention trying to decide if they're the right decisions. Give yourself time to cope with the reality of it all, and listen to your doctor's advice as to how quickly you need to take action.

My diagnosis was in late October, and the doctor said I could wait for surgery until after the holidays. I was looking at a very full speaking schedule the next year and realized the longer we put it off, the more it would affect my obligations. So we scheduled surgery several days after my last speaking engagement in November and a week before Thanksgiving. It made for a very unusual and different kind of holiday season, but my family rebounded beautifully, and it was good having them home at Christmas to help.

Most people will be quite resilient and understanding that plans need to change and priorities shifted to focus on your fight for life. "Fight for life" rather puts it all into perspective, doesn't it? So now you have decisions to make. I pray it won't be too difficult for you. Bathe yourself in prayer, and use the "Peacekeeping Worksheet" in appendix B.

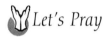 *God's Love Letter to You*

Dear_____, (fill in your name)
  I will instruct you and teach you in the way you should go; I will counsel you and watch over you (Psalm 32:8).
Your Decision Helper, God

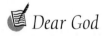 Let's Pray

Prayerfully personalize with me Hebrews 13:20–21.

Lord, we come together before you in prayer . . .

May the God of peace, who through the blood of the eternal covenant brought back from the dead our Lord Jesus, that great Shepherd of the sheep, equip _____ and Janet with everything good for doing his will, and may he work in us, _____ and Janet, what is pleasing to him, through Jesus Christ, to whom be glory for ever and ever. Amen.

More Waiting

BE STILL BEFORE THE LORD AND WAIT PATIENTLY FOR HIM. —PSALM 37:7

I had to go back yesterday for more biopsies. I was supposed to hear from them today, but they called and said the report was not in, so I'll have to wait until Monday. —Edna

Dear God

Dear God,

I called and told Dr. West the family decision to have the lumpectomy and diagnostic lymph nodes removed. Then came the flurry of phone calls back and forth to set all the dates. So many tests and procedures before the surgery date in one month. I laughed at the irony of the surgery date falling two days after the scheduled date for the original mammogram with the center that forgot to send out the letter. I would just be discovering all this. Surgery instead of a routine mammogram that week!

Lord, I know it was you prompting my gynecologist, Dr. Carter, to think he felt something in the right breast, when all along the problem was in the left. When I called and thanked him for being so diligent, he seemed a little surprised but grateful for the acknowledgment. He assured me I was in the best of hands and would do well. I needed to hear those reassuring words as many times as possible.

Then came the scary phone call that the consultant radiologist at the surgery hospital wanted more mammograms of the left and right sides. "Do they suspect more cancer?" I asked. "Maybe," they hedged. "On the other side?" "Yes." Back for more pictures, at the hospital breast center. All new faces. Then the dreadful waiting for the phone call with the results that could possibly change all the plans and disrupt my peace. Here we go again . . . in Your waiting room. Adding to the drama, the consultant radiologist got food poisoning and could not read the x-rays and give a report for two days. Trying to live life as normal, I headed out with the ministry team for our annual fall retreat, my cell phone nearby. The car grew silent when the phone rang. Anticipation filled the air. Good news! No new spots. We would proceed as planned. That was a tough retreat. I wanted to cry all the time, but the women were looking to me for direction. Their love and compassion was healing and calming. They helped me with the wait.

Returning from the retreat, I continued with scheduled speaking trips. Interestingly, many who previously had heard me speak said I was different this time. The waiting and awareness of my vulnerability brought out a new boldness and sense of urgency to make my message understood. They seemed to get it. Lord, thank You that my schedule was so full—it helped with the wait. Our grandsons came home early for the holidays, and I held new baby Micah the day before my surgery. New life quickened my desire to enjoy every moment with these precious grandbabies . . . so young, innocent, and loving. Their unconditional love and joy was the best antidote for waiting—just what the doctor ordered!

Waiting with You, Janet

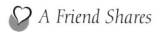 A Friend Shares

[An e-mail I received after a speaking engagement one week before surgery]
Janet,
When you walked into the room and sat down, I looked up and smiled at you. I noticed there was something different about you; I didn't know what it was, but there was a different look on your face and in your eyes. After the conference was over and everyone had gone home, Chris and I were cleaning up the mess! She shared with me your new journey.

I got in my truck and thought about you all the way home and it finally came to me that what I saw on your face was the glory and the strength of the Lord. You really did look different, even your smile was different. Your eyes, as you looked at me and greeted me, were softer. Reflecting back on that day and knowing what I know now, the silent testimony you gave me was hope. Hope that when my trouble comes, He will provide all I lack. I saw His strength and His glory on you, and when you spoke, I heard in your voice complete trust and peaceful joy. Thank you for showing me the provision of the Lord. I am praying for you daily.
Grace and peace, Lucinda Rountree

Mentoring Moment

I don't know about you, but I have been impatient my whole life—to be filled with patience is my constant prayer. Since waiting takes patience, keeping my normal schedule is my preferred waiting technique. It's good therapy for me. I wait best staying busy. I really wasn't sick; I looked normal. I felt the picture of health and energy. So carrying on as usual left little time to dwell on the circumstances or worry about life after breast cancer. God blessed my speaking during that time by taking it to a new depth.

I am sure your breast cancer found you in a similar situation—life. Right in the middle of all you do every day, a bomb drops. It consumes your thoughts. Maintaining normal activities, when you wonder if life will ever be "normal" again, may seem impossible right now. Let me assure you, it is the best therapy. While we can never go back to the days before breast cancer, we can maximize the ones still available before treatments or surgery commence. Our families and friends also will cope much better if they see us doing the things we did before. Waiting periods allow everyone to adjust to changing lives, but for now we live our lives one day at a time. This is not denial. This is living in the present.

📖 Gods Love Letter to You

Dear_____, (fill in your name)
Wait for me; be strong and take heart and wait for me (Psalm 27:14
paraphrased).
Waiting with you, God

🐰 Let's Pray

Prayerfully personalize with me Psalm 33:20–22.

We, _____ and Janet, wait in hope for the LORD; he is our help and our shield. In him our hearts rejoice, for we, _____ and Janet, trust in his holy name. May your unfailing love rest upon us, O LORD, even as we, _____ and Janet, put our hope in you. Amen.

Being a Good Witness

THE WORLD'S A HUGE STOCKPILE OF GOD-WONDERS AND GOD-THOUGHTS. NOTHING AND NO ONE COMES CLOSE TO YOU! I START TALKING ABOUT YOU, TELLING WHAT I KNOW, AND QUICKLY RUN OUT OF WORDS. NEITHER NUMBERS NOR WORDS ACCOUNT FOR YOU.
—PSALM 40:5 MSG

I WILL PRAISE THE LORD AT ALL TIMES. I WILL CONSTANTLY SPEAK HIS PRAISES. I WILL BOAST ONLY IN THE LORD; LET ALL WHO ARE DISCOURAGED TAKE HEART. COME, LET US TELL OF THE LORD'S GREATNESS; LET US EXALT HIS NAME TOGETHER.
—PSALM 34:1–3 NLT

✍️ Dear God

Dear God,

As I filled out the initial patient application for the BreastCare Center, You were revealing the purpose and plan for my breast cancer. I began writing "self-employed" for the answer to "Who is your employer?" You gently nudged, "Janet, you are not actually self-employed. I AM your employer. After all, your ministry name is *About*

His Work Ministries." *Oh, yes, You are right, Lord,* I thought. So I wrote in "The Lord," as my employer. Little did I know how many places that application would travel. As I meet all kinds of people—doctors, technicians, nurses, fellow patients—my prayer is, "Lord, let me be a witness to any who do not know You, and let those who do be a comfort to me."

Lord, You answered that prayer big time! It was so reassuring when someone would pop in while I was having a mammogram or procedure and with a smiling face announce, "Just wanted you to know I have the same Employer you do!" Nurse Barbara, the head of the hospital breast center, saw who my Boss was and introduced herself by saying she shared the same Boss. Wow! Oh God, another sign—this was the right hospital. Barbara was a sister in Christ who would be following my case carefully in the days to come.

I also knew people would be watching to see how Dave and I handled a crisis in our life as Christians. I prayed we would be a sincere witness there too. From the responses we received, it truly seems we accomplished that. Lord, it is easy being happy when things are going well, but the true test of our faith is when they aren't. Dave and I want others to see we have a peace and joy that could never come from our own resources. Thank You for giving Dave and me evangelistic gifts and a heart to use them. We are grateful and pray others draw closer to You because of my breast cancer.

Evangelically Yours, Janet

 ## Janet Shares

Please forgive the group e-mail; but all of you have been so faithful and loving to pray, I know you are anxious to hear the results. First, I have felt every single one of those prayers! Thank you so much! God has faithfully answered them and given us peace that passes understanding. Well, there is good news and bad news. Bad news, it is the big C. Good news! It is noninvasive, meaning it is contained and surgically removable. Radiation should result in 100 percent cure. We will let you know the surgery date in November. We appreciate continued prayers as we all adjust to this new character-building experience. Also, asking for prayers of focus as I have three speaking engagements in November and three Woman to Woman Mentoring Ministry events. My prayer is that none will be disappointed, and I can honor all of the speaking engagements.

Also, Dave and I planned to spend Thanksgiving in Sun Valley (tough duty, right?) with Kim and Toby and Toby's parents, and we are still hoping to make the trip. Here is a quote from Warren Wiersbe I keep on my computer, and some have heard me say it before: "Whenever God is blessing a ministry, you can expect increased opposition as well as increased opportunities." Like my godly son-in-law, Toby, so beautifully put it, "The ministry must really be doing some great things for you encountering this attack!" Amen to that! You all are such a blessing to us, and I am anticipating new opportunities.

We love you all, Janet

Mentoring Moment

Staying strong in the face of a cancer diagnosis is tough—even for a Christian. But our call is to live out our faith. If others see we go to pieces just as they do, then they wonder what good is our God? Where is He in our life now? They at least have drugs, alcohol, food . . . and myriad coping mechanisms. Why would they choose God over those numbing choices? The answer can be revealed in us. Wow, that's a lot of pressure, but never fear, the Holy Spirit will work through us. Galatians 5:22 says that when the Holy Spirit controls our life, "the fruit of the spirit is love, joy, peace, patience, kindness, goodness, faithfulness, gentleness and self-control." When we're punctured, literally or figuratively, what pours out is the evidence of what's in us.

This does not mean we cannot be sad or cry or grieve. Those are *real* feelings requiring expression, but our witness becomes what we do with those emotions and feelings. Do we try dealing with them ourselves, or do we let Jesus carry our burdens while we focus on getting well and using our circumstances to glorify God? The choice is ours—it's not easy, and we can't do it alone.

God's Love Letter to You

Dear_____, *(fill in your name)*
You will receive power when the Holy Spirit comes on you; and you will be my witnesses . . . to the ends of the earth (Acts 1:8 paraphrased).
Your Strength, God

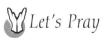 Let's Pray

Prayerfully personalize Philippians 4:11–13 MSG.

Lord, You are so worthy of our prayers . . .

Actually, I, _____, don't have a sense of needing anything personally. I've learned by now to be quite content whatever my circumstances. I'm just as happy with little as with much, with much as with little. I've found the recipe for being happy whether full or hungry, hands full or hands empty. Whatever I, _____, have, wherever I, _____ _____, am, I,_____, can make it through anything in the One who makes me who I am. Amen.

Your Letter to God

How did you make the tough decisions, or are you currently in that process? Have you leaned on God for comfort and strength, or are you still struggling? If there are or were times of haunting anxiety and fear, can you release them to the Lord today? In a time clearly all about you, can you notice who God is bringing into your life that He might want to reach *through you*? It's a tough job, but one that brings relief and change of focus. Ask Him to help balance the reality of the disease with the potential of eternal life for both others and yourself.

Dear God,   *Date:*

_____

_____

_____

_____

_____

_____

_____

_____

_____

_____

_____

_____

CHAPTER SEVEN

Starting Treatment

YOU'RE MY GOD; HAVE MERCY ON ME.
I COUNT ON YOU FROM MORNING TO NIGHT.
GIVE YOUR SERVANT A HAPPY LIFE;
I PUT MYSELF IN YOUR HANDS!

—*Psalm 86:3–4 MSG*

Someone's Praying

"The peace that passeth all understanding" is what I had the day I arrived at the hospital for surgery. God granted me what I'd prayed for since July—the grace to face whatever might come. From the time of diagnosis, the prayers of my family and friends truly sustained me. —Anita

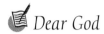 Dear God

Dear God,

Driving to the hospital the morning of surgery, it felt as if we were on our way to the airport to drop me off on a speaking trip. I was that calm. No anxiousness or flurries in my stomach—none of my usual signs of nervousness. I knew my strength came from You, dear Lord. Many people had been praying and were at that very moment lifting me up to You.

Peacefully Yours, Janet

A Sister Shares

Janet, hope all is well with you and your family. You're in my prayers as you minister to others. I count it a special blessing to have met you and Jane. Please keep my family and me in your prayers. My cancer seems to be spreading. Prayer is one of the most powerful tools we have, and I am a living testimony that it works. "To God be the glory!" Take care and keep looking to the One who cares for us all.
Blessings to you and yours, Edna

Mentoring Moment

Have you asked others to pray for you as you undergo treatment? If not, will you start right now? I know it's scary, because it means telling others about your breast cancer, but those willing to pray probably should know anyway. There will be days when you cannot pray for yourself . . . it's just too hard. I have those days too. It's OK. God knows the burdens of our hearts. Seize any opportunity for others to pray over you and for you before surgery or a treatment. Ask a pastor from your church or a friend's church to pray with you. If this is your first time to ask a pastor to pray for you, it might seem daunting and vulnerable, but this is their profession—just as your doctors administer medical care, pastors administer spiritual care. Put yourself on as many prayer chains as possible. Prayer is good medicine. Even medical studies are proving that patients receiving prayer have better outcomes.

However, God's will and timing always prevails. As we pray for restored physical health and wellness, God might be using our sickness to heal our own or someone else's spiritual ills; and those, my friend, are more terminal than cancer. A spiritually sick person made well in Christ is the ultimate answer to prayer.

📖 God's Love Letter to You

Dear_____, (fill in your name)

Are you in trouble? Pray. Are you happy? Sing songs of praise. Are you sick? Call the pastors or elders of the church to pray over you and anoint you with oil in my name. The prayer offered in faith will make the sick well, and I will raise them up. If they have sinned, they will be forgiven. Therefore, confess your sins to each other, and pray for each other so that you may be healed. The prayer of a righteous man or woman is powerful and effective (James 5:13–16 paraphrased).
Your Answerer of Prayer, God

Why Prayer Could Be Good Medicine
Dianne Hales

Hundreds of scientific investigations into faith and healing present a new frontier for medical research. With funding from the National Institutes of Health (NIH), investigators at Johns Hopkins are studying a group of women with breast cancer who say a meditative prayer twice daily. "We are not out to prove that a deity exists," says Professor Diane Becker of Johns Hopkins, recipient of two NIH grants for research on prayer. "We are trying to see whether prayer has meaning to people that translates into biology and affects a disease process." Medical acceptance has grown along with solid scientific data on prayer's impact, says Dr. Dale Matthews of Georgetown University, author of *The Faith Factor*. He estimates that about 75 percent of studies of spirituality have confirmed health benefits. "If prayer were available in pill form, no pharmacy could stock enough of it," he says.

Prayer—whether for oneself (petitionary prayer) or others (intercessory prayer)—affects the quality, if not the quantity, of life, says Dr. Harold Koenig, Director of Duke University's Center for the Study of Religion/Spirituality and Health: "It boosts morale, lowers agitation, loneliness, and life dissatisfaction and enhances the ability to cope in men, women, the elderly, the young, the healthy, and the sick. . . . While I personally believe God heals people in supernatural ways, I don't think science can shape a study to prove it," says Dr. Koenig, "But we now know enough, based on solid research, to say that prayer, much like exercise and diet, has a connection with better health."[1]

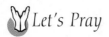 Let's Pray

Lord, help us enter prayerfully into our treatment phase. Remind us to pray for every person who has a part in our care. Give them wisdom, and guide their hands and minds as they treat us. For those who do not know You as their Savior, please let them see Jesus in us. Guard our mouths and hearts as we interact with them. Remind us that even in our illness, You use us to draw others to eternal life. Help us remember on the dark days that eventually the light of eternity awaits us. Until then, we remain in Your hands. Amen.

We're Not Just a Number

In the past three months Leslie has endured more pain and sickness, more toxic drugs and invasive medical tests, and more physical indignity, scary talk, and just plain sadness than any human being should have to suffer in a lifetime. Yet she has borne it all with such stoicism and grace. I have not seen her cry. Nor has she uttered a single word of self-pity. Not one. —Bernard Wolfson, speaking of his wife, Leslie Furth[2]

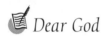 Dear God

Dear God,

The first procedure on surgery day was a wire insertion to mark the incision spot. That seemed simple enough. As Dave and I sat holding hands in yet another waiting room, I noticed each patient was called by a number—not a name. How impersonal. Patient confidentiality is one thing, but a first name is comforting. When they called my number, Dave verbalized my thoughts: "So now you are just a number!"

It got worse. The cancer was against my breastbone and hard to locate. My sore breast, still very tender from the needle biopsy, was repeatedly shoved into the excruciatingly tight machine, to no avail. As each technician failed, there was a flurry to find another to give it a try, leaving me clamped in the machine in the company of a stoic female technician. Uncontrollable tears trickled down my face; she silently handed me a Kleenex. My mind screamed, "Lord, I need human contact." I asked her name. It broke the ice. Our names are so important. They are our identity.

After an hour the tension thickened. I felt faint. Finally, the fourth technician found the spot. To insert the needle, the doctor had to get down on his knees underneath me. What a bizarre sight and experience! Staggering out to the waiting room, I told Dave that was the worst thing I ever encountered awake! He knew something must be wrong and was praying through the psalms and reading his *Power of a Praying Husband* book. Thank You for my godly husband.

Lord, help the busy technicians and doctors never reduce patients to "a number," "a case," "another DCIS," "a double mastectomy," "a procedure." Remind them of their humanness . . . our humanness. You made us man and woman, and You gave each of us a name.

Namely Yours, Janet

 ## A Sister Shares

On one particular treatment day . . . the nurse couldn't find a vein that worked, so she had to "go shopping for one," as she put it. . . . I had to get up and go to the bathroom to splash cold water on my face. I felt faint and nauseated by the pain. While I was in there, Doug, my dear, sweet husband, who stands about six feet four inches tall, was talking to my nurse. He said, "You aren't going to hurt Brenda any more, are you?" . . . He wasn't threatening, just trying to strongly encourage her to get it done with the least amount of pain possible. . . . I opened the door and smiled at my knight in shining armor. . . . Then the nurse smiled and said, "Let's get this over with." I wasn't sure if she would punish me for bringing my bodyguard or get the vein on the next poke. I said the Lord's Prayer silently to myself. And it's a funny thing . . . she found the right vein. . . . And I have to mention that at the next chemotherapy session, she got the vein on the first try. —Brenda Ladun[3]

 ## Mentoring Moment

In addition to asking for prayers for yourself, ask for prayers for all the people you encounter during your treatment. We need to pray for a softening of their hearts and a true appreciation that they are saving lives—it's not just a job. Many focus on just doing their job, forgetting the people and the reason they are doing it. Try not to get angry or judgmental, because it only makes you feel worse. When the opportunity arises, gently let them know their words or actions are hurtful, or that you don't appreciate being referred to as a case number or diagnosis. Express what you feel. Many times we are afraid to confront healthcare professionals, fearing it might compromise our treatment. If you present your concerns in a loving, nonjudgmental way, they probably will be grateful.

📖 God's Love Letter to You

Dear_____, (fill in your name)
*   I call my own sheep by name and lead them out. . . . I am the good shepherd; I know my sheep and my sheep know me (John 10:3, 14 paraphrased).*
Your Good Shepherd, God

Let's Pray

Lord, we are Your sheep, Your children, Your friends, Your followers! It couldn't get any better than that. Help us remember we are special. Each, one of a kind. The apple of Your eye. Even when some forget our earthly names, call us unkind names, or label us with our disease, that is not who we are. We know that someday when those of us who believe in Your Son, Jesus Christ, get to heaven and spend eternity with You, we will find our names written in the Lamb's book of life . . . *our names* . . . not numbers. Praise our heavenly Shepherd! Amen.

It's Time for Surgery

The surgery went well, but two days later the surgeon phoned to say the final pathology report showed more cancer cells in my breast. I had a second lumpectomy the following day. This time the pathology report was "all clear"! Thank You, Lord! —Anita

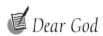 Dear God

Dear God,

The walk from the needle insertion to the surgery suite gave me a chance to regroup. Interestingly, the stoic technician walked us over. She was much more relaxed now; so was I. The wind was blowing outside, and it occurred to me looking out the windows that the rest of the world was going on about its day not even noticing I was having surgery. A surgery that would change my life forever. Something so earth-shattering to me didn't affect the gardener mowing the lawn or the parking attendant or the maintenance men scurrying through the halls. They were part of this healthcare scene too. Profound thoughts for impending surgery.

Your patient, Janet

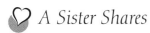 A Sister Shares

The Saturday before my surgery, I attended our church's ladies' retreat. During the evening singing, I heard God speak to my heart, "Your dad had cancer and died. You have cancer but will not die." I asked God if that impression in my heart was Him or me? If it was Him, would He please confirm it? He did. The night before surgery, at 4:00 a.m. in my hotel room, I felt God's hand guiding my decision regarding reconstruction. He didn't give it to me days ahead but right on time. That was over eleven years ago! God had me face my greatest fear with Him at my side. —Darlene M.

Mentoring Moments

Some of you might be like my friend Cindy who had chemotherapy and radiation to reduce the tumor before surgery. Others of us had surgery first. We all follow the game plan best for us. However, eventually surgery day arrives, settling the internal tug of war between wanting the day never to get here and putting it all behind us. Breast cancer is surreal—so personal—so abnormal. It challenges our femininity. It confuses us. To eliminate the bad, we must sometimes eliminate the good. Our *breasts*, Lord. Could it get any worse?

As much as we know surgery is necessary, there still is an impending sense of dread. I think we fear the unknowns more than the pain. What will they actually find in surgery? How will we look afterward? What will the scar look like? Will there be complications? How will recovery go? The list is endless.

I countered those concerns by being grateful that technology had progressed so far. God has gifted men and women, like my doctors and yours, to help rid our bodies of unhealthy parts. Everyone working at the hospital has one goal—to help us get well. That was a comforting thought to me, and I hope it is to you too.

God's Love Letter to You

Dear_____, (fill in your name)

I am near. Do not be anxious about anything, but in everything, by prayer and petition, with thanksgiving, present your requests to me, and my peace, which transcends all understanding, will guard your hearts

and your minds in Christ Jesus. Finally, breast cancer sisters, whatever is true, whatever is noble, whatever is right, whatever is pure, whatever is lovely, whatever is admirable—if anything is excellent or praiseworthy—think about those things, and I will give you peace (Philippians 4:5–9 paraphrased).
The Great Surgeon, God

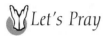 ## Let's Pray

Lord, we hoped and prayed surgery would not be our destiny. Part of our bodies deceived and turned against us. You gave us breasts with so many purposes and functions, and they became the enemy. Comfort us that we made the right decisions and that the doctors and surgeons will do their best to save our lives and put our bodies back together again. We ask for endurance to withstand however many surgeries and procedures await us and the assurance that You are present in every surgery, recovery, and treatment room . . . watching over and loving us. Thank You. Amen.

Being Strong for Our Loved Ones

I started trying to cheer up my family. —Grace Bell

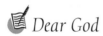 ## Dear God

Dear God,

What a relief to arrive at the surgery suite. They were expecting me. There stood my precious daughter, Kim, greeting me with a big, comforting hug before the nurses whisked me into a cubicle to prep for surgery. I could read the fear and sadness written across Dave's and Kim's faces. A couple of months ago our biggest problem was what color to make our new kitchen cabinets! Now they asked me to sign a form giving Dave permission to determine if the hospital should take unusual means to keep me alive. "Hey, I'm just having breast surgery. You aren't expecting me to die on the operating table, are you?" A formality, they assured me.

"Let's pray," I said. I was afraid the drugs would kick in before I knew what we were praying about. Dave prayed. I peeked to see how they were doing. There stood my towering, six-foot-four husband hovering over me. Tears streamed down Kim's cheeks as she sat next to the bed holding my hand. The threat loomed that our time together might be shorter than we hoped. I still had more grandchildren to enjoy and more mentoring of my "baby" in taking care of her future babies. Please, Lord, say it isn't time to take me yet. Let me give her confidence; no, better yet, You give her confidence it is going to be OK. Mom will be fine.

A loving wife and mother, Janet

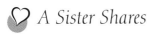 A Sister Shares

"It's cancer." My heart sank, and I held my breath with disbelief. My husband's eyes filled with tears, and so did mine. I asked God to give me strength, and He did. I looked at my surgeon and asked, "What do we do next?" Three days later, I had a lumpectomy, but the pathology report brought more bad news. There were still cancer cells in the margins! I was terrified and asked God for strength again. With this report my husband was not handling the news well at all. He cried and said he wasn't ready to lose me. At that moment, God gave me the right words to comfort him. The next day I still wanted to give my husband more encouraging words, so I mailed him a card telling him I was going to be OK. —Gloria

Mentoring Moment

On surgery day our loved ones gather round, taking their cues from us. We feel weak in our own strength and want to jump off the surgery table and run away. Let me suggest praying together is the best cue you can give them, whether or not your family members are believers. God will provide the comfort you all seek. They will see your trust is in the Lord, and the Holy Spirit will provide assurance that you can do this and so can they.

If you are still investigating God or are a new believer, trust takes time to develop. Trust is a process in human relationships, as well as with God. God will prove to you He really does have your best interest in mind, even when it's not visible to human eyes.

God's Love Letter to You

Dear_____, (fill in your name)

You are blessed when you trust in me as Lord, when your confidence is in me. You will be like a tree planted by the water that sends out its roots by the stream. The tree does not fear when heat comes; its leaves are always green. It has no worries in a year of drought and never fails to bear fruit (Jeremiah 17:7–8 paraphrased).
Your and Your Loved Ones' Source of Strength, God

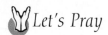

Let's Pray

God, we feel weak and want to curl up in Your lap with Your strong arms encircling us. We don't want to be brave or courageous . . . we want to break down and pour out our hurts and fears. But looking into the eyes of our families and friends, we see fear, panic, remorse, dread . . . and we feel compelled to comfort them. Reassuring them reassures us. We don't want to match their sense of gloom, but only You can keep a contagious smile on our faces and peace in our hearts to mirror to others. Unleash our hidden reserves. We trust You will come through for us in a new and refreshing way. Praise You, Lord, for who You are. Amen.

We Need Friends

For decades Leslie has nourished her friendships, phoning us frequently, choosing perfect quirky gifts and sending handwritten note cards long after they went out of fashion. And, more than anyone I've known, she rejoiced when her friends became each other's friends. Now many of us stream to her side, and turn to one another, in simple testament to what Leslie created. —Janet Gornick, friend of Leslie Furth

WHEN GOD'S CHILDREN ARE IN NEED, BE THE ONE TO HELP THEM OUT. . . .
WHEN OTHERS ARE HAPPY, BE HAPPY WITH THEM. IF THEY ARE SAD, SHARE THEIR SORROW.
—ROMANS 12:13, 15 NLT

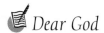

Dear God

Dear God,

When we first arrived at the surgery suite, I asked if my friends could find me. "Yes," the nurses assured, anyone asking would receive directions. OK. Jane and Cathy, the friends who brought me the balloon, plant, and snacks on needle-biopsy day, were coming. Another friend assured me she would be there too. That was just enough. I didn't need a large group—just my family and dear friends, and, of course, You, Lord. As Dave finished praying, around the corner came Jane and Cathy, and there was Lorna! What a special treat. But where was my other friend who had promised to come?

The doctors arrived. My surgeon is a very nice-looking, mature man. Standing next to him was a tall, dark, handsome anesthesiologist. The girls went silent, mouths hanging open, as the doctors asked about my entourage. I introduced my friends and family and assured the doctors of their prayer covering during surgery. They nodded in acknowledgment and said in unison, "We'll see you in there."

They were ready for me now. Where was my late friend? Oh, dear, she always has good intentions but overbooks. I was disappointed. "I love you, honey! I love you, baby! I love you, my Enaj!" were my last words trailing down the hall as I lifted up my hand in a feeble wave good-bye.

Your friend, Janet

A Friend Shares

My best friend, Janet, had breast cancer. What a difficult word to say. Four days after her diagnosis we flew to Virginia to present a Woman to Woman Mentoring Training. Sitting in the audience while Janet was onstage training, I kept thinking, *Wow, Janet has breast cancer.* A silencing, humbling thought. On our plane ride home, I shared my thoughts of not knowing what to say because I never experienced breast cancer up close and personal. I felt sad and confused, and my heart hurt badly. Then I simply reached over the armrest and patted her knee, saying, "I'm here for you."

The day after surgery I called my dear friend. As she chatted, I interrupted, "Janet, I love you. God told me this morning this is what it feels like to lay down your life for a friend. My tears yesterday came from a place deep in my heart screaming, 'Oh no, Lord, I don't want to nurture and care for her. I'm not ready; it hurts so much. That should be me on the gurney, not her.' The Lord comforted me, 'Jane, you are ready.'" —Jane "Enaj" Crick

Mentoring Moment

First, let me explain that I am dyslexic, so my friend Jane and I have pet names for each other, which are our names backward. She is Enaj. I am Tenaj. Friends often have nicknames or certain ways of communicating only they understand. Jane and I have that kind of friendship. God calls us His "friends" too. Amazingly, He chose the familiar term *friend* and sent His only Son, Jesus, to earth to die for His friends—us!

Supporting another woman during a life crisis is laying down our life by . . .

- Giving our time

- Putting her needs before ours

- Loving someone else more than we love ourselves

- Being willing, if necessary, literally to risk our own life for our friend

Not everyone understands this concept, and some will disappoint us—just as we probably have disappointed others. For everyone who lets us down, someone else pleasantly surprises us. Celebrate those *surprise* people, and tell them how much you appreciate them.

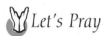God's Love Letter to You

Dear_____, (fill in your name)
This is my command: Love one another the way I loved you. This is the very best way to love. Put your life on the line for your friends. You are my friends when you do the things I command you (John 15:12–14 MSG).
Your Loving Friend, God

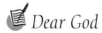Let's Pray

We do want overflowing joy, and we know that comes from serving others and not ourselves. Right now we really need to be served, but make us aware of how we can help others even through our illness. When a friend disappoints us, we will remember we have the Best Friend in the whole world—You! Help us be the kind of friend we long to have. Amen.

What Did They Do to Me?

HOW FAINT THE WHISPER WE HEAR OF HIM! —JOB 26:14

They didn't have to tell me. I already knew. God told me. —Izzy

Dear God

Dear God,

The first words I remember speaking in the recovery room were, "What did they take?" Even though surgery was to be a lumpectomy, I signed papers giving the surgeon permission to do what he deemed necessary while still in surgery. Or, maybe, I gave Dave authority to make that decision. I remember saying something like, "They are his breasts too." The nurses assured me the surgery went as planned. Even though quite sore, I still had both breasts.

Gratefully Yours, Janet

A Sister Shares

I am seventy-five years old. Thirty-five years ago I had breast cancer. I had a lump and woke up from surgery with a breast removed! In the recovery room, I overheard the nurses asking, "Who should tell her?" They didn't have to tell me. I already knew. God told me.

In those days no one talked about breast cancer. Before my surgery I didn't even know what a mastectomy was. Those terms didn't become public conversation until famous people started getting breast cancer. There were no extensions, so I didn't have radiation or chemotherapy. I really have no regrets. —Izzy

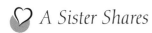 Mentoring Moment

During those first fuzzy moments as the anesthesia wears off and the nurses try to wake us up, all our thoughts were probably similar: *What did they do while I was asleep?* In our sluggish state, we try focusing on people's words as they attempt to explain what happened. Then the questions flood our mind . . . *How long was surgery? What did they have to take? What are the lab results? What is my prognosis? What can I have for the pain? Maybe I just need to sleep this off, and we can talk later.*

God's Love Letter to You

Dear_____, (fill in your name)

Cry out to me, the LORD, in your trouble, and I will bring you out of your distress. I still storms to a whisper; the waves of the sea are hushed. You will be glad when it grows calm, and I guide you to your desired haven. My love never fails (Psalm 107:28–31 paraphrased).
I Am watching over you, God

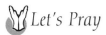 Let's Pray

Prayerfully personalize with me Psalm 107:19–22.

Lord, we offer You our prayer . . .

Then _____ and Janet cried to the LORD in their trouble, and he saved them from their distress. He sent forth his word and healed them; he rescued them from the grave. Let _____ and Janet give thanks to the LORD for his unfailing love and his wonderful deeds for men. Let _____ and Janet sacrifice thank offerings and tell of his works with songs of joy. Amen.

The Hospital Stay Is a Relief

While the hospital is a dreary, isolating, and dispiriting place, there is something about being so removed from worldly concerns that leaves ample room for building and enjoying meaningful relationships. —Leslie Furth[5]

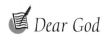 ## Dear God

Dear God,

Kim and Dave came into the recovery room. My girlfriends, having kept the vigil until surgery, had long since left to care for their families. It was a mutual decision for me to spend the night in the hospital. In fact, a room was waiting. What a relief. Getting dressed and into a car was an unfathomable thought! I don't remember much about transferring to the room, but I still visualize that room today. Oh, the hospital bed felt so good. All the position adjustments offered some semblance of comfort, and medication dulled the pain . . .

Sleepily Yours, Janet

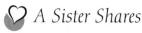 ## A Sister Shares

I was one of the youngest patients on the oncology floor. I played bingo with the older patients and won! They were upset, so I gave them all the gifts people had given me. I didn't get bouquets—I got sprays! I had so many beautiful flower arrangements and gifts, and I just spread them throughout the hospital. —Izzy

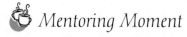 ## Mentoring Moment

My original plans were to come home the night of surgery if I felt like it. I didn't feel like it. I am so glad I took a day to adjust. I needed the pain shots, adjustable bed, and someone helping me. My husband needed time to adjust to my home care. Indulge yourself. This is not the time to be tough or to ignore your needs. In our roles as workers, wives, and mothers, we often put everyone else's needs before our own. We are so very practical. Now it's payback time—our turn to be on the receiving end of TLC. Not that I enjoyed the hospital, but at this point, the hospital staff is much better equipped to deal with us than our families.

Whether in the hospital or recuperating at home, let yourself enjoy a welcoming sense of relief from coordinating and organizing your world. Nothing is more important than getting well. Doctors' orders to stay in bed, rest, and let others wait on us give us permission to do just that. When friends and family come to visit, we can linger over conversation, not worrying about all our to-dos because the only significant to-do is "doing better than we did yesterday."

Allow your body to reap the benefits of some downtime while adjusting to the recent trauma. Don't worry . . . no one will think you're slouching. Everyone wants you well. If you must go home because of insurance or scheduling conflicts, be prepared:

- Have plenty of pillows in your bed for propping and resting your arms and back.

- Clear off your bedside table or place a TV tray next to your bed before going to the hospital, and put on it things you'll want at easy reach.

- Have pajama tops or nightgowns that button up the front. It is almost impossible and inadvisable to put anything over your head.

- Loose fitting and comfy is the fashion of the day.

- If they told you to wear a special support bra after surgery, purchase it before you go to the hospital so you can wear it right away. It helps with the pain.

- If you are already in the hospital, give this list to someone and ask him or her to take care of everything before you come home.

God's Love Letter to You

Dear_____, (fill in your name)
    Be still, and know that I am God (Psalm 46:10).
Calmly yours, God

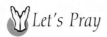 ## Let's Pray

Prayerfully personalize with me Psalm 143:1.

Our Father in heaven, we cry out to You in our pain . . .

O LORD, hear _____'s and Janet's prayer, listen to _____'s and Janet's cry for mercy; in your faithfulness and righteousness come to _____'s and Janet's relief. Amen.

The Lonely Oncology Ward

I ALWAYS LOOK TO YOU, BECAUSE YOU RESCUE ME FROM EVERY TRAP. I AM LONELY AND TROUBLED. SHOW THAT YOU CARE AND HAVE PITY ON ME. MY AWFUL WORRIES KEEP GROWING. RESCUE ME FROM SADNESS. —PSALM 25:15–17 CEV

YET I AM NOT ALONE, FOR MY FATHER IS WITH ME. —JOHN 16:32

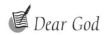 ## Dear God

Dear God,

I didn't want Kim and Dave to leave the hospital. Afraid they would be gone if I drifted off, I struggled to talk and stop my eyes from closing. What an overwhelming desire to sleep, but what comfort opening my eyes and there they were. I remember one conversation about my daughter-in-law's Aunt Bonnie, who completed a three-day breast cancer walk. I commented that Bonnie walked for me too. Kim lovingly said, "Next time you and I will walk together, Mom." Tears came to both our eyes.

As the sun slowly set and the room darkened, my eyes drooped uncontrollably. Kim was hugging me with a good-bye kiss and "I love you, Mom." I sent Dave to get himself some dinner. I cried and slept. Tears were a mixture of pain, sadness, stress, relief, and freedom from pent-up fear about the surgery. I was alive. Thank You, Lord.

When Dave returned with his dinner, he said I should not expect any flowers. "Why not?" "Because you're on the oncology ward, and they don't allow flowers," he explained. There was that dreaded word again, *oncology.* What a shock! I hadn't considered they would put me on that floor. While working as a dietitian in hospitals, I always felt sorry for patients on the oncology ward; now I was one of them. Oh Lord, it is simultaneously humbling and frightening.

Lonely Yours, Janet

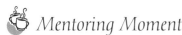 A Sister Shares

I have been in the hospital for seven weeks. It's been a long time and sometimes feels like my whole life. Some moments have been surprisingly upbeat, but some have been grim. The first time my children came up to my room was blissful. And I've had some wonderful times with friends and family who have visited from all over the country. . . . But other times, when I'm between visitors—and we get the depressing news that my sight is diminishing without sign of return—it's really, really difficult. The dark afternoons as my vision deteriorates have been mournful.

While the hospital is a dreary, isolating, and dispiriting place, there is something about being so removed from worldly concerns that leaves ample room for building and enjoying meaningful relationships. My visits with friends and family are uninterrupted by demands of work, e-mail, errands, and childcare. While I miss those everyday experiences, I have let myself enjoy the luxury of unrushed time for conversation, reflection, and intimacy. My visitors have helped me to continue enjoying books by reading to me, bringing me audio books, or sitting with me for hours. . . . Jo sent me a prayer that I find comforting, though I'm uncertain of its provenance: *"May I be safe. May my heart be filled with loving kindness. May my body be filled with health. May I rest in my beingness."* —Leslie Furth[6]

Mentoring Moment

We all handle pain and illness differently. Some want to be alone; others want people around. Many who say, "Leave me alone," secretly hope people ignore their protests. Usually, I don't want to be fussed over and prefer to be alone when sick. This was different. I didn't want to be alone . . . alone with my thoughts in a strange place. But I was not really alone. God's presence filled every area of that room, which was such a comforting reality.

Let your loved ones and friends know your preferences. Maybe certain family members and friends are exhausting, or you are not comfortable having people see you at your worst. That's OK. Ask a spokesperson to lovingly inform others that you appreciate their prayers and concern and someone will let them know when you are ready to receive visitors. When our pastor's wife, Kay, was in the hospital with chemo treatments, Pastor Rick said from the pulpit that sometimes Kay was so sick, she even didn't want him in the room. He was kindly telling the congregation that Kay appreciated their prayers, but right now company was not appropriate.

If, on the other hand, the doctor says it's OK to have company and you're lonely, let the word get out that you welcome healthy visitors. Darlene Gee says she enjoyed having visitors and looked at those first few days when everyone was coming to visit as one long opportunity to party with her friends! We all have different personalities. There is no right or wrong way. Just be sure others know your wishes.

God's Love Letter to You

Dear_____, (fill in your name)
I will never leave you nor forsake you (Joshua 1:5).
Your Constant Companion, God

Let's Pray

Lord, You promise never to leave or forsake us. Your presence surrounds us; we are never truly alone. But in our humanness we long for a physical touch, a voice uttering words, and ears to hear our cries. We want "Jesus with skin on"—Your tangible presence expressed through another human being. Please help us recognize when it's good to be alone and when we need the comforting presence of others. Bring to our side those who will be a healing balm for this time of sorrow and pain. Thank You in advance for providing human comfort as well as the Holy Spirit's constant soothing of our physical and emotional pain. Amen.

Your "C-A"

Janet came home today around 4:00 p.m., and we left the cancer at the hospital, hopefully forever. —My husband, Dave, in an e-mail to friends and family

Dear God

Dear God,

In those first days after surgery everyone around me was speaking a different language—one that would soon become mine but I was not prepared to accept yet. Like after the shift change in the hospital, when the new nurse's aide asked what side my C-A was on. "My what?" "Your C-A!" Just initials. What was she talking about? "I don't know what you mean," I answered frustrated. "Your cancer!" she explained impatiently. "What side is your cancer on?"

No one had ever referred to this as "my cancer." Is this how we would talk about it? Would other patients on the oncology ward understand her? But hadn't the doctor told us he got it all? He went back during surgery to take more than he'd expected because the margins were not clear; but the second time, all was good to go. So wouldn't it be more appropriate to ask what side my cancer "used to be on"?

Distressfully Yours, Janet

 ## A Sister Shares

The infantilizing experiences of being dependent upon others for my most basic needs makes it hard to retain my identity as a competent, autonomous adult. When I listen to the nurses laughing and talking outside my [hospital] room, I feel a deep envy and think of how ungenerous I am about other people's happiness. . . . I know overall my care has been immeasurably enhanced by the constant presence of family and friends, who have been a source of support and advocacy. My friend Isaac noticed I was hesitant to tell the nurses if I was in pain or having a new symptom. He took it upon himself to report these details, so nothing went undetected or untreated. I continually struggle with feeling like a burden to my friends, family, and doctors. It is really helpful to be reminded of the importance of articulating my needs, so I can get appropriate care. —Leslie Furth[7]

 ## Mentoring Moment

The nurse's aide was routinely doing her job—with no idea she was being insensitive. You may be quite comfortable with quickly taking ownership of your breast cancer. Whether asking people to use our names, not letting others hurt our feelings, or making known our physical and emotional needs, we all arrive at *our* way of coping. Eventually we face the reality that no one else can bear this affliction for us. It is ours. Don't be devastated by that thought, because God can and will help us bear it. Soon we are no longer embarrassed by having breast cancer, or in denial, or wanting to ignore it. The physical, mental, and emotional healing begins when we face it, not on our own strength but relying on the Lord's supernatural power.

📖 God's Love Letter to You

Dear_____, (fill in your name)

When all you owned was taken from you, you accepted it with joy. You knew you had better things waiting for you in eternity. Do not throw away this confident trust in me, the Lord, no matter what happens. Remember the great reward it brings you! Patient endurance is what you need now, so you will continue to do my will. Then you will receive all that I have promised (Hebrews 10:34–36 NLT paraphrased).
Your Confidence, God

🙏 Let's Pray

Lord, our hearts hurt and cringe. *Cancer* is not a word we want in our vocabulary . . . especially not applying to *our* bodies. However, a nameless, faceless enemy is impossible to fight. So we must identify, name, and learn about the enemy, cancer, in order to wage the best battle without shame or hesitation. We are soldiers in this fight, and we beseech You to help us be *victors*, not *victims*. Amen.

✍️ Your Letter to God

Ask for the power of prayer to flood your life during surgery and treatment. Have you had painful and anonymous moments? Don't bury them. Explode in your journal. What was surgery like? What was the hardest part? What were the blessings? Who made your day doable? If you still await surgery, journal the wait. Can you allow yourself comfort and relief without feeling guilty? Have you accepted your C-A? Ask God, Your Creator, to help you adjust to this new life.

Dear God, _____ *Date:* _____

_____

_____

_____

_____

_____

Enjoying the Good Days

On a good day,
enjoy yourself.

—*Ecclesiastes 7:14 MSG*

There Are Humorous Moments

I lost ten pounds, and Dave found them. —Janet

Both breasts are equal and reactive to light and accommodation. —A medical record

I used to be a 36B! Now I'm a 36 long. —Heard in a mammogram waiting room

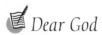 Dear God

Dear God,

That same dear nurse's aide who jolted me into accepting my "C-A" brought a smile to my face the next morning as she helped me with a sponge bath. Shakily standing at the bathroom sink, still hooked up to an IV pole and feeling very lightheaded, I almost fell over when she boldly announced she was envious of my figure. Oh my! She was at least twenty years younger, and while not overweight, I am definitely not a model. Laughingly, I said, "What?!" "Yes," she said admiringly. "You have curves. I wish I had curves."

Lord, You used this one young lady to teach me a life lesson! Are we ever happy with what we have? I had breast cancer, which no one wants, but still this healthy young woman was envious because I had curves! Go figure. I was thinking, *Curves are some trade-off for breast cancer!* It did, however, give me a lift to realize that even though I look pretty bad this morning, no makeup, hooked up to an IV, in a hospital gown, pale and exhausted, she still saw something valuable about my body, which had endured so much in the last twenty-four hours and still had a beating to take. She made me laugh. She lightened my mood. She gave me value. She definitely helped me forgive her for the previous day's C-A comment.

Laughingly Yours, Janet

 Two Sisters Share

Martha is a quick thinker. She tells a story of going for a mammogram and the technician's commenting, "'Oh, you only have one breast.'" Martha writes, "I assured her I was a 'late bloomer.' The laughter filled the halls and we became good friends."[1]

Linda M. laced her update e-mails with humor. The doctors discovered that the origin of her bone cancer was from a metastasized spot in her breast. In one e-mail she explained, "The chemo kills the cancer, and it will shrink up and die. I will still have holes in my bones where the cancer was. Do you think God will send special messages through these holes? Think I'll have a better connection now?" In another e-mail she discusses the necessity for a mastectomy to remove the cancer at its origin. After explaining the medical details, she launched into, "Insurance would cover reconstruction—double Ds, here I come. I will put Dolly Parton to shame. I won't be able to stand up. You have to think about the lighter side, you know." Then she puts it all into perspective. "It's a good thing all this wasn't discussed on the day of my original diagnosis, or I might have gone over the edge. It's a lot easier to handle now that I have a mental grip on the disease."

 ## Mentoring Moment

Cherish those funny times—there will be some. Often they go overlooked or minimized by the seriousness of the situation, but laughter is good for healing and for the soul. It helps keep everything in perspective. The Bible assures us we will laugh again. "The nights of crying your eyes out give way to days of laughter" (Psalm 30:5 MSG). For years my pastor, Rick Warren, taught life was like a roller coaster, where you have good times, go down into bad times, then come out into good times; and so the life cycle repeats. However, the same year his book *The Purpose Driven Life* became an overnight bestseller, his wife, Kay, experienced breast cancer. Simultaneously having the best and the worst year of his life, he realized the roller-coaster scenario was not accurate. I agree. Life is never all bad and then all good. Both are happening side by side. Our job is not to let the bad overshadow the good. Don't let the serious eclipse the humorous.

Often I recall a situation during those foggy treatment days and think, *That was really funny.* Like when I focused so intently on only shaving under my right arm and avoiding my left armpit because of the lymph-node surgery, I also was only shaving my right leg! I just burst out laughing in the shower. Sometimes I do some crazy things—how about you? I have found that instead of chastising myself, I just have to laugh about it and share with others in a humorous way. It gives them something to smile about instead of frowning when we talk about our cancer.

Children always lighten the mood. My grandchildren were visiting for Christmas during my surgery and radiation, and they were so sweet and considerate of Grammie's "owie." Although after several days they did want to know when my owie was going to be better and I could roughhouse with them again.

Izzy tells a cute story about her son, who was six years old when she had her mastectomy. Their miniature dachshund, Tammy, had puppies and was having trouble nursing them. Her son announced at school, "Tammy is having problems with her *gickles*, just like mommy is!" Shirley wrote that after learning she needed surgery, her nine-year-old grandson, Nick, sang a jingle to his own tune: "God is bigger than the boogeyman, the surgeon's knife, and the stitches too!"

God's Love Letter to You

Dear_____, *(fill in your name)*

There is a time for everything, and a season for every activity under heaven: a time to weep and a time to laugh, a time to mourn and a time to dance (Ecclesiastes 3:1, 4). A cheerful heart is good medicine, but a crushed spirit dries up the bones (Proverbs 17:22).
The Author of Laughter, God

Let's Pray

Father, You gifted us with laughter as well as tears. Let us keep a healthy balance of both during these difficult days. We can always find something to laugh at or see the humor in. Let our eyes not become so clouded with fear and trembling that we miss the joy of a young child's laughter or the opportunity to laugh at a good joke on ourselves. Please grant us that balance between hysteria and humor. Give our spirits a lift—let us feel the healing power of laughter and lightness in our lives. We ask this, too, Lord, for our dear friends and families who are so worried and burdened with our illness. Help us celebrate joy wherever it presents itself. Amen.

Feeling Like a Little Girl Again

Lifting the lid, I could see nappy white fur filling the space. "Oh," I smiled, pulling the small stuffed animal from the box, "it's a little lamb. How darling."... "It's a music box.... How perfect... I wound the ring tight and let it go... Jesus loves me this I know.... It's perfect," I replied, winding the lamb up one more time, letting the simple tune remind me that Jesus did love me. —Anne[2]

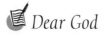 Dear God

Dear God,

Wow! Did You ever surprise me with Your presence and comfort in a tangible way. Sleeping so much those first twenty-four hours in the hospital, I seldom wore my glasses and am blind without my contacts. I thought there was a gift bag on the counter across the room but dismissed it as something from the hospital. After all, I was only here overnight.

No visitors had come to my room, other than Dave and Kim, and I wouldn't be receiving flowers on the oncology ward!

Before Dave left to go home and get some sleep, he remembered the bag. "Oh," he said, "you have a gift from Nurse Barbara" (the Christian nurse I mentioned who headed up the breast cancer center at the hospital). Dave explained that Nurse Barbara saw him sitting in the waiting room outside surgery. She went into the hospital gift shop, came out with this bag, and instructed him to give it to me. My curiosity was piqued. I love surprises, and this was so unexpected. Well, the oncology-ward patients probably all woke up with my shrieks of delight as I reached in and pulled out a darling, white, fuzzy stuffed sheep with a nametag on his ear, "Fleece."

How amazing! The call You gave me to go into full-time ministry came through the verses in John 21:15–17, where Jesus, in effect, says to Peter, "If you love me, feed My sheep." You know, "Feed My sheep" is my testimony! What immediate comfort as I hugged Fleece. Barbara could not have known the significance of giving me a sheep. The next morning, she visited my room, and I explained the "Feed My sheep'" story to her. She commented there were also stuffed bears in the shop, but something (Lord, I know it was the Holy Spirit) prompted her to buy Fleece. Again, such a reassuring way to show me You were with me throughout it all. Fleece was a constant reminder of Your unceasing presence in my life as my Abba, Father, Daddy, Comforter.

Your little girl, Janet

A Sister Shares

A year later, I smiled when our local newspaper ran a series of articles about Leslie Furth's battle with breast cancer. I did a double take and laughed to myself as I opened the paper one week and there smiling out at me was Leslie in her hospital bed cuddling a black stuffed sheep. "Lamby" had become a surrogate of sorts when Leslie and her husband were trying to conceive their first child, Oliver, now five. After being "kind of forgotten," Lamby became an important part of Leslie's stay in the hospital.[3] That was an "Aha!" moment for me that this was a universal need, not just mine. —Janet

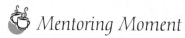 *Mentoring Moment*

That little guy, Fleece, brought so much comfort. I carried him everywhere. He was seldom far from my side. I slept with him, hugged him, took him on a plane trip, tucked him under my arm like a pillow to rest on, and treated him like my favorite pet. I regressed back to childhood and felt the same comfort that a blankie or favorite stuffed animal provides.

Lisa Whelchel, former *The Facts of Life* star, now conducts weekend conferences called MomTime Getaways. She commented in an interview in *Today's Christian Woman* magazine, "The women seem to need to be little girls again and just play. . . . So often we feel guilty about tending to our own needs, which of course we need to do to avoid burnout and in order to have something to offer those who depend on us."[4] I read that and thought, *that is exactly what I just wrote in the book.* If I didn't convince you, maybe hearing from another grown-up woman will give you permission to indulge the little girl in all of us.

During those dark nights or painful times, embrace the softness of your favorite comfort object. Strangely, I never felt foolish as a grown woman carrying around and hugging a stuffed animal. Instead, I felt the arm of the Lord comforting me in all my senses. Martha was a grandmother with adult children, and yet she wrote during her cancer experience, "I needed my parents [who were deceased] so much at this time."[5] She also was given a little baby-size pillow from a friend who had the same type of breast cancer. Martha said, "That pillow became a part of my wardrobe for eighteen months."[6]

Maybe your comfort isn't a stuffed animal or a pillow, but I encourage you to find *something* dear to keep near. Don't be embarrassed or apologetic about it. These are tough times. We need to acknowledge our child side. You don't have to be a grown up through the whole process. Often in adulthood we lose the childhood awareness of what meets our innate needs. These inner yearnings are God-created to serve as warning lights of a void in our lives. Only God can fill our deepest spiritual yearnings, but He will also satisfy our human senses with "Jesus with skin on" or, in my case, "fleece on."

God's Love Letter to You

Dear_____, (fill in your name)

I, the same Lord, who scattered my people, will gather them together and watch over them as a shepherd does his flock. . . . You will be radiant because of the many gifts I have given you—. . . Your life will be like a watered garden, and all your sorrows will be gone. The old and young will dance for joy in the celebration. I will turn your mourning into joy. I will comfort you and exchange your sorrow for rejoicing (Jeremiah 31:10, 12–13 NLT paraphrased).
Your Abba, Daddy, Papa, God

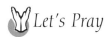 Let's Pray

Sometimes, Lord, we know You as our Daddy and come to You as little children hungry for a hug and kiss from our beloved Papa. We are so in need right now of that kind of solace. We don't always feel like grown-up big girls these days, and we just want the pain and anguish to go away for a while, so we cling to things that bring peace and rest to our souls.

Lord, we know that Your Word, the Bible, is what You want us clinging to, and it will provide comforting answers to our questions. Thank You for inspiring every word and telling us in 1 John 3:1 that we are Your children: "How great is the love the Father has lavished on us, that we should be called children of God!" And that we are! Amen.

Lots of Love

I don't know how we would have gotten through this difficult time without the outpouring of love and support from so many. I have not felt alone at all . . . which is such an amazing gift! —Kay Warren

Love is more than a characteristic of God; it is His character. —Anonymous

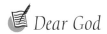 Dear God

Dear God,

Thrilled and *grateful* seem inadequate words to express the love I have felt! I never knew how much my friends and family loved me. It was as if the floodgates of love sprang open, and everyone rushed through with cards, meals, help, rides, hugs, and prayer. When I looked into my husband's and children's eyes, I saw love mixed with compassion and a touch of fear—an abrupt realization I was not the only one dealing with my mortality. Sometimes, we don't realize how important something or someone is until threatened with loss.

Lord, I must admit, I could bask in this love forever. There is a way to do that, I know, by extending that same love to everyone I meet. What I give out, I get back tenfold. Father, help me never to forget this feeling. Keep me ready to offer love whenever I see another person sick in heart or body.

Lovingly Yours, Janet

A Sister and Friend Share

From the diagnosis on, I was surrounded by the love of friends and family so I still feel their reverberation inside me; like the silence when the organ stops playing in a church, it's going to echo and stay a part of me for a very long time.[7] I am propelled forward by hope, the love of others, and a deep, primal determination to be with my children.[8] —Leslie Furth

Even though Leslie and Bernard have lived in Southern California for only five years, new friends and local acquaintances have given so much. Leslie's and Bernard's coworkers, the parents of their children's friends, and a dizzying array of local people have contributed food, carpooling, play dates, gifts, and late-night company. [Bernard refers to them as the "local brigades" and affectionately calls Natalie Peterson his "director of volunteer services."[9]] And why this urban barn raising? Because many of these people met Leslie and fell in love with her at first sight, as I did. Because Leslie and Bernard have graciously accepted it all, understanding instinctively that allowing people to give—and to take part in this impromptu community—is itself an act of generosity. And because there is more kindness in this world—straightforward, uncomplicated kindness—than I knew there to be before Leslie became ill.[10]—Janet Gornick, writing about her friend Leslie Furth

 ## Mentoring Moment

Many breast cancer ladies reported feeling showered with caring and love. Nancy Tuttle wrote, "I think love has a lot to do with my healing."[11] Darlene Gee said, "I have never felt more loved in my whole life! Everyone came to visit, and being a social person, I loved having them around. Sometimes it actually felt like a party. They all wanted to help, so I had to think of things for them to do." Darlene needed the "Bless You! Here's Where I Need Help" list provided for you on page 374.

Of course, there are always those who disappoint us. Where were they when we needed them? Was this too hard to go through with us? Try not to focus on them. God will have to do His work in softening their hearts. There is probably at least one person who has been there for you like you never expected. What we all learn from this is to be the friend we want to have. When we are feeling better, the best way to pay back the kindness of others is to pass it on to someone else. Several years ago the movie *Pay It Forward* depicted this theme. Every selfless act of kindness needs no more than a thank you and a promise to go and do likewise.

For now, though, our place is on the receiving end of all that love and kindness. You may find it far easier to extend than receive love. Some of us feel embarrassed to be on the receiving end or maybe even unworthy. Nothing could be further from the truth. Proverbs 31:10 tells us we are "worth far more than rubies." Our letting others show how much they love us is really our gift to them. They feel so helpless to ease our pain or remove our fear, and the one thing they can freely extend is *love*. We have all heard there is nothing greater than to love and be loved in return. "There are three things that will endure—faith, hope, and love—and the greatest of these is love" (1 Corinthians 13:13 NLT).

God's Love Letter to You

Dear_____, (fill in your name)
I give you a new command—to love one another. Just as I have loved you, so you must love one another (John 13:34 paraphrased).
Love always, God

Let's Pray

Prayerfully personalize Psalm 63:1–8.

O God, you are my, _____'s, God, earnestly I, _____, seek you; my soul thirsts for you, my body longs for you, in a dry and weary land where there is no water. I, _____, have seen you in the sanctuary and beheld your power and your glory. Because your love is better than life, my lips will glorify you. I, _____, will praise you as long as I, _____, live, and in your name I, _____, will lift up my hands. My soul will be satisfied as with the richest of foods; with singing lips my mouth will praise you. On my bed I, _____, remember you; I, _____, think of you through the watches of the night. Because you are my help, I, _____ _____, sing in the shadow of your wings. My soul clings to you; your right hand upholds me. Amen.

Your Letter to God

Were you able to laugh at humorous situations, even with stitches? Thank God for the lighter moments. Have you discovered a comfort item, or are you thinking, *If only I had something to comfort me*? Ask God to reveal what you long for. If it is to know Him more fully, then ask God into your heart if you have not already done that. If you found a comforting item but didn't recognize it as a gift from God, acknowledge that before Him now. This is a good time to remember all those acts of kindness and love on your behalf. As you write them, let the Lord replace any sorrow with joy at how He has shown His love to you through others.

Dear God, _____ *Date:* _____

_____

_____

_____

_____

_____

_____

_____

_____

_____

_____

_____

_____

_____

_____

_____

_____

_____

_____

_____

_____

_____

_____

_____

CHAPTER NINE

Making It through the Bad Days

If God hadn't been there for me,
I never would have made it.
The minute I said, "I'm slipping, I'm falling,"
your love, God, took hold and held me fast.
When I was upset and beside myself,
you calmed me down and cheered me up.

—Psalm 94:17–19 MSG

It's Hard Being Brave

Dear God, I'm tired of illness, depression, and old things. I crave lightness, hope, health, and future. Help me to get rejuvenated and to pass my energy on to those about me. —Nancy Tuttle[1]

BLINDED BY TEARS OF PAIN AND FRUSTRATION. I CALL TO YOU, GOD; ALL DAY I CALL. I WRING MY HANDS, I PLEAD FOR HELP. —PSALM 88:9 MSG

I TRY TO MAKE THE BEST OF IT, TRY TO BRAVE IT OUT. —JOB 10:16 MSG

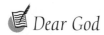 Dear God

Dear God,

Some days I just want to cry and cry. This is such a new emotion for me. I always longed for compassion. It seems like anything and everything reduces me to tears. I've never been one to cry in public, so this is quite an adjustment for both my family and me.

Radiation brought its own challenges. Tears flowed during the CAT scan and all through the tattooing procedure. When the tech doing the tattoos asked why I was crying, I had no answer. I understood the purpose of the tattoos was to show them where to radiate without having to measure each time, but why something permanent? "So if you ever need radiation again and something happens to our files, we, or other doctors, will know the area previously radiated. You can't be radiated in this area ever again," they explained. That made sense. The tattoos were smaller than a pinprick and hidden under my clothes, but my heart wrenched at things happening to my body I had no control over. I didn't like it one bit!

I know You say in Ecclesiastes 3:4 that there is "A time to cry and a time to laugh. A time to grieve and a time to dance" (NLT). Help me adjust to the time-to-cry-and-grieve part and not feel guilty about it. Help those around me not worry or try cheering me up with platitudes or make me feel less spiritual. Right now, I think crying is healing.

Tearfully Yours, Janet

Three Sisters Share

Then I had to tell my other coworkers. . . . "Hey Steph," I said, "I have to tell you something. I have breast cancer." To my surprise I wasn't crying. I was OK! Dr. Winchester told me that when I could look someone in the face and say I have breast cancer and not cry about it, I'd know I'd come to terms with it. But instead of me crying, tears were rolling down Stephanie's cheeks. —Brenda Ladun[2]

I will have this chronic bone pain always—I'll have some good days and some fair days. I don't plan on having any *bad* days. No such thing now. I have actually seen worse conditions than my own, even if the stage may be better than mine. Please keep some good thoughts and prayers for a friend of my sister's. She had breast cancer surgery, chemo is terrible for her, and her bone scan came back with a couple of lesions. She has four children, oldest in junior high and youngest is two. Now, God knew I could never be that *brave*. I think my road has been a bed of roses compared to that, and I really don't feel like I can complain at all. —Linda M.

I know I'm low; I have to be as it's not every day you hear that big bad word . . . CANCER. You don't stop to think how you may have gotten this big tormenting gorilla into your body . . . wherever it may be. The truth is, I have to hear it again today and can I do it and how *brave* will I be? I know I'm tired but I know I'm strong and have an army of strong ones right by my side. . . . Please, Lord, give me needed strength. I love you and I feel your presence. —Martha[3]

 Mentoring Moment

We are going to have bad days—times of sadness and tears. It just goes with the territory. Often, as Christian women, we think the world expects us to be so strong and brave. We fear it might show a lack of faith if we are sad. As long as we understand God never leaves us or forsakes us and we are not living in a perpetual pity party, we should feel free to express our natural feelings.

Tears are cleansing and healing. They also are God's plan for letting pent-up emotions escape, much like the valve on a pressure cooker or poking potatoes before we put them in the oven lets off steam. If those outlets are not in place, the pressure cooker or baked potato explodes and makes a huge mess. Likewise, if we don't have outlets for our emotional pressure and tension, we eventually "lose it," and that is not a pretty picture.

I like how Martha puts it: "Tears are safety valves of the heart when too much job, suffering, hope, excitement, and pressure is put on a person."[4] It is not healthy to walk around in a constant state of denial, with repressed feelings, or guilt. Tears are God's gift to us. He provided them for our use, as needed. The world looks cleaner and brighter after a good soul-cleansing cry.

We also need a time and place where we feel completely free to yell, scream, cry, and maybe throw a few things, as long as we don't hurt anyone or ourselves emotionally or physically. Our family and friends, especially our children, may be scared when we cry or have outbursts, so try to find a secluded refuge, even if it's just locking yourself in the bathroom. Our loved ones need assurance that when we cry or don't feel like being cheery, that is when we need their compassion and love the most. This, too, will pass.

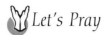 God's Love Letter to You

Dear_____, (fill in your name)

Be brave. Be strong. Don't give up. Expect me, God, to arrive soon (Psalm 31:24 MSG paraphrased).

Catching each tear, God

Let's Pray

Prayerfully personalize Psalm 56:8 (NLT).

You keep track of all my, _____'s, sorrows. You have collected all my, _____'s, tears in your bottle. You have recorded each one in your book.

Lord, we long to be like Job, who told his wife, "We take the good days from God—why not also the bad days?" (Job 2:10 MSG). We want to be godly representatives, but right now, we are hurting. This is so hard, and our hearts break just thinking of all we must endure before this is over, and we always wonder if it really ever will be over, and that makes us unhappy too. Help us be strong when we need to be. We are literally *crying out.* Thank You for understanding us and giving us the blessing of tears. Amen.

The Journey Can Be Lonely

"Be strong and courageous. Don't be afraid, for I will be with you." Clinging to that promise of His presence, I embarked on the process and whirlwind of decision making with my doctors, in the turmoil finding stillness and guidance to go through the necessary steps, tests, and procedures. His promised presence was there as I experienced and discovered the unique loneliness of the journey. —Grace Marestaing

BE STRONG AND COURAGEOUS. DO NOT BE AFRAID OR TERRIFIED BECAUSE OF THEM,
for the LORD your GOD goes with you; HE WILL NEVER LEAVE YOU NOR FORSAKE YOU.
—DEUTERONOMY 31:6

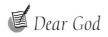 *Dear God*

Dear God,

Realizing no one could go through breast cancer for me, or even always be with me, sent a cold chill through my heart. While everyone supported and loved me, I alone had to have dye shot into my veins for the lymph-node mapping . . . endure the excruciating needle biopsy and wire placement . . . painful surgery. I alone carried the heavy weight of fatigue, dizziness, and sleepless nights.

The ultimate alone time was when everyone exited the radiation room and bolted shut a thick steel door, leaving me lying on a metal bed in a steel-encased room while poisonous destroying rays assailed my breast. I never got used to it. Others made light of it, saying things like, "It's just like going to work every day. You come in at a scheduled time—actual treatment takes only about fifteen minutes—then you're on your way." It's painless. Piece of cake. Why so sad?

To me it was not painless. I sensed the killing rays entering my body, doing their dirty work. Necessary work, but with what long-term effects? What a paradox, that to live, part of me had to die. Had they done their calculations properly? Were they missing my heart and lungs? Daily these thoughts plagued my mind, while the only sound in the cold, sterile room was the whirring of the machine. I had no choice but to trust, pray, and express my frustrated feelings in tears rolling down my face.

Mercifully, Lord, as I lay on my back on the narrow radiation table, my eyes fixed on the cross that was cut in the ceiling to let in laser beams, a constant reminder I was not alone. You will never leave me nor forsake me. My prayer each day was, "Lord, please protect my body from any harm from this radiation."

I also sometimes feel alone watching friends going on with their lives. They leave from visiting or hang up the phone and continue about their day as usual. My life never will be "usual" again. I pray for their protection from breast cancer, and that in itself brings feelings of isolation and loneliness. A constant prayer that I will be the only one. Lord, did You need me closer to You—away from the noisy crowd? Was your intention to draw me in even as I looked up at that cross in the radiation-room ceiling? Fulfill Your purpose in me, and let me never forget that with the Holy Spirit in my soul, I never walk alone.

No longer lonely, Janet

A Sister Shares

Occasionally I felt a "pity party" coming on. These are the kind of parties you don't plan; they just happen. They're *lonely* too, because you don't have time to mail out invitations and no one shows up but you. No streamers, flowers, or cakes at pity parties. They're of short duration and successful if you recognize enough of the symptoms to end this type of self-pity before it really takes hold . . . on your fragile inner self. These are my symptoms of needing to share and be with people. —Martha[5]

Mentoring Moment

I know you have lonely times too. Many phases of this breast cancer journey trigger a devastatingly empty, alone feeling. Maybe it comes while lying in bed at the hospital . . . or sitting for hours receiving chemotherapy . . . or hugging the toilet while throwing up—no one can do that for you. Maybe it shows up while you're putting on that little gown preparing for your diagnostic mammogram . . . or while you're shivering on the exam table waiting for the doctor to swing open the door and finally make his appearance . . . or when you eventually look in the mirror and realize you are *truly* bald or your breast is *actually* gone. Whenever and wherever it comes, we all have those moments of excruciating, intolerable loneliness. It is natural. It happens. Your friends have to leave, and your family hasn't arrived home from work or school yet. You sit in the living room or bedroom or hospital room watching the invasion of shadowy darkness . . . and you just feel *so alone.*

You've heard we're never alone with Jesus in our lives, but you long to experience His presence. Well, alone is the perfect time and place to do that. Being by ourselves or feeling all alone is when God can really get our attention. No distractions—just God and us. If you have not already experienced this, the next time loneliness grabs your heart, picture Jesus sitting right next to you. What is the conversation you would have with Him if He were there in person? Remember He is *always* with you in Spirit.

God's Love Letter to You

Dear_____, (fill in your name)
    You can be sure of this: I am with you always, even to the end of the age (Matthew 28:20 NLT paraphrased).
Your Constant Companion, God

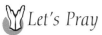 *Let's Pray*

Prayerfully personalize Psalm 139:1–12, 23–24 MSG.

GOD, investigate my, _____'s, life; get all the facts firsthand. I'm an open book to you; even from a distance, you know what I'm thinking. You know when I, _____, leave and when I, _____, get back; I'm never out of your sight. You know everything I'm going to say before I, _____, start the first sentence. I, _____, look behind me and you're there, then up ahead and you're there, too—your reassuring presence, coming and going. This is too much, too wonderful—I, _____, can't take it all in! Is there anyplace I _____, can go to avoid your Spirit? To be out of your sight? If I, _____, climb to the sky, you're there! If I, _____, go underground, you're there! If I, _____, flew on morning's wings to the far western horizon, you'd find me in a minute—you're already there waiting! Then I, _____, said to myself, "Oh, he even sees me in the dark! At night I'm immersed in the light!" It's a fact: darkness isn't dark to you; night and day, darkness and light, they're all the same to you. Investigate my life, O God, find out everything about me, _____; Cross-examine and test me, _____, get a clear picture of what I'm about; See for yourself whether I've done anything wrong—then guide me on the road to eternal life. Amen.

Elusive Sleep

I GO TO BED AND THINK, "HOW LONG TILL I CAN GET UP?"
I TOSS AND TURN AS THE NIGHT DRAGS ON—AND I'M FED UP!
—JOB 7:4 MSG

RISE DURING THE NIGHT AND CRY OUT. POUR OUT YOUR HEARTS
LIKE WATER TO THE LORD. LIFT UP YOUR HANDS TO HIM IN PRAYER.
—LAMENTATIONS 2:19 NLT

Dear God

Dear God,

Will I ever sleep the night again? This never has been a problem, but now I find myself tossing and turning and waking up several

135

times during the night—every night. I wonder . . . *Are You trying to get my attention? Am I just uncomfortable from surgery? The night sweats? Medications? Or all of the above?* Sometimes I am crying . . . sometimes praying . . . And sometimes just plain irritated about being awake! Oh Lord, how long will this go on? I feel sleep deprived, and I'm sure that's why I'm so ditzy and dizzy during the day. When will I feel rested and refreshed from a good night's sleep?

Sometimes I just don't feel like doing anything. Before cancer, people called me the Eveready bunny . . . full of energy, on task, multitasking, never admitting to a limit. I see concern in Kim's eyes when she relates that people ask if it's driving me crazy being down, and she responds, "No, it isn't, and that's worrying me. Mom is OK with just lying there or taking a nap!" The relief was evident on her face the first day she saw me dressed in something besides lounging clothes.

Sleepily Yours, Janet

Two Sisters Share

I think 4:00 to 4:30 in the morning must be a time when God speaks to us or we need to be sharing our hearts with Him. Often I awaken at that early-morning time—sometimes with God's voice unraveling something I've been thinking about, or encouragement, or sometimes just praying for one or more of the people on my prayer list. It is a good time to do battle. There seems to be clarity about that early time when everything is still and quiet, including my brain. —Grace Marestaing

I was awakened at 4:30 a.m. by a voice whispering my name, "Nancy." The Lord was gently waking me from a deep sleep by speaking my name inside my head. Although God has awakened me in the middle of the night on several occasions and I have been led to pray for specific things that later proved to need prayer, I had not heard Him speak my name before. I fell to my knees beside my bed. I did not need to take off my shoes in his holy place, because my feet were already bare. —Nancy Tuttle[6]

Mentoring Moment

The above quote from Grace Marestaing was a response to an e-mail I wrote her at 4:00 a.m. I was having a tough time starting Tamoxifen and found myself wide awake looking at the clock every night at 3:00 a.m., tossing and turning till 4:00, then just getting up. It was so frustrating until I decided to stop fighting it and go with it. I remembered David wrote to God in Psalm 17:3, "Go ahead, examine me from inside out, surprise me in the middle of the night" (MSG). Then awake, in Psalm 63:6 he spent the time thinking back on good things: "If I'm sleepless at midnight, I spend the hours in grateful reflection" (MSG).

Another psalmist used the night hours to thank God: "I get up in the middle of the night to thank you; your decisions are so right, so true—I can't wait till morning!" (Psalm 119:62 MSG).

Grace Marestaing, Nancy Tuttle, David, the psalmist, and I found the middle of the night an excellent time to talk to God—maybe praying or reading the Bible will comfort you back to sleep too. I do know getting angry and frustrated with insomnia doesn't help. Sleeplessness due to surgery, medication, and hormonal changes is perfectly normal; however, not sleeping because of worry or anxiety isn't going to help your recovery.

In those early days after surgery or in the midst of radiation or chemotherapy, take naps during the day if you are tired, because exhaustion is not going to help you heal. What freedom not to feel guilty or make excuses for taking a nap . . . doctor's orders, so let yourself indulge! The following tips might help at night:

- My oncologist suggested 400 units of vitamin E twice daily for night sweats, and in about three weeks the night sweats practically disappeared.

- Avoid caffeine, sugar, and chocolate in the evening.

- Be sure tea is caffeine free.

- Herbal sleepytime teas are helpful to sip before bedtime.

- Don't watch the late news; it will keep you up for sure.

- Turn off the television at least an hour before bedtime. Many studies show watching television before going to sleep actually stimulates the brain instead of resting it. You might fall asleep, but chances are good you will have bad dreams or wake up later in the night.

- My favorite—talk someone into giving you a relaxing backrub with an aromatherapy oil or lotion.

- A nice warm bath or shower. Don't have the water too hot, though, because that gets the blood pumping and can keep you awake or make you too hot when you climb into bed and thus trigger a night sweat.

- Try reading a few comforting scriptures.

- Journal to God in this book. Get it all out of your mind and on paper.

- Following surgery, use pillows to prop yourself up in a comfortable position in bed.

- Say a nighttime prayer, asking God to bring nourishing, comforting, essential sleep.

A great scripture to pray before going to sleep is the one below under "Let's Pray" . . . especially the last sentence. The good news is this sleepless phase usually passes once your surgery site starts to heal, your body adjusts to whatever medication you are taking, and the treatments subside. So hang in there and take advantage of every sleep opportunity you get, day or night.

God's Love Letter to You

Dear_____, (fill in your name)
My presence will go with you, and I will give you rest (Exodus 33:14). You'll take afternoon naps without a worry, you'll enjoy a good night's sleep (Proverbs 3:24 MSG). Creator of Sleep, God

Let's Pray

Prayerfully personalize Psalm 3:4–5 and 4:8 NLT.

Lord, I am weary and tired and I need Your help . . .

I, _____, cried out to the LORD, and he answered me from his holy mountain. I, _____, lay down and slept. I, _____, woke up in safety, for the LORD was watching over me. I, _____, will lie down in peace and sleep, for you alone, O LORD, will keep me safe. Amen.

It Still Hurts

NIGHT PIERCES MY BONES; MY GNAWING PAINS NEVER REST. —JOB 30:17

I traded cancer pain for arthritic-type pain. I think every joint in my body is stiff most of the time. —Linda M.

I was not getting any rest and very little sleep. I just withdrew into a shell and tried to live with my pain. —Martha

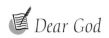 *Dear God*

Dear God,

Terror gripped my heart six months after surgery when my surgery breast became swollen and sore. My shoulders ached with the weight, and I could not even stand a bra strap. What was going on? Why was this happening? Even scarier, no one seemed to have answers. My oncologist said to check with my surgeon. The surgeon said, "Yes, you sure are swollen, but everything else looks fine. Why don't you go to our shop and see if they can fit you for a more comfortable bra?" An hour and at least fifty bras later, we finally found one I could tolerate that had pockets for an insert on the smaller right breast side.

Still, the nagging thought, *Why is this happening?* Finally, at Your prompting, I made an appointment with the radiation oncologist. He took one look and said, "Perfect. This is a good thing. The swelling is from fluid going to the damaged cells to cushion them as they heal. A year after radiation your breast will shrink. Since it is swollen now, it might just shrink down to normal size!" "Why didn't someone tell me this in the first place?" I asked him. "Why don't the other doctors have this information so they would know to expect this?" He responded that he did need to get an explanation letter to them. I hope he does, so that someone else won't have to worry needlessly.

Lord, I needed that reassurance. I received so much valuable information, but nothing prepared me for this event. The swelling has since gone down, and I wear that comfy bra almost every day. Now if my frozen shoulder would just go away. It seems, again, no one can determine the actual cause or cure. Give me the will and the endurance to keep doing the exercises through the pain. If this is to be my thorn in the flesh, my constant reminder, then so be it. If it is curable, help me persevere to complete recovery.

Painfully Yours, Janet

 A Sister Shares

I did not have all the debilitating effects of chemo. My hair thinned but did not all fall out. Luckily, I had plenty to spare. I suffered minor malaise for a few days, but nausea was easily managed with a wonderful drug called Zofran. My Sjogren's Syndrome [a chronic autoimmune disorder] was actually helped by the chemo. . . .

Most of the worst trouble I had was with the radiation. One of the characteristics of Sjogren's is inability to tolerate the ultraviolet rays of the sun. The radiation treatments exacerbated my fatigue and caused more severe burning of the breast than is typical. It was expected with my history and unavoidable. I had retained my breast and therefore radiation was of utmost importance. It was a painful Christmas for me. The burns intensified and got infected. Luckily, I had planned for this eventuality and got most of my Christmas preparation out of the way. My husband prepared dinner. It was the quietest and least festive Christmas we have ever had, but yet very poignant. The kids were happy with their loot. Paul and I were happy the worst of the radiation was behind me. —Bonnie[8]

 Mentoring Moment

If something does not seem right, pursue it. Don't let doubt and worry consume you. Making the rounds of doctors was worth it to receive assurance that everything was OK. As it turned out, while doing research for this book, I discovered my radiation oncologist had discussed the possibility of breast swelling in the literature he gave me when I first started radiation. Of course, I was in a fog then, as probably you were, too, when you started radiation or chemotherapy. I might have read it in the beginning, but six months later I had long since forgotten. The doctor was so gracious and kind not to point this out to me but instead patiently calmed my fears.

If you have radiation treatment or lymph nodes removed, ask your doctor about exercises for your arm. Five to twenty percent of women experience a swelling of the arm, called lymphedema. Do everything the doctors suggest for preventing side effects of treatment. During radiation I followed instructions so carefully not to get any cuts, lift anything heavy, or in any way harm my left arm that my shoulder actually froze. I tried acupuncture, physical therapy, exercises, and heat, but my shoulder still does not have full mobility without pain. If you had a mastectomy, there is a regime of exercises, wound care, and suggested support bras for reconstruction. With a prosthesis, make sure you have a proper fit to prevent neck and shoulder pain. Most doctors will give you written instructions, but ask them or their assistant to go over everything with you to ensure you understand. Ask questions. Take notes on the "Appointment Notes" (page 353), and call if you have any questions after you get home. Also check out "National Contacts" (page 345).

Very likely, there are areas of tenderness or soreness you just want to go away. Sometimes the cure doesn't feel worth the effort or pain. I found it helpful to have someone keep me accountable by asking, "Did you do your exercises today?" I also asked the Holy Spirit to keep after me. Nag me! Prod me! Push me! Remind me! Heal me!

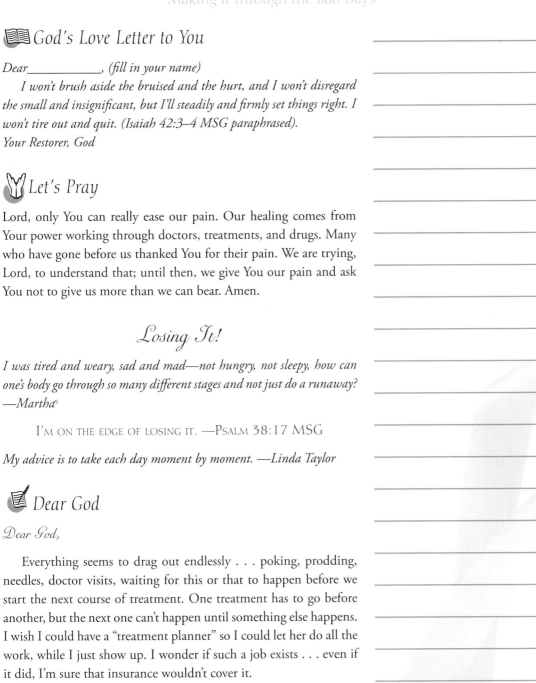 God's Love Letter to You

Dear_____, (fill in your name)

I won't brush aside the bruised and the hurt, and I won't disregard the small and insignificant, but I'll steadily and firmly set things right. I won't tire out and quit. (Isaiah 42:3–4 MSG paraphrased).
Your Restorer, God

Let's Pray

Lord, only You can really ease our pain. Our healing comes from Your power working through doctors, treatments, and drugs. Many who have gone before us thanked You for their pain. We are trying, Lord, to understand that; until then, we give You our pain and ask You not to give us more than we can bear. Amen.

Losing It!

I was tired and weary, sad and mad—not hungry, not sleepy, how can one's body go through so many different stages and not just do a runaway? —Martha

I'M ON THE EDGE OF LOSING IT. —PSALM 38:17 MSG

My advice is to take each day moment by moment. —Linda Taylor

Dear God

Dear God,

Everything seems to drag out endlessly . . . poking, prodding, needles, doctor visits, waiting for this or that to happen before we start the next course of treatment. One treatment has to go before another, but the next one can't happen until something else happens. I wish I could have a "treatment planner" so I could let her do all the work, while I just show up. I wonder if such a job exists . . . even if it did, I'm sure that insurance wouldn't cover it.

Most of the doctors are good about communicating with each other, but my heart always stops when one of them says, "Oh no, that is not what you should have done." Or, "Why did they have you do that?" I want to scream, "I don't know. Why don't you ask them?"

My nerves are on edge. I want so badly for everything to be over, but I look on the calendar and see months before we are finished. Then, I guess, we never are completely done, are we? Follow-up appointments—did they say for the rest of my life? Never again answering "routine" to the nurse's inevitable question when setting mammogram appointments, "Diagnostic or routine?" A constant reminder, over is never really over.

Lord, help me assimilate this season into my life. Let me deal with the continuous need for treatment and watching, without doubt and fear. Using the information presented to me to determine the best outcome, I chose a course. Now I must put it all in Your capable hands, knowing that at some point it is just beyond the doctors and me. You will be the final judge when enough is enough.

Continue to bring opportunities for me to witness as I trudge on through the treatments. Thank You that technology exists to treat my cancer. In the midst of the drudgery, help me not lose sight of how fortunate I am living in an era where they know so much about treating breast cancer. Father, I pray the research goes on to discover a complete cure.

Sometimes losing it, Janet

A Sister Shares

Chemotherapy was like a marathon for me. The long, hard period took much perseverance and prayer. I had eight treatments—one every three weeks. In all those months, I missed work only two and half days due to the side effects of chemotherapy. God is so good!

Radiation was the final sprint toward the finish line. I had only a light reddening of the skin with the thirty-three radiation treatments. The worst thing about these treatments was the scheduling five days a week, but the best thing was getting to know the people I saw every day in the waiting room at the cancer center. As I look back on this experience, I see the countless ways that God was arranging and working in my life. He taught me to be a little less proud, more receptive of help from others, and a lot more trusting in Him.
—Cheryl

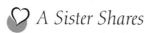 Mentoring Moment

While each of our journeys might be different and some require more surgeries, more chemo, more radiation, and others sail through, at some point the process just gets to you. Vacations, getaways, holidays, even everyday routine life has to fit into your new "everyday life." Eventually we all pray, "Oh Lord, when will this ever end? I'm losing it!"

Some of you find checking off milestones and charting your course is helpful. You write down the entire journey—all the dates, length of treatments, rechecks, and expected prognosis. Then, just like on a trip, you check off where you have traveled. It gives you a feeling of accomplishment and moving forward. Don't be discouraged, though, if you have to go back and revisit a couple of those stops . . . maybe another surgery, or more chemo later. Even on trips we often retrace our route back to a junction to get to the next destination. In the "Sanity Tools" (appendix B), you'll find "My Breast Cancer Journey Map" (page 371) to chart your treatment course; you may find that helpful. Highlighting where you have traveled will be an encouragement as more highlights appear on the page.

However, if looking at the whole trip in one glance overwhelms and depresses you, then just take it one day at a time. Maintain a treatment calendar and only look at the current day's schedule. The days fly by, whether you are having fun or not. Four months, six months, or even a year sounds like a long time up-front, but even the longest day has an end. Soon the passed days of treatment outnumber the ones you still have ahead of you.

God's Love Letter to You

Dear_____, (fill in your name)

What a gift life is to those who stay the course! You've heard, of course, of Job's staying power, and you know how I, God, brought it all together for him at the end. That's because I care right down to the last detail. And since you know I care, let your language show it. Don't add words like "I swear to God" to your own words. Don't show your impatience by concocting oaths to hurry me up. . . . Are you hurting? Pray. Do you feel great? Sing (James 5:11–13 MSG paraphrased).
Your Staying Power, God.

Let's Pray

Prayerfully personalize with me Lamentations 3:18–26 CEV.

I, _____, tell myself, "I am finished! I can't count on the LORD to do anything for me." Just thinking of my troubles and my lonely wandering makes me miserable. That's all I, _____, ever think about, and I am depressed. Then I, _____, remember something that fills me with hope. The Lord's kindness never fails! If he had not been merciful, we, _____ and Janet, would have been destroyed. The Lord can always be trusted to show mercy each morning. Deep in my heart I say, "The Lord is all I, _____, need; I can depend on him!" The LORD is kind to everyone who trusts and obeys him. It is good to wait patiently for the LORD to save us. Amen.

Your Letter to God

Is sleeplessness driving you nuts and affecting your attitude and tolerance level? Write down ideas of how to rest your mind and body. If you are sleeping well, express your abundant gratitude. Journal the words you would say if God were sitting next to you. Be bold. Let Him know how you feel. He can take it, and He prefers you unload on Him rather than on those around you. Listen. Be quiet. Is He speaking back to you in your heart and mind? Write down what He says. Then the next time you feel alone or losing it, read His comforting words to you.

Dear God,   *Date:*

_____

_____

_____

_____

_____

_____

_____

_____

_____

_____

_____

_____

CHAPTER TEN

Getting Needed Support

ALL PRAISE TO THE GOD AND FATHER OF OUR MASTER, JESUS THE MESSIAH!
FATHER OF ALL MERCY! GOD OF ALL HEALING COUNSEL!
HE COMES ALONGSIDE US WHEN WE GO THROUGH HARD TIMES,
AND BEFORE YOU KNOW IT, HE BRINGS US ALONGSIDE SOMEONE ELSE
WHO IS GOING THROUGH HARD TIMES
SO THAT WE CAN BE THERE FOR THAT PERSON JUST AS GOD WAS THERE FOR US.

—2 Corinthians 1:3–4 MSG

A Mentor Helps

There are actually women who I believe have been put in my path to talk about this. I know that I have saved other women from going through treatment they didn't need. —Renne[1]

The Lord sure blessed me with my Bosom Buddy. —Jamie

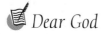 Dear God

Dear God,

I still marvel at Your presence through all of this. In the beginning of the journey when Dave, Kim, and I were at the family planning conference, You brought the hugest blessing into my life—my very own mentor. When Dr. West finished explaining all our surgery and treatment options, he introduced us to Grace Marestaing. Grace floated into the room like an angel. I noticed Grace talking to a couple in the waiting room when we arrived at the BreastCare Center that morning. Her kind and gentle countenance was calming and caring when she asked them, "So how are you doing?" I later learned she was talking to parents of a very young woman with aggressive breast cancer.

Joining us at the conference table, Grace explained she was a volunteer at the BreastCare Center. She'd had a mastectomy last year and would be available to answer questions. Glancing down at the spot on my application where I had put "the Lord" as my boss, she laughed. "Interesting employer!" "Yes," I responded, leaning in and looking her straight in the eye. "Is He yours too?" "Absolutely!" An instant bond.

Grace was a sign of Your presence throughout this battle. My mind wandered for a moment to the Woman to Woman Mentoring conference, and the mentoring game skit. The mentee selects "Grace Abounds" as her mentor. Looking into Grace's sympathetic eyes, I smiled back, knowing I had my very own Grace Abounds! Thank You, Lord, for Grace.

Gratefully Yours, Janet

Two Sisters Share

The last procedure is a tattoo to give color to the reconstructed nipples. The day after that, I felt the need to talk to Karen Jackson. She had been my mentor throughout the cancer experience. Her surgery and chemotherapy preceded mine by a matter of weeks. . . . This teacher offered me strength and hope all along the way. When I was terrified of the chemotherapy, she said, "Hey, it's not so bad, just a lot like morning sickness when you're pregnant." That made it seem doable. When I was in my hospital bed after surgery, Karen showed me, even though my arm was sore, that soon I'd be able to lift my arm just like she could. And when my hair was about to fall out from the chemotherapy, she gave me tips for buying a wig and counseled me on how it would feel emotionally. Karen was a perfect stranger before I had cancer. Now I feel like she's a sister. —Brenda Ladun[2]

At Queen's Hospital, where I went for radiation treatments, they offer a free one-year Healing Touch program as part of their pain-management program. I filled out a questionnaire asking personal questions like career background, marital status, medical history, ethnic background, and so forth. Then the program director matches the breast cancer patient with a "Bosom Buddy" who is a former breast cancer patient with the same type of treatment and similar diagnosis as the current patient. My Bosom Buddy and I have become close friends outside the program, too, and we share many things over the phone and through e-mail. The Lord sure blessed me with my Bosom Buddy. —Jamie

 Mentoring Moment

Jamie was a mentor in our Woman to Woman Mentoring Ministry at Saddleback Church when I first started the ministry. She has since moved to Hawaii, and I was surprised to receive a Christmas card telling me she had the same type of breast cancer I had. As we corresponded, she mentioned the Bosom Buddy and Healing Touch program, and it sounded so much like our mentoring ministry.

Often, I lamented that God used me to create and lead a mentoring ministry but I never had a mentor myself. God graciously answered those laments with Grace Marestaing. Even though our breast cancers and treatments differed, I knew she would understand my thoughts and fears. We connected immediately and have remained close friends. She prays for my writing and reminds me, "He who began a good work in you will be faithful to complete it."

We may need different mentors for various phases of our treatment. I didn't realize that at first. The radiation center suggested talking with their patient advocate, Liz, who had the same type of breast cancer and treatment as I had. My first response was, "No, thank you." I was thinking, *I have Grace. Even though she didn't have radiation, I don't need anyone else right now.*

Then on the first day of radiation, there was Liz. I couldn't believe it! "It's you they were talking about?" I exclaimed through my tears. I knew Liz. I trained and guided her in being a mentor in the mentoring ministry, and now she was offering her experience to help mentor me through radiation. How could I turn that down? As Liz and I began chatting, a floodgate unleashed, and out poured my questions and fears about radiation and what lay ahead. Liz ushered me into a conference room and calmly and lovingly answered my many questions about this phase of treatment like no one else could—she had been there. Knowing exactly what I was feeling, she offered tangible suggestions and advice.

Many things can only be understood by another woman who has walked in our shoes. Our loved ones do their best, but it is important to find someone who has had breast cancer and is willing to encourage and talk with you. Caution: be sure this person is ready to focus on you and isn't still in the throes of her own cancer. Today, I am there for others in the same way Liz and Grace mentored me. Just last week, I had the opportunity to meet with Kay Warren, our pastor's wife, who had just finished her course of chemotherapy and radiation. It was a blessing to share tips I learned about nutrition and regaining our seemingly lost energy. Titus 2:3–5 is the basis for the Woman to Woman Mentoring Ministry, and I paraphrase those verses as, "Mentoring is teaching what you've been taught so you can train others." God does not let things happen in our lives just for our own character building, even though that is an important part of it. He is going to put someone else in our path with a similar situation, and He asks us to reach out, step out, and speak out what we've been taught to help other sisters in need.

If your doctors or hospitals do not provide mentors, find them for yourself. They are invaluable. Suggested ways to find a mentor are:

- Visit a breast cancer support group.

- Ask at your church.

- If your church has a Woman to Woman Mentoring Ministry or another mentoring ministry for women, contact them.

- Call the American Cancer Society, and look at their Web site (see "National Contacts," page 345).

- Keep your ears open for someone who knows a woman who has gone through breast cancer. Ask your family and friends to do the same.

- Ask your doctors if they know someone with a similar case as yours who is willing to meet with you.

- There are several toll-free phone numbers for chat lines and twenty-four-hour hotlines on the National Contacts list.

- Of course, this book is my opportunity to mentor you.

Mentoring is simply sharing those "been there, done that" experiences. With God's help you made it through, and she can too! I have given that definition numerous times and written it in my books, but never did it become more real than when I had Grace and Liz in my life. They gave me wise counsel and a loving, listening ear. Doesn't that sound like something you need too?

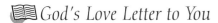 God's Love Letter to You

Dear_____, (fill in your name)

I, God, am able to make all grace abound to you, so that in all things at all times, having all that you need, you will abound in every good work (2 Corinthians 9:8).
Your Mentor, God

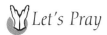 Let's Pray

God, this is such new and foreign territory. We never imagined needing this kind of a mentor. It is humbling and humiliating to feel so inadequate. We know You don't want us being lone rangers in this fight for life. We need help and training from someone who has experienced this battle and knows the enemy's tactics and how to survive and thrive. We give You praise for all who help us and ask that You use us to do the same when we are on the other side of this crisis. Lead us, direct us, guide us, and love us through another breast cancer sister. We earnestly ask Your help. Amen.

It's All about You

This process has made me more intentional about leaving space and margins in my life . . . time for quiet, for walking and exercise, for precious relationships with friends and family, time to enjoy new friendships . . . time for fun . . . time for me. —Grace Marestaing

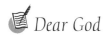 Dear God

Dear God,

Wow, a tough concept to grasp—"it's all about me." How can this be, when it is all about You, Lord? Pastor Rick's book *The Purpose Driven Life* came out right before my diagnosis, and my friends often

---

Grace Abounds
by Janet Thompson

Feelings flow.
Stories told.
Waiting answers.
Ah, it's cancer.
Unshed tears.
Over years.
Held inside.
Ah, such pride!
Building, building.
Yielding, yielding.
Now release.
Ah, such peace.
Pain, sadness.
Grief, madness.
Not fair.
Ah, many care.
"I'm Grace."
Kind face.
"Interesting employer."
Ah, "I'll mentor."
"I cried.
But survived."
Dr. West,
Ah, "the best."
Life's dear.
No fear.
God surrounds.
Ah, Grace abounds.

© 2002 *AHW* Ministries

I wrote this poem for our Christmas card during the "cancer" Christmas. It's in gratitude for Grace.

quoted the first line to one another, "It's not about you." Now everyone is telling me that it is all about me?

The first day Liz and I talked, she said, "Janet, you look so tired. Are you getting sufficient rest? Are you eating enough?" I shared my frustrations of trying to make Christmas nice for my family, the saga of our house remodel with no functioning kitchen, ministry demands that don't stop just because you stop—and on I spewed. Liz gently cautioned, "Janet, it's all about you right now. You have to let everyone know that, and you must accept it yourself. Let others do things for Christmas and the ministry." Certain that Liz had read our pastor's book, I protested, "But Liz, the first line of Pastor Rick's book says it is not about me! I can't reconcile this in my mind. A war is going on inside me trying hard not to make it about me."

Then Liz gave me wise counsel. She said, "Janet, it has to be all about you now, so you can get well and regain your energy. It *is* all about Him, but you have to be in shape to spread that message." Of course. Why hadn't I seen that clearly myself? Liz reminded me that the longer it took me to recover, the longer it would be before I was on the road again for You.

My next question was, how does a wife, mother, and grandmother who has capably taken care of the family and all their needs tell everyone she can't do it right now? How do I help them see it has to be all about me without frightening or burdening them with the load?

Again, Liz's advice was wise. "Be honest. Tell them you are tired and need to rest. You don't even have a kitchen sink or counters, so continue using paper plates and plastic utensils right through the holidays. Let others bring food and grocery shop and Christmas shop for you. Lower your expectations of Christmas and household duties."

Every day the radiation therapists echo the same message: "Don't overdo. Let others do for you. It's all about you." Any resistance out of my mouth is quickly squelched with, "Your body needs to rebuild itself. Daily we are tearing it down, and it needs food, energy, and rest to rebuild. Listen to our words." I'm trying.

Wearily Yours, Janet

A Sister Shares

[After retiring] I now had more time to concentrate on getting healthy. I went to two different nutritionists and began to eat a low-fat diet with lots of fruits and vegetables, and whole grains. I bought "organic" whenever possible. My teacher friends purchased a juicer for me so I could make juices and smoothies out of whole fruits and vegetables. I took vitamins and drank herbal teas and lots of water. I gave up caffeine and wine. I took daily walks and long relaxing warm baths. I spent time in prayer and meditation. I joined eight Bible studies, but soon cut back to two weekly studies that required lots of homework. I also attended biweekly and monthly covenant groups and spent hours reading the Bible and other inspirational books. I kept a journal of my feelings and the things for which I was grateful. I even went to a psychologist to deal with some unresolved anger and guilt. Most importantly, I learned to fully trust God. He is the provider for all my needs. His grace is sufficient. —Nancy Tuttle[3]

Mentoring Moment

As moms, wives, employees, employers, ministry workers, housekeepers, cooks, and all the many hats we twenty-first-century women wear, we often think no one can replace us. Certainly we are the ones who set the pace for Christmas and other celebrations, run the home, and maybe, like me, even handle the finances. Suddenly both the family and you must adjust to your not doing what you so capably did for years.

In the past if I was tired during the day or evening, I just drank a cup of coffee or took a walk, then plowed through, sometimes to exhaustion. With breast cancer, that all stopped. *Now,* when I am tired, my body shuts down. I turn off the light and the computer. No one expects us to be superwomen through this—we can't set that expectation on ourselves. The more we physically and emotionally pamper ourselves, the more quickly our old self is going to return— well, maybe not the same old self, but a new definition of us.

Let me give you Liz's advice: now is the time for everything to be about you. When your body says take a nap, don't push through it. Our bodies are designed to regulate us, and God made little warning signs to alert us when it's time to sleep, eat, exercise, recreate, be alone, or be with people. Remember, Father always knows best.

God's Love Letter to You

Dear_____, (fill in your name)
Then my Son, Jesus, said, "Come to me, all of you who are weary and carry heavy burdens, and I will give you rest. Take my yoke upon you. Let me teach you, because I am humble and gentle, and you will find rest for your souls" (Matthew 11:28–29 NLT paraphrased).
Your Burden Carrier, God, and My Son, Jesus Christ

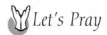 *Let's Pray*

God, putting ourselves first is a foreign concept. We are nurturers and caretakers accustomed to putting others' needs before our own. Now we can't keep up our usual responsibilities, but we fear taking a break to recuperate. Help us put our trust in You as our very capable Provider and Caretaker. Teach us to humbly swallow our pride, receive help, and recuperate. Please heal us and restore our health . . . and when You do, let us never forget the lessons we learned from stopping to smell the roses . . . the coffee . . . the ocean air . . . listening to the sounds of children playing . . . babies crying . . . or loved ones pouring out their undying love for us just as Your Son, Jesus, did for us on the cross. For that, we are ever grateful. Amen.

Should You Join a Breast Cancer Support Group?

Having worked in the medical field for many years, I really didn't think I needed to attend a support group but eventually did. I found that no one has the same story. From this I developed a friendship with Norma, and we walk together every other day. We will be taking part in the Susan G. Komen walk/race together. We also participated in exercise programs provided by local health clubs—they provide them free to cancer patients. —Shirley

BY YOURSELF YOU'RE UNPROTECTED. WITH A FRIEND YOU CAN FACE THE WORST. CAN YOU ROUND UP A THIRD? A THREE-STRANDED ROPE ISN'T EASILY SNAPPED.
—ECCLESIASTES 4:12 MSG

REAL SURVIVORS LEARN WISDOM FROM OTHERS. —PROVERBS 28:26 MSG

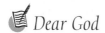 *Dear God*

Dear God,

Why do I hesitate to join a support group? Is it because I am still coming to grips with even needing one and acknowledging I am, indeed, "one of them"? Does that make it all too real? Am I worried I might not be able to handle hearing about those who are dying or worse off than I? A few weeks after surgery I got a call from the BreastCare Center asking if I was going to join their next six-week support group. They said most women in the group had a new diagnosis or were in treatment like me. They met at night at the BreastCare Center, and I wasn't up to driving all that way in the dark. I wondered how other women did it. I told them I was already going to several small groups and there was no energy for another night out.

Then there it was in the church bulletin—Saddleback's Breast Cancer Support Group. Should I go there, Lord? Do I need it? How would it help? I feel almost guilty not going.

Will I regret it later? Could I be of help to someone or she to me? I don't seem to feel peace either way. Father, direct me in the path You want me to take.

Questioningly Yours, Janet

 ## Two Sisters Share

A Stanford study of women with metastasized breast cancer showed that participating in support groups improved their quality of life and doubled their length of life. I began attending a spiritual wellness group at church for cancer patients going through treatment. There are many types of cancer support groups, and I tried several before I found this one where I felt at home. This group has helped me see that a complete healing includes spiritual and emotional healing, as well as physical healing. As we share our journey with cancer, we get strength and hope from each other, from the Bible, and from praying for each other. Strange as it may seem, it is one of the most joyful groups I have ever been involved in. —Nancy Tuttle[4]

My moral support came from a Reach for Recovery monthly breast cancer support group sponsored by the American Cancer Society. Here they share their chemo, radiation, diagnosis, etc. experiences. A woman can attend whenever she wishes, free of charge. We also share one another's phone numbers and addresses in case we want to talk and/or meet for additional moral support whenever we feel the need. It is a great way to share side effects of medication and talk about what your boyfriend or spouse thinks about what you are going through. This group is still so important to me. —Jamie

 ## Mentoring Moment

I did not join a breast cancer support group, although in researching this book, I attended the one at our church after reading this description on Saddleback's Web site: "Our support group is run by breast cancer survivors. They have been diagnosed with breast cancer, received treatment, and are currently in remission. Saddleback Church's Breast Cancer Support Group encourages women with breast cancer to use this time to seek God and His will for their lives, encourage and build one another up in the Lord, and discuss concerns and fears while we see one another through this difficult time."

I appreciated that the support group was led by women who had experienced breast cancer and now were offering to mentor others. The group members seemed to find comfort in being around women who had shared the same journey and experiences. Darlene Gee said of her participation, "I go to help and encourage others and let them know there is an abundant life after cancer. I have hiked the Grand Canyon and gone on a mission trip to Kenya. However, sometimes it is sad at how young some of the new girls are, and it's scary when you hear about recurrences."

At their group I noticed women in all steps of the journey, from newly diagnosed and contemplating choices, to fully recovered, and every stage in-between. You may feel there is so much going on during the treatment stage that you can't fit in another thing; on the other hand, it might be just what you need to get through it! You might also appreciate a support group if you experience a letdown when treatment ends, much like postpartum blues or after you have completed any intense project. All your energies and time are spent on treatment, then one day you are finished, and you wonder, *Now what?* The answer might be the fellowship and conversation of a group.

There are also support groups for women with the same type of breast cancer or in the same age category. Go to the "National Contacts" on page 345 for phone numbers and Web addresses. Linda M. joined a support group for women with advanced breast cancer. She said, "It is a small group, and I really enjoyed being with women who are in the same place I am. I have come to know that I have had it quite good so far, so I consider that answered prayers. It is a very positive group as well, so that will keep my spirits high."

Many of the Reach for Recovery programs also provide in-home assistance from former breast cancer survivors. Martha had a friend who volunteered for the program in her area, and she recalls this woman showing up one day at her door with her first bra and temporary breast form to use until the doctor wrote a prescription for a permanent prosthesis. This same woman brought Martha a small pillow that became her constant companion. In my area the Reach for Recovery volunteers visit ladies who have just had surgery and help them with using their arms after lymph-node resection and surgery.

Some groups form informally. My husband gave me a gift of a massage and facial for my birthday, and the massage therapist, Carol, had had breast cancer similar to mine only two years prior. She'd had to go daily in a van with other cancer patients to a Kaiser Radiation Center, an hour and a half from home. Carol said at first she dreaded the trip but soon began looking forward to it as she developed friendships and relationships with other patients in the van. They formed their own support group and still meet once a month for lunch.

I also read in the paper of a breast cancer survivor who formed a dragon-boat race team as a support group for other cancer survivors. The participants feel embowered with self-confidence by physically teaming together in their battle against cancer as well as winning races!

Here are some ways to locate a support group in your area:

- Ask at your doctor's office or treatment centers if they recommend one.

- Call your local American Cancer Society branch. If you don't know their number, call the American Cancer Society (see "National Contacts," page 345).

- Call your church and ask if they have a breast cancer support group, and if not, ask if they know of one in your area or at another church.

- Go to the names you put down under the "Who Will I Call or Where Will I Go When I Am Feeling . . ." form (page 375), and call them on those days when you need support.

- Ask a friend to go with you to your first support group if you need a ride or feel uncomfortable going by yourself. At the breast cancer support meeting I attended, there was a woman who accompanied her newly diagnosed friend "just to be there and give her support." Looking back, I am sure my friend Jane or Grace would have gone with me in a heartbeat if only I had asked—but I didn't.

- Some have found counselors helpful, but make sure they are Christian, biblical counselors who will advise you from the Bible.

- If you are in a quandary about whether or not a support group is helpful, use the "Peacekeeping Worksheet" (page 349).

God's Love Letter to You

Dear_____, (fill in your name)

Don't give up meeting together, as some are in the habit of doing, but encourage one another—and all the more as you see the Day approaching (Hebrews 10:25 paraphrased).
Your Constant Supporter, God

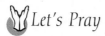 Let's Pray

Lord, please give us the courage and energy to seek out wise counsel and support. We do have many questions, and it would be nice to talk to others who understand our feelings and emotions. Help us find the group where we can be blessed and be a blessing. Thank You for all the support we receive from You and others. Amen.

My Family Needs a Support System Too

A positive diagnosis for cancer is a shock any way one looks at it. It not only affects the person diagnosed, but the whole family system. —Grace Marestaing

I don't envision having the luxury of a nervous breakdown anytime soon. —Bernard Wolfson, husband of Leslie Furth[5]

To provide friendship, understanding, education, and support for kids who have a parent with cancer. —Mission statement, Kids Konnected

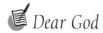 Dear God

Dear God,

I am a bit concerned because my family is not seeking support. I so appreciated the men from Dave's small group coming to the hospital to wait with him during surgery and actually standing by while he met with the doctor after surgery. But what about now? Should I research someone for Dave to meet with? I asked him if he wants to talk to other breast cancer husbands, but he says he doesn't need it. I know the wife of one of his Bible study fellowship leaders died of breast cancer. Lord, is that weighing on Dave's mind and heart?

On top of everything, I awoke one morning and found Dave on the phone talking to someone about a job. "What happened to the job you have?" "It's ending next month," he said. "I didn't want to tell you while you were going through surgery." Oh Lord, my poor husband has a sick wife, a torn-up home, is losing his job in the midst of all the bills for both, and the holidays are quickly approaching. Please protect Dave. Comfort and give him strength. Help him shoulder the concerns of our life as I focus on surviving.

Our children are scared. No one in our family has had cancer. Michelle is sad, and Shannon, shocked! Kim is fearful I will die. Sean keeps asking how Mom is doing. My sister, a doctor herself, is worried. She probably knows too much about what could happen to me. Lord, comfort them all. Bring people into their lives to talk with, and let them turn to You more than ever before for solace and comfort.

Seeking support, Janet

A Sister Shares

My husband, of course, is quite upset, and will be stuck in the thought of it for a while as he lost his father to cancer and his mom has it now. I think it takes me being up and around more normally for him to come around. He is not one for group therapy, so I am relying on his friends and church to comfort him. —Linda M.

A Husband Shares

Many people tell me they can't imagine where I find the strength to deal with two small children and a gravely ill wife, while holding down a job. But that's easy: I have no choice. I love Oliver and Caroline [his young children] more fiercely than I ever could have imagined, and I know that they need me badly right now. Luckily, they are pretty well insulated from all this insanity, at least during the week. Between kindergarten and day care, they both lead full and happy lives. However, I don't envision having the luxury of a nervous breakdown anytime soon. I do have my moments, though. I blow off steam by throwing mini-tantrums when I'm alone. I throw things and curse my rotten luck at being a 'prisoner' of this lousy situation—forced into the role of caregiver and sole provider.

But as much as Oliver and Caroline need me, I think I need them more. They keep me focused and in the moment, which is the only way to live under these circumstances. They force me to think of the pragmatic, daily stuff: They're hungry and thirsty, they want to play, they need books and toothpaste on their brushes . . . and lots of cuddling at bedtime. They jump on the bed and throw pillows and make an awful mess. It's craziness—and I think I'd go crazy without it. —Bernard Wolfson, husband of Leslie Furth[6]

Mentoring Moment

It seems everything should stop when you get the breast cancer news, because your world surely does. Without warning, all the attention shines on you, and the family has to catch up as best they can. Husband and wife are biblically one, so what happens to one body figuratively happens to the other. His wife's breast cancer affects every husband. If you are married or engaged, talk openly with your husband or fiancé about his fears and concerns. Encourage him to seek someone at church or a buddy he can talk to, cry in front of, and pray with. Our church has a Breast Cancer Caregivers group, which is a support group led by men whose wives have had breast cancer.

Your children are going to be scared, no matter what their age. Mine were adults, but the impact was still the same. Young children might not grasp the seriousness of the situation, which is actually good protection for them. Helping them cope takes creativity that you probably won't have. Teens often don't want to deal with it, which can seem hurtful, but it is perfectly normal for their age group. The Kids Konnected program is national and offers group support and a twenty-four-hour hotline for kids of all ages as well as parents. Contact information for Kids Konnected and Gilda's Club, another family support group, are on the "National Contacts" page (page 345).

Try to engage your extended family and church family to be there for your immediate family. When asked where you need help, a response might be, "Could you take the kids to the movies with you this weekend?" or, "My husband just needs a night out or a day off. Would your husband call mine and invite him to go to a baseball game or play golf?" Every family reacts differently. Often they surprise us in ways we would never expect—good ways and, sometimes, bad ways.

So many are lifting prayers and thoughts for you right now, take a moment to ask God to comfort your family from their fears or concerns. Recognize that any negative behavior probably stems from either fear or not knowing how to react.

God's Love Letter to You

*Dear*_____, *(fill in your name)*
    Go home to your family and tell them how much I, the Lord, have done for you, and how I have had mercy on you (Mark 5:19 paraphrased).
Supporting your family, God

Let's Pray

Father, You know our family is hurting, scared, and often doesn't know how to help. Please bring a supernatural peace to their souls. Give us patience with them and them with us. Protect the little ones from the turmoil that encircles our house. Provide an extra portion of love and shelter from any repercussions of our disease. Help us find joy in each other's company and make the very best of all the days You give us together. We are family, and You are the Head of our family. We look to You now to lead us safely through this uncharted desert experience. Thank You, Lord. Amen.

Creative Ideas for Family

A Treasure Hunt to the Hospital

One newspaper story about Leslie Furth told how her five-year-old son, Oliver, didn't want to see her in the hospital because she didn't come home with them. It was easier for him to avoid the hurt of leaving her. A friend of the family found a creative way to engage Oliver in a treasure hunt that ended at the hospital. Oliver went willingly to the hospital as part of the treasure hunt, and Mom turned out to be the sought-after treasure. After this fun experience, Oliver was able to visit more regularly.[7]

A Bedside Picnic

Margaret Kelly's coworkers brought the family home-cooked meals every night, and the owners of the business brought lunch once a week just to let her know they hadn't forgotten her. "Even better, my family came upstairs and laid down a blanket, and we had a picnic dinner every night in my bedroom," she says. "That support made all the difference to me." Margaret says that while immense support through all five surgeries didn't ease the pain, it did ease her worry and allowed her to focus on healing.[8]

Send Them Cards Too

The folks at Kids Konnected mentioned that kids often say as they receive the program-provided gift package: "Wow, this is so great. My mom gets cards every day. But I am sad too . . . it sure would be nice if someone sent me a card." Ask family and friends to send your husband and kids cards too. I am sure you will notice quite a change in their attitude and countenance as they feel the love and warmth expressed in those cards.

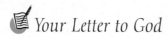 *Your Letter to God*

Has a mentor helped you, or how could you find one? Have you had a tough time making life "all about you"? Ask God for help accepting energy and emotional limits and courage and humility to receive help. Was joining a breast cancer support group a blessing or uncomfortable? If you didn't join one, how did you receive support? Does your family have support through this uncharted territory? Journal ideas of what might relieve some of their fears and pressures and afford them extra amounts of joy, peace, relief, and comfort.

Dear God,   *Date:*

_____

_____

_____

_____

_____

_____

_____

_____

_____

_____

_____

_____

_____

_____

_____

_____

_____

_____

CHAPTER ELEVEN

Knowing Who Is in Control

No test or temptation that comes your way is beyond the course of what others have had to face. All you need to remember is that God will never let you down; he'll never let you be pushed past your limit; he'll always be there to help you come through it. So, my very dear friends, when you see people reducing God to something they can use or control, get out of their company as fast as you can.

—*1 Corinthians 10:13–14 MSG*

Spinning Out of Control

Cancer has taught me to trust. I was always trusting myself instead of God. But I find that God provides for all my needs. When I get overwhelmed by circumstances, it's because I'm trying to do it again, and not turning it over to Him. When I release my cancer to God, He works everything out for good. —Nancy Tuttle[1]

It took a lot of soul searching before I discovered my fears and anger were rooted in the loss of my independence and control. I felt like a failure. —Brenda N.

I was willing to let the Lord take control of everything except my children, and, of course, I had no peace. —Darlene Gee

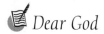 Dear God

Dear God,

You know how much I love being in control of my life circumstances. Now I must let go and let You orchestrate the many facets of my treatment. I can't believe the things I am allowing them to do! The words *radiation* or *chemotherapy* always brought to mind images of killing part of my body. I could never let that happen to me. Yet here I am, saying, "Yes, put dye in my veins." "Yes, take out lymph nodes that could result in side effects." "Yes, radiate me daily and destroy good cells along with bad cells."

Lord, if it were not for that cross in the ceiling above the radiation table, I would feel abandoned. I hate that to live, part of me must die. Then You so kindly remind me that to live is death. Death to myself, as You live anew in me. Maybe this is a word picture You want me to share. That helps, Lord. You are using my breast cancer and using me. Things aren't spinning out of control after all.

Controllably Yours, Janet

A Sister Shares

Something wonderful happened before dawn on the day of my surgery. This type-A personality, who had to be in control and make the house, the kids, the husband, the career, even the dog run smoothly, had to let go. I realized I was not really in control of anything. God was in control. What a freeing feeling! God was in control of everything in my life. On this morning of major surgery I put all the worry and fear on Him and allowed the Lord to take away my fear. I felt as if He wrapped His arms around me. God really was in control that day. —Brenda Ladun[2]

☕ *Mentoring Moment*

Our day is all about control. The family depends on us to keep everyone where they are supposed to be on time. We keep the cupboards full of food, soap, toothpaste, toilet paper, paper towels . . . the works! We oversee clean clothes, clean house, schoolwork, social calendars, school calendars, and dentist and doctor appointments.

The short-circuiting words, "You have cancer," plunge us spinning out of control. Yes, we have choices all along the way, but they are not in areas in which we ever wanted to make decisions. We had life planned out—well, at least the next week. One doctor appointment throws our world into a tailspin. My friend Linda Ferrigno, whom I mentioned earlier had lung cancer, was all dressed up for a party when she and her husband went to the memorable "out-of-control doctor appointment." Just a routine physical, but the doctor's office called her to come back in later that day. Not expecting a problem, their plan was to stop by the doctor's office and then go on to the party. The diagnosis—"You have lung cancer"—canceled the party and changed their plans for the rest of their lives. In one instant time stands still, the reins jerked from our hands.

Actually, we never really have the reins. God just lets us *think* we do. He, of course, is in ultimate control of our destinies. How humbling it is to realize we cannot stop this on our own. There is no going back, changing things, praying it away, wishing it away, yelling, and screaming—nothing is going to reverse a positive diagnosis. There is that occasional miracle where positive turns to negative, but we have no control over that, do we? God gets all the glory when that happens—or at least He should.

Cancer forces us to *cooperate* rather than *control*. Some of us might actually feel relief no longer being organizer of our universe. Slowly the realization seeps into our psyches that life was actually out of control all along. We gladly drop the reins, get off the runaway horse of our "in-control life," and surrender fully to God and His plans for us. We seek His wise counsel for the next step. Others of us hang on with all our might. The horse runs even faster, dragging us behind—bruised, bloodied, and beat up. There comes a point in all our lives where we have to let go and let God.

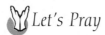 God's Love Letter to You

Dear_____, (fill in your name)

You are not controlled by your sinful nature. You are controlled by My Holy Spirit if you have My Spirit living in you. . . . If Christ lives within you, even though your body will die because of sin, your spirit is alive because you have been made right with me (Romans 8:9–10 NLT paraphrased).

In control of the universe, God

Let's Pray

You know, Father, how hard it is for us to surrender control to You . . . or anyone. Speak to us in ways we can hear. Remind us we are not looking at the whole picture, but You are, and You want us healthy more than we want it ourselves! Give us confidence in all those who treat us. Maybe someone will gain eternal life by accepting Your Son, Jesus Christ, because of our illness. When we look at things in that light, it helps us see how really in control You are. Thank You for Your Son, Jesus Christ, who gave His life for ours. We are so grateful, and we willingly surrender our life to Your control. Amen.

Controlling the Controllable

I want to control the controllable and leave the uncontrollable to God. —Kay Warren

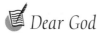 Dear God

Dear God,

I have come to grips with the reality that in order to gain control, I have to give it up. To save my life, I must let go of it. To regain strength and wholeness, I must admit weakness and brokenness. I must bare my breast in front of strangers who are treating me—including some men. Oh Lord, such vulnerability engulfs me at each radiation day and every doctor appointment. Slowly, these people are not strangers anymore, but that doesn't make it any easier. While I made the initial decisions for surgery, testing lymph nodes, and radiation, once the treatments commence, someone else tells me what to do and when. Someone else takes control over my going and coming—my very life. Lord, how I prayed for You to give them wisdom, accuracy, and discernment, and give me a sense of trust in their expertise.

Still, I struggled with where I might take a more active part in my treatment. You helped me see, Father, that it was by doing everything they instructed. Taking care of my skin during radiation was one area I could control. I followed their instructions religiously, and today there is no scarring. "Don't lose weight, because you'll lose it in your breast, and it will change the mapping we did for the radiation," the radiation therapists warned. I could control that. So I weighed every day to stay in a safe range. They also cautioned, "Don't get any cuts on your left arm, and don't lift anything heavy during radiation." I actually went overboard on that and ended up with a frozen shoulder. You know me, Lord, obsessive sometimes.

"Ask questions if you don't understand something," they all assured me. Ah, power in information. I could do that, and I did. "Rest when you are tired. Eat healthy." Wow, I realized, there really were controllable areas of my care where I could make a positive impact.

Regaining some control, Janet

Two Sisters Share

Probably the most useful advice I have had is from my acupuncturist . . . (the fact that I have one still makes me chuckle at how a once-mighty skeptic has broadened her mind through desperation). She counseled me to think more about what I emanate in the way of energy, or aura, and less about what I may or may not be taking in from outside. I cherish that advice because it turns my passive/victim tendency on its head and puts me in even greater control. It may all be illusory, but I don't care. I want to craft just the right illusion to feed my optimism, because I am convinced now that *what my mind thinks ever so quietly to itself, my body overhears.*
—Leslie Furth[3]

I remember taking a nap one afternoon shortly after losing my hair and breast. My husband woke me up because it was time to go to my parents' for dinner. I started to cry, saying, "I feel like Humpty Dumpty. I have to put myself back together again." I pulled on my wig and stuck my "boob" in my bra and left, not in a very good mood. Shortly after, God revealed to me how I may not be able to control what was happening to my body, but I could control my attitude toward it. I then began to think of the wig as "my helmet of salvation" and the prosthesis as my "breastplate of righteousness," and it actually empowered me to put on God's armor! —Darlene Gee

165

☕ Mentoring Moments

If we are not cautious, breast cancer and its treatment can shift our attitude to that of victims with no control over what happens in our lives. Maybe we even slip into blaming everything we do or can't do on the cancer. We don't ever want to give this disease the power to turn us into victim personalities. Our goal is to be *victorious*, not *victims*! Start looking for safe areas to take action. It will help you feel less afflicted and more assertive and active in your health plan. However, be cognizant of areas that impose on authority you gave the doctors, unless you feel the need to question a procedure he or she suggests.

Don't be surprised if you find yourself doing strange things to gain back control in some area of your life. I mentioned earlier that we took a Thanksgiving ski trip one week after my surgery. Oh, did I forget to mention it was a *ski trip*? Don't worry; I didn't ski. The day before the trip, as you can imagine, I had very little energy for packing. All day I was thinking about what to take and trying to rest so I would be up to helping my husband pack for us when he got home from work. To his great surprise, he walked into the closet and found me sitting on the floor sorting my sock drawer! It was almost a compulsion to take control and organize this unruly drawer—throw out old socks and put the keepers in neat, efficient rows for ease of selecting just the right color. Insane, you say—or are you laughing because you did something similar?

Desperately seeking regained health, I found that controlling my diet was one area where I could actively participate with my treatment. Soon after radiation I met Robyn Boyd, author of *RawSome Recipes*, at a writers' conference, and she helped me learn ways to detoxify by eating completely organic foods, switching from cooked to mostly raw fruits and veggies, taking greens supplements, and eliminating sugar. Dave and I threw out our microwaves—we had two—and we both went through withdrawal, learning how to cook, or uncook, without them. I made field trips to stores in our area that offered organic foods and did comparative shopping analyses to find which ones offered the best prices and choices. I learned about juicing, dehydrating, and new recipes to incorporate all our new foods and preparation. Taking on our healthy nutrition project was empowering. It also resulted in great joy and a sense of accomplishment when only six months later, both Dave and I lost weight and had glowing physicals and test results.

In addition to diet we can take control over our exercise, rest, relaxation, following of doctors' instructions, or perhaps starting a project we can complete with a sense of accomplishment—even if it is just organizing our sock drawer! Our thought life is the control center for our actions. We probably never will discover the elusive "fairness" in having breast cancer, but we can *consciously* decide it will not ruin our lives. Now, that's control!

Don't feel you have to do everything mindlessly without asking questions. It is your prudent right as a patient to be well informed. Write down your questions on the "Questions-and-Answers Note Page" (page 357). Be sure to note the answers. Knowledge is powerful. Know about the treatment your body receives. You might find it helpful to search for information in the books I recommend in "Books Janet Found Helpful" (page 346) or online—but again, I caution, stay balanced. Don't put yourself in information overload, which leads to paralysis rather than empowerment.

📖 God's Love Letter to You

Dear_____, (fill in your name)

My grace is sufficient for you, for my power is made perfect in weakness (2 Corinthians 12:9).
Your Stronghold, God

🐰 Let's Pray

Prayerfully personalize 2 Corinthians 12:9–10.

You, Oh Lord, are omnipotent . . .

Therefore I,_____, will boast all the more gladly about my weaknesses, so that Christ's power may rest on me. That is why, for Christ's sake, I, _____, delight in weaknesses, in insults, in hardships, in persecutions, in difficulties. For when I, _____, am weak, then I, _____, am strong. Amen.

Seeing God in Control

No matter what I'm going through, I can commit it to God, knowing He's in control. He always sees me through. It's the tough times that grow our Christian character. He just asks that we depend on Him, trust Him, and allow Him to be what He's promised to be. —Edna

Seems I can feel a tear drop on my heart when I hear "have a nice day."
—Martha[4]

✍ Dear God

Dear God,

Oh, how I cringe when someone says to me, "Well, you know, God is in control!" Surely they don't mean it this way, but I receive it like, "Have a nice day." It is such an oft-repeated, thoughtless, don't-know-what-else-to-say platitude. It feels like they are discounting and minimizing how my life really is at this moment. It's a shutdown. It closes my spirit. It says to me, "You can't talk about anything bothering you because that shows a lack of faith and I really don't want to get involved."

God, I see You in control all around me—a nonexistent problem in my right breast leading to detection of cancer in my left one; meeting my excellent team of doctors; the companionship of Grace, Nurse Barbara, Fleece, Liz; the cross cut in the ceiling above the radiation machine; the witnessing opportunity with the radiation staff throughout the Christmas season; sitting next to "RawSome Robyn" the first lunch of the writers' conference, where I met Howard Books; writing *Dear God, They Say It's Cancer*; the opportunity to speak from the platform about my breast cancer. Only You, Lord, could have the same movie playing on the televisions in the waiting room at the BreastCare Center that infamous first biopsy day and in the dentist's office as I had my teeth cleaned on the last day of radiation. What a miraculous sign to me that You were there in the beginning and the end of my treatment—the Alpha and the Omega!

Lord, please help me respond lovingly. I know people don't mean to come across legalistic, insincere, or condescending, but often they do. So many remind me of the friends of Job, trying to fix it, or affix blame, or come up with a reason or remedy, or do what I call a "hit-and-run Scripture drop." Lord, help me learn from this.

Knowingly under Your control and loving it, Janet

A Sister Shares

Thank You for my cancer—You are in control, and You do love me. You know what is best for my loved ones and me. You have a plan. Help me to trust in You and be part of Your plan. . . . Thank You for using cancer as a teacher for me—to slow me down and put me in touch with You. Help me see cancer as . . . an adventure to learn from and then go on. Bless my husband and my son and my supportive family and friends as they go through this adventure with me. Make us strong through our weakness and our dependence on You. —Nancy Tuttle[5]

Mentoring Moment

I am sure people have said to you, "God is in control" as a response to discussing your breast cancer. It is very common in the church and among Christians. You probably have some of the same reactions to it I do. God helped me see how to circumvent this comment or insinuation, rather than reacting or withdrawing. Try this: when people ask, "How are you doing?" answer, "You know, I have seen God in control of every area of my breast cancer (or every area of my treatment, or every area of my family, and so forth)." Then give them an example, followed by your current situation, such as, "But today, I am very tired. I could sure use prayers for energy." With this type of a response, you have:

- Assured them *you know* God is in control *before* they can say it

- Reinforced both your faiths by giving an example of God's divine presence

- Told them how they can pray for you

- Witnessed God actively working in your illness, while honestly conveying how you feel right now

This replaces their casually spoken "God is in control" with your testimony of His control in action. What a reassurance to them and you every time you tell another story of God's great presence in your life and illness.

God's Love Letter to You

Dear_____, (fill in your name)
I have told you these things, so that in me you may have peace. In this world you will have trouble. But take heart! I have overcome the world (John 16:33).
My Son, Jesus Christ, God

Let's Pray

Prayerfully personalize the apostle Paul's reassuring words in Ephesians 1:19–20 NLT.

I pray that you, _____, will begin to understand the incredible greatness of God's power for us who believe him. This is the same mighty power that raised Christ from the dead and seated him in the place of honor at God's right hand in the heavenly realms. Amen.

Your Letter to God

Have you seen God at work in your cancer? Are you struggling with the seeming lack of control in your life? Pour it all out to God. Ask for tangible ways to see He is in control. Try to surrender to Him the control of your illness. Have you discovered areas for input or help in your treatment and recuperation? If so, what are they? It will help to write them down to read on those days when everything spins out of control.

Dear God,   *Date:*

_____

_____

_____

_____

_____

_____

_____

_____

_____

_____

_____

_____

_____

_____

_____

_____

_____

_____

_____

_____

CHAPTER TWELVE

Adjusting to a New Normal

On that day the sources of light will no longer shine,
yet there will be continuous day!
Only the Lord knows how this could happen!
There will be no normal day and night,
for at evening time it will still be light.

—*Zechariah 14:6–7 NLT*

"Normal" Isn't Normal Anymore

Many cancer survivors refer to a "new normal" life. For me, part of this "new normal" life is the persistent knowledge of my own mortality. —Nancy Tuttle[1]

After a while, life with cancer begins to seem strangely normal. The unspeakable becomes the routine—the new mundane. —Bernard Wolfson, husband of Leslie Furth[2]

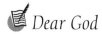 Dear God

Dear God,

One line from the many breast cancer books I read penetrated my heart: "You have to come up with a new definition of normal for your life." Overnight! One day I was an active author, speaker, ministry leader, mother, wife, and grammie balancing all my roles with energy and fortitude. Suddenly I was reduced to a "patient" with limitations, treatments, and losses: energy, use of body parts, modesty, dignity, and a life without breast cancer. Breast cancer is now a permanent part of my history . . . testimony . . . health . . . decisions . . . interactions . . . legacy . . . faith . . . and my relationship with You and others.

As days passed, it became progressively apparent I would not pick up where I left off before my diagnosis. Today I struggle with what "normal" is. After fifty-five years of becoming "me," suddenly someone unrecognizable lives in this body. Muddled thinking and confusion worsen my dyslexia, causing emotional—sometimes irrational—behavior. I look in the mirror and wonder, *Who is this woman?* I never cried at sad stories before. Worship songs seldom brought on tears. I busied myself fixing my children's problems, not crying over them. With one swift surgeon's blade, You cut out the callousness, pride, and lack of empathy and replaced them with a heart that bleeds. I feel others' pain, sadness, and brokenness. I have a new awareness of what breaks Your heart.

Newly normal me, Janet

 Two Sisters Share

"New normal" means I can no longer put off that trip, or writing my memoirs for the grandchildren, or passing along my faith to my children, or telling my family, "I love you." "New normal" also means a full calendar with many scheduled visits to the doctors for treatments, blood tests, and scans. It sometimes means less energy, but the luxury of afternoon naps. It means limiting some physical activities like lifting groceries and laundry, carrying grandkids, leaning over the tub to bathe the dog, or running downstairs. It can mean a missed meeting or visit with family due to a low white blood count, which means my immune system is down, and I would probably catch whatever bug is going around. It also means becoming more humble. I have lost my hair three times. . . . I have learned to live in the moment, and each moment has become precious.

It's easier to do the important things, like going to a museum and having lunch with a friend, and let the unimportant things, like housework, go. Relationships with loved ones and friends become very important, and I have developed a deeper relationship with God. —Nancy Tuttle[3]

I have read that breast cancer and its aftermath are like a broken mirror—once you have had it, your life never fits back the way it went before. I see the struggle differently. For me it was an enforced unburdening. I had to let go of a great deal that had to do with the material world, to pare down, in order to muster the energy to fight the disease. My job slipped away; my unfinished dissertation gathered dust; everything that was not about tending and being tended by loved ones fell away. My connection with the outside world—through the cultural institution where I worked, with the preschool where my son, Oliver, goes, with my own school—receded. My one and only institutional affiliation, my new place of hope and healing and trials-by-fire and down-on-your-knees nausea, was my oncologist's office and the nurses with their chemotherapy lifelines. —Leslie Furth[4]

 ## Mentoring Moment

Initially, I fought the "new normal." I would think, *I am only having breast cancer and radiation, then I'll get back to life.* Have you had those thoughts too? We hope breast cancer is just a bump in the road, but it is more like a *detour*. BC often stands for breast cancer, but for me it meant "before cancer"—BC, I had a memory for detail, was a multitasker and organizer, and my husband balanced me with his calm, laid-back personality. At first, neither of us knew how to adjust to the changes in me. Out of necessity, we quickly learned to shift and change some roles. I always balanced the checkbook and paid bills, but now it took hours, and I made mistakes. Dave took over bill paying, and I readily relinquished it.

Another "old normal" that had to change was my role of social coordinator, planner, and hostess for our family gatherings. New traditions replaced the old. Since I had radiation at Christmas in the middle of the house remodel, we didn't have our annual party or a Christmas tree, and I didn't decorate. Instead, we made a manger scene with a washtub, straw, a borrowed doll, a hanging star, and a few stuffed sheep, and we put our presents around the manger. This actually became a "new normal" tradition for us.

The next step after accepting the new normal is helping family and friends understand and adjust to your new reality. Frequently I had to sit everyone down and explain I could not do the things I did before. When they became impatient with my forgetfulness or limitations, I patiently reminded them again . . . it was our new *normal*.

Are you feeling better now about your "new normal"? There is no point in fighting it, because we can't. I would set deadlines based on BC energy and couldn't meet them, which made me feel defeated. I had to drop out of some things—good things. I learned to delegate, cast off, say no, take rests, and refuse to feel guilty about the changes. You are going to have to do the same. Maybe this is God's definition of normal.

Here are a few universal, basic "new normal" tips:

- Simplify, simplify, simplify—meals might just be a big salad and fruit.

- Save your energy for things you value most.

- Lower expectations of others and yourself. This relieves stress—theirs and yours!

- Say no and mean it.

- Write things down—humbling but necessary.

- Use the "Sanity Tools" in appendix B.

- Prioritize your schedule, and eliminate low-priority, high-energy projects.

- Budget getting the house professionally cleaned, even if only twice a month.

- Remember people are coming to visit you, not to do a House Beautiful tour.

- Delegate, delegate, delegate—let someone else do something you have always done, and learn to be satisfied with the results.

- If you are a night owl, go to bed earlier.

- If you are an early-morning riser, try to catch another half hour of sleep.

- Buy something you "normally" would not buy.

- Wear something you "normally" would not wear.

- Explain to your family your "new normal"—as many times as it takes.

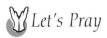 God's Love Letter to You

Dear_____, (fill in your name)

I live in the high and holy places, but also with the low-spirited, the spirit-crushed. And what I do is put new spirit in you, get you up and on your feet again (Isaiah 57:15 MSG paraphrased).
Your Normal-Maker, God

🙏 Let's Pray

Lord, it's difficult adjusting to and accepting this new normal. Please bring encouragers into our lives who welcome the "new us" and step into the roles we can no longer perform. Refine us. Let us stop bemoaning the loss of the old selves and relish the new selves. With You as our stronghold and enabler, we can and will do it! Open new doors, and we will walk through with our heads held high and giving You all the glory. Amen.

Where Did Your Energy Go?

You feel like you will never have energy again! —Darlene Gee

When you're going through radiation or chemotherapy, just doing the ordinary is extraordinary. —Janet

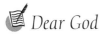 Dear God

Dear God,

People used to call me the "Eveready bunny," but no one would call me that now. My new chant is, "I'm so tired. Oh, I am so tired. I am exhausted . . ." I wonder where my energy went, and will it return? Will I ever be able to do the things I did before in a day? When am I going to feel like going back to the gym? Taking a walk around the lake? Reading? Sometimes it just seems too exhausting to lift a book. Answering e-mails? They are piling up, and for once in my life I don't care. Cooking? Oh Lord, just thinking what to cook makes me want to take a nap. I can't stand the idea of going to the store. Deciding what to buy is too much work. I went into the grocery store I shopped in for seventeen years and was so overwhelmed at all the choices and the people, I actually turned around and walked out!

What is happening to me? Lord, I am too young to be acting this way! I can see the fear in my children's eyes. Friends have been gracious to give me rides everywhere because I don't trust myself driving, especially at night. Oh, I feel so needy and vulnerable right now. Just writing this makes me want to take a nap.

Running on empty, Janet

A Sister Shares

I had aggressive chemotherapy and radiation followed by a year of Tamoxifen. I reacted so violently to chemotherapy that I had to have a MUGA scan to see if my heart could take it. They gave me a sedative that lasted forty-eight hours in which I could dress myself and act almost normal, but could not remember anything, and then I would "wake up" and wonder things like, *Who opened my mail?* Wow, it was me!

Once after a chemo treatment my husband said I saw a barn and told him the motel had a vacancy and I was tired. Very scary. With radiation I felt extreme fatigue and slept a lot. I swelled up as big as my breast had been [she had a mastectomy] and became very sick with flulike symptoms. A surgeon removed the burned tissue that was causing the sickness. During this time I took a psychology class at Penn State University to keep my mind from going to mush from all the drugs. But you know, I can do everything I did before the cancer. I am strong and healthy. —Karen

Mentoring Moment

Have you had some of those exhausted moments yourself? If you haven't, don't be surprised if they come. Some people sail through chemo with minor discomfort, and others are so sick, they need hospitalization. Some gain weight; others lose weight. Some go to the gym after radiation; others, like me, are exhausted most of the time. I've heard of women shopping several days after surgery or working right through treatments. Don't compare.

Be particularly aware of this difference in breast cancer support groups and doctors' waiting rooms. It is easy to wonder why your treatment or reaction is not like someone else's. A good group facilitator will steer away from this discussion. Otherwise, doubt creeps in: Do they have a better doctor? Why aren't you experiencing these side effects? Or why are you when others aren't? Keep everything in perspective—you are one of a kind, as unique as a snowflake.

📖 God's Love Letter to You

Dear_____, (fill in your name)

   May your strength match the length of your days! There is no one like me, the God of Israel who rides across the heavens to help you, across the skies in majestic splendor. I, the eternal God, am your refuge, and my everlasting arms are under you. (Deuteronomy 33:25–27 NLT paraphrased).

Your Refuge and Strength, God

🙏 Let's Pray

Oh, Father, we aren't what we used to be. Everything takes so much energy, and we often look at people through glazed eyes. We want to push on—so sure our old energy will return, disappointed when it doesn't. We cry out to You for fortitude, stamina, energy, and balance to know when we need rest. Stop us from pushing beyond healthy restraints. Retrain and retire us when necessary. Don't make us go through another illness to understand Your will is accomplished in our lives by *being* more than *doing*. We are listening. Amen.

Chemo-Radiation Brain

Some patients have referred to this side effect [chemotherapy-induced changes in cognitive function and memory] as "chemonesia." —Dr. John Link[5]

One of my patients in treatment made three separate commitments for Christmas dinner. —Dr. Marisa C. Weiss[6]

🖊 Dear God

Dear God,

   Forgetfulness and error plague me. This Type A, on-top-of-it-all, multitasking, phenomenal-memory woman is now forgetful and riddled with mistakes. Every time I write down a wrong number or spell a name incorrectly or forget something at the store or walk into a room and don't know why I'm there, a self-doubt knife turns inside me, and I feel a little bit of me dying. I liked who I was; didn't You,

Lord? I used to get frustrated with people who were forgetful. "Don't you remember?" I often asked my husband and children as they looked at me with blank faces. Did You need me to walk in their shoes to be more tolerant and understanding?

It is frightening, because they depend on me. Now I must humbly admit I am not the woman I used to be. Perhaps, in Your eyes, I am more the woman You want me to be: less prideful, arrogant, and know-it-all; more patient, giving, receptive to help, tolerant, understanding, forgiving . . . Wow, the mores far outweigh the lesses. I think I'm getting it now! And this lesson, trust me, I will remember!

Clarity and recognition gradually beam through of why a new definition of normal is necessary. I must pace my day so as not to deplete my energy before nighttime—that brings a new sense of organization. I write down everything and rely on a notebook organizer. Lamenting about my forgetfulness and confusion, I often receive the response, even from Dave, "Oh, that's how I always am, and I don't even have radiation or Tamoxifen as an excuse. At least you have an excuse." I laughingly reply, "But I was never like that before."

Remembering You, Janet

A Sister Shares

I do different things to keep myself occupied. I was even able to read a book in December. If I could remember the full name, I would recommend it. Stupid Chemo brain. I have problems when I walk to the back of the house to get something and can't remember what I went for, but I am hearing from so many of my friends that they have the same problem and aren't even on chemo! But they haven't asked me to lie down and give up, so I am still pushing forward. I am mentally sound and I feel good. I am just a little slower than I used to be. So keep up the prayers for us. —Linda M.

Mentoring Moment

Are you learning to laugh at the silly things you do? In rereading this page just now, I noticed that I wrote "*beast* cancer." I chuckled and said aloud, "Well it is a *beast* for sure!" I spend a great deal of time alone at home writing. It became evident we needed to take precautionary measures to ensure I didn't burn down the house by forgetting something on the stove or turning on the wrong burner under an empty skillet or leaving a toaster oven or coffeepot on all day. You get the picture; in fact, you probably are saying, "I do that too. This is normal? Yeah!" Dave took charge of replacing all our appliances so everything has an automatic shutoff.

It took a long time to multitask again after radiation and the onset of Tamoxifen. Previously I could do twenty things at once and know right where I was in each task. People marveled at how I did that! No more. The Lord truly humbled me. For months I was lucky to make *one* thing for dinner from beginning to end without losing it. Full dinners were out of the question.

Over the years, I had tried notebooks and organizers but always found them more cumbersome than just keeping everything in my mind. Humbly and proactively, I found an organizer that works for me and now use it as my memory. When things come to mind, I write them down in one place—grocery lists, phone calls to make, questions to ask, what to do every day . . . everything is there. I designed *Dear God, They Say It's Cancer* to be your breast cancer organizer as well as a journal. Use the "Memory Notes" on page 337 and the "Sanity Tools" in appendix B. If you are writing notes all over the house or office, that only adds to your frustration and that inner voice chastising, "You are so scatterbrained." "You always forget things." "You should have known that already." "You can't do anything right anymore." Ladies, that voice is not the Lord's; His voice is uplifting and encouraging.

I blame everything on Tamoxifen! Chemotherapy also affects memory and cognitive thinking. Many women refer to this as "chemo brain." Brenda N. actually thought she was going crazy until another breast cancer sister assured her this was normal. Brenda says gratefully, "Speaking with this woman gave me new hope." Radiation affected my clarity—it was probably just from the exhaustion and blood going to repair my body cells rather than to my brain. I felt dizzy most of the time. If you are not sleeping well or if you are having night sweats, sleep deprivation definitely affects memory and, I might add, attitude.

When treatment is over and your energy returns, you may find your mind returns with it. For those who must continue on chemo indefinitely, take Tamoxifen or another drug, or are experiencing menopause symptoms, there are things we can do. We must use our brains, or we will lose them. Some creative ways to do that are:

- Do crossword puzzles.

- Read literature—I found just focusing on the newspaper helps.

- Watch educational television, and try to follow what they are teaching.

- Do technical projects that require reading instructions—that is a huge stretch for me!

- Work with your hands—knit, crochet, play a musical instrument, garden, paint, cook, stamp, put pictures in an album, type, write, journal.

- Change your routine—this is scary, I know, because routine gives you some stability; but see if you can change the way you do something or a route you usually take to force your brain to think. (Be sure to take your cell phone with you.)

- Visit new places—going to health-food stores and learning the products and comparative prices was a huge brainteaser for me. I wanted to quit, but now I see it was God's way of helping me strengthen my brain. If you have never gone to plays or concerts, make a reservation and go. Try a new restaurant where you don't know the menu. Sit in a different area of church. Be adventuresome!

- Take a vacation to a place you have never been. New sights, sounds, and activities are very stimulating to the brain.

- Take a class—learn something you always wanted to know. (I sat next to an elderly couple on a plane who were taking Spanish lessons.)

- Exercise—it gets the blood flowing to your brain. Many times writing this book, I would take a walk and the next chapter would just fall into place or a new creative thought would come to mind.

- Eat healthy—Studies show that blueberries, strawberries, and spinach, along with other deeply colored fruits and vegetables, are high in antioxidants, which may help protect brain cells from damaging molecules called "free radicals."

- Sleep—nothing replaces a good night's sleep, which might be difficult right now. If you are not sleeping well, a daytime fifteen- to twenty-minute power nap refreshes your brain. Anything over ninety minutes may leave you groggy and make it difficult to sleep at night. I love waking up with the answer to a question or a way to word something in the book now crystal-clear. The night before, sitting tiredly at the computer, it was clear as mud!

- Lighten up—I have to tell myself daily: Don't be too hard on yourself. Let others help—it gives them a chance to shine.

- Pray daily for God to help you remember the things that are most important to Him—He will remember to do that.

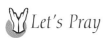 God's Love Letter to You

Dear_____, (fill in your name)

Do not conform any longer to the pattern of this world, but be transformed by the renewing of your mind. Then you will be able to test and approve what is my, God's, will—my good, pleasing and perfect will (Romans 12:2 paraphrased).
Transformer of your mind, God

Let's Pray

Prayerfully personalize Psalm 103:1–5 NLT.

My Lord and Savior . . . Restorer of my body and mind, I will remember to . . .

Praise the Lord, I, _____, tell myself; with my whole heart, I, _____, will praise his holy name. Praise the Lord, I, _____, tell myself, and never forget the good things he does for me. He forgives all my, _____'s, sins and heals all my, _____'s, diseases. He ransoms me, _____, from death and surrounds me, _____, with love and tender mercies. He fills my, _____'s, life with good things. My, _____'s, youth is renewed like the eagle's! Amen.

Learning to Receive

I've always been so independent, not wanting to ask others for help too often. I've had to get over that! I've discovered giving others a chance to help is as much a blessing to them as it is to me. —Cindy

I am a "giver"; therefore, it was hard for me to "receive." However, one of my friends shared with me, when you don't let someone do something to help you in these times, you are robbing them of a blessing! —Linda Taylor

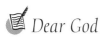 Dear God

Dear God,

I have always been the doer, giver, independent, do-it-myself woman . . . as You well know. Nothing could have prepared me for how much I would need other people's help and how willingly they would give it. It has been humbling to watch others do things for my family and me. Yet I am beginning to realize it is a blessing to them too. It allows them to step out of themselves and give from their hearts. I know it's a reflection of their love and care for Dave and me, and my heart swells and overflows. I feel the stretch as some people help in areas they might not be comfortable. But that makes it even more cherished.

I have fond memories of starting the day with my neighbor Eti bringing over scones and lattes and sitting in a chair beside my bed chatting away like we did this every day. Of course, Jane was there to organize the food brigades, answer e-mails, blow dry and style my hair, wrap our grandkids' Christmas presents, take over the ministry, go with me to radiation, or talk on the cell phone as I drove there . . . that always made it so much easier. I could never recapture or thank her enough, and the wonderful thing is, she doesn't expect it! Yet she knows I would be there for her in a heartbeat.

That's what it's all about, right, Lord? You don't want us living independent of each other. Your plan is for us to take care of our neighbors and them of us. You are our example to follow of the One who gave the most.

Learning to receive, Janet

A Sister Shares

We started reaching out to others for support. It's hard to be dependent on others and to ask for help, especially when you're used to being very independent. However, a neighbor who drove us to an appointment when neither my husband nor I could drive said, "You have given us a blessing." So I tried to accept help and give blessings. —Nancy Tuttle[9]

Mentoring Moment

Many of the women sharing their stories in this book said, "It was hard to let others do things for me, because I am so used to doing things for myself; but when I did, they thanked me. They said it blessed them." God made us with an innate desire to give of ourselves to others. Most people want to give; we don't know how to receive. Being on the receiving end is a new normal, and it takes time to adjust.

I quickly learned that being ill is not the time to be tough; people really do want to help. Our role is to let them! One day at church, friends asked how I was doing. The wife said she wanted to do something—clean my house, run errands—where did we need help? While I stammered around, my husband popped in with, "A meal would be great!" I knew that this woman did not like to cook, but she didn't miss a beat. She asked what we liked and what night would be best. Both she and her husband arrived with our meal on the designated night, and we had a chance to sit and visit.

Often we realize how many times we could have helped someone else and didn't, so we don't feel deserving to receive help ourselves. Let it be a learning experience. When well and back on our feet, we then look for ways to help others. After my recovery the wife of the couple who brought us dinner had shoulder surgery, so Dave and I took them dinner and ate it with them. We were doubly blessed.

Fear of rejection can stop us from asking for help. We are afraid they . . .

- Won't want to give it

- Will give it begrudgingly

- Will disappoint us by flaking

- Will feel we're imposing on them

On the other hand, because so many of us don't receive help well, people don't ask if we need assistance because they don't want to receive our rejecting, "No thanks, I can do it myself" attitude. That is definitely a lose-lose situation. Fear of rejection is rooted in pride, and the Lord says, "I hate pride" (Proverbs 8:13). So instead of *saying*, "Let me know if you need any help," just *do* something helpful. Conversely, when people ask where we need help, tell them; or better yet, hand them the "Bless You! Here's Where I Need Help" form on page 373.

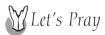God's Love Letter to You

Dear_____, (fill in your name)

If you give, you will receive. Your gift will return to you in full measure, pressed down, shaken together to make room for more, and running over. Whatever measure you use in giving—large or small—it will be used to measure what is given back to you (Luke 6:38 NLT). Your Love Giver, God

Let's Pray

Lord, thank You for all who come to our aid. Forgive us if we spurned anyone wanting to help. We're new at this. Sometimes people weren't there for us, and maybe that's because we weren't there for them in their time of need; again, we ask forgiveness. We want to change and graciously receive kind offers of others and boldly do kind deeds in return. You are our perfect example of giving. The more we learn about You and read Your Word, the more pliable and vulnerable our hearts are. We are an ever-ready work in progress. Amen.

A New Need for Peace and Calm

I WANT SOME PEACE AND QUIET. I WANT A WALK IN THE COUNTRY, I WANT A
CABIN IN THE WOODS. I'M DESPERATE FOR A CHANGE FROM RAGE AND STORMY WEATHER.
—PSALM 55:7–8 MSG

HOW BLESSED . . . GOD, THE WOMAN YOU INSTRUCT IN YOUR WORD, PROVIDING A CIRCLE
OF QUIET WITHIN THE CLAMOR OF EVIL. —PSALM 94:12–13 MSG

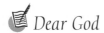 Dear God

Dear God,

Recovery seems slow . . . two steps forward, one back. My breast swelling and shoulder hurting nags at my energy and challenges my sense that "all is well." I search for ways to make my daily life calm. This seems laughable. Pounding and sawing prevail as we continue the completion of our remodel. Father, please give me ideas to bring calm to my spirit like the balm of Gilead. The Tamoxifen creates its own array of problems. Menopause symptoms assault me with sudden onsets of sadness, sleep sweats, confusion, and anxiety. New feelings to me. I have no coping techniques. This constant state of chaos cannot be good for healing. My state of mind is so important to recovery. You know my continuous prayer for relief. Thank You, Lord, for Your ever-present help and guidance in my life.

Calmly seeking You, Janet

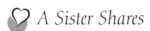 A Sister Shares

Cancer taught me to use other healing tools, such as relaxation and visualization. . . . My favorite time to use visualization was during radiation. Unlike chemotherapy, where you can read, watch TV, listen to tapes, sleep, or talk to others, radiation is a solitary and somewhat scary experience, where you are unable to move or sleep. During my daily radiation treatments I visualized the Seven Dwarfs marching up and down my spine with their picks, picking out the cancer and filling in the holes with their shovels as they sang, "Hi ho, hi ho, it's off to work we go!" MRI scans were a similar experience, without the pounding x-rays. My doctors used the MRI to determine the location and size of my lesions. I endured the long sessions in that claustrophobic tube by visualizing Jesus lying next to me holding my hand. —Nancy Tuttle[10]

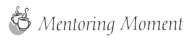 *Mentoring Moment*

Even today, I need order. If my office or house is messy, anxiety builds and I can't start a task in the midst of it. When I remove clutter, it unclutters my mind. This was new to me, but I embraced it. When I feel peace fleeing, it is time to straighten my surroundings. If you don't have the energy yet, go to someone on the "My Support and Help Team" list you will make on page 371, and give someone a call. Many people love to throw out things and all the better when it is someone else's!

Previously I thrived on activity, so I did not have a repertoire of relaxation tricks up my sleeve. The need for quiet and calm was definitely a new normal—actually a new requirement, a necessity to my daily survival. Your mind is an important part of the healing experience, so do what works best for you. Here are some tips on relaxing that continue to help me:

- Continuously play music. Loud, lively praise music if you need cheering up. Soft, melodious instrumentals if you're anxious or nervous. I especially enjoy praise instrumentals, sounds of water, and spa-type music.

- Light candles, even in the daytime. Walk into every room to extinguish them before leaving the house. Aromatherapy lamps are also nice.

- The sound of running water, as in a brook or creek, is relaxing. We placed fountains throughout our house and yard.

- Give up some things others can do. I delegated all my Woman to Woman Mentoring Ministry duties and trained myself to be satisfied with the results.

- Allow time to do things you enjoy.

- Exercise. Studies prove that daily walking helps in breast cancer recovery.

- Allow yourself time to rest without feeling guilty.

- Make sure every appliance has an automatic turnoff to eliminate worrying about the risk of fire.

- If possible, sleep until you wake up. If you must rise at a certain time, try waking up to soft music—no radio news or talk shows. Wake up gently, not with a sinking feeling in the pit of your stomach or your heart racing to a loud sound.

- Set doctor appointments at times convenient for you and not during peak-traffic rush hours. My standing daily radiation appointments were late morning.

- Do things that make you happy, and surround yourself with what is pleasing to your eye! We painted the rooms in our house happy, bold, and cheerful colors. When it's time to redecorate, give yourself permission to be adventuresome.

- Reward yourself. I always wanted hardwood floors. I got them. Though they were impractical, we even put them in the kitchen and our bedroom. Why not?

- Find young children to play with, read to, and enjoy. Spend as much time as possible with grandchildren.

- Take regular, relaxing, leisurely bubble baths. Get a bath pillow, turn on soft music, light candles, turn off the lights, mix in detoxifying bath granules, and relax—even in the middle of the day!

- Avoid negative people or those who bring you down.

God's Love Letter to You

Dear_____, (fill in your name)
Speak to one another with psalms, hymns and spiritual songs. Sing and make music in your heart to me, the Lord. (Ephesians 5:19 paraphrased).
Calmly, Gently, Peacefully Yours, God

Let's Pray

Lord, You tell us to have a calm and gentle spirit, and in today's fast-paced world that seems foreign. We are women used to getting things done, and we set high standards. Now some of us can't do that anymore. Our minds and bodies don't function like they used to. Are you removing us from the fast lane? Is Your dream for us to stop and enjoy the sunset, the sound of a babbling brook, the cry of a baby wanting a hug, the smell of a freshly mowed lawn, the glory of a new dawn? Help us, Lord, to relax, reflect, refresh, and restore. Let us rebuild both our bodies and our relationship with You. You are our calm in the storm. Amen.

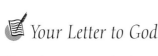 *Your Letter to God*

Where have you cut back or know you should? What is your new normal? If you struggle with low energy, appetite, joy, tolerance, memory, or however current treatment zaps you, how could you find times of peaceful assurance to refill and refresh? Do you sometimes feel like you are losing your mind? Ask the Lord what would bring calm and peace into your particular situation, according to the way He uniquely created you.

Dear God,   *Date:*

Chapter Thirteen

Adapting to Body Changes

For we know that when this earthly tent we live in is taken down—
when we die and leave these bodies—we will have a home in heaven,
an eternal body made for us by God himself and not by human hands.
We grow weary in our present bodies, and we long for the day when we
will put on our heavenly bodies like new clothing. For we will not be
spirits without bodies, but we will put on new heavenly bodies.
Our dying bodies make us groan and sigh, but it's not that we want to
die and have no bodies at all. We want to slip into our new bodies so
that these dying bodies will be swallowed up by everlasting life.
God himself has prepared us for this, and as a guarantee he has given us
his Holy Spirit. So we are always confident, even though we know that
as long as we live in these bodies we are not at home with the Lord.
That is why we live by believing and not by seeing.

—2 Corinthians 5:1–7 NLT

The Miraculous Creator

Dear God, I am what I am, and yet You love me. Thank You for creating me. —Nancy Tuttle[1]

I CREATED YOU AND HAVE CARED FOR YOU SINCE BEFORE YOU WERE BORN. —Isaiah 46:3 NLT

KNOW THAT THE LORD IS GOD. IT IS HE WHO MADE US, AND WE ARE HIS. —Psalm 100:3

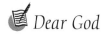 Dear God

Dear God,

How could anyone not believe in You as the Creator of the universe? The Bible says You knew us before we were created in our mothers' wombs and You have every hair on our heads numbered! I know that last part is helpful for women in chemotherapy. You know exactly how many hairs they lost and how many will grow back! What incredible love!

Dave and I marveled when the radiation oncologist explained the process of radiation. During our first visit he told us how You, God, made the good cells to completely repair themselves within twenty-four hours after each radiation treatment, while less and less of the bad cancer cells regenerate. He said physicists have it figured out to exactly how many treatments ensure that they eradicate all of the bad cells. For me, they calculated thirty-five treatments. Oh Lord, how could anyone not believe in You as the Great Creator when they hear something like this? You created the human body with incredible ability to reproduce and repair itself, down to the smallest cell. How could any radiation doctor or technician not believe in You, Lord?

This cell death and rebuilding process caused my exhaustion. It takes a lot of energy and calories to rebuild those cells. That helped reinforce the need for rest and eating right to do my part in helping and not hindering Your miraculous life process. Thank You, Lord, my Creator, my Savior, my Source of life.

Your miraculous creation, Janet

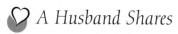 A Husband Shares

If I were religious, I'd be asking myself a lot of questions about the meaning—and character—of God. Is God some vindictive creature who finds entertainment picking on mortals or does everything—the good and the bad—happen for a reason, as part of some divine plan? I'm largely agnostic, and yet I must confess I find great comfort in knowing that so many people—close friends and perfect strangers alike—are praying for us. It doesn't matter whether they're Catholic, Evangelical, Jewish, Buddhist, or nondenominational. It's all positive, healing energy. I find considerable appeal in the "divine plan" theory, even though

I don't believe it. I can't help but notice the many good and surprising things that have happened because of Leslie's cancer—and because of our decision to write about it. We have received an outpouring of love and support from friends, family, and readers. We've made new friends, renewed contact with old ones, and discovered long-lost relatives. —Bernard Wolfson, husband of Leslie Furth[2]

Mentoring Moment

I know the cancerous destruction of your body may make it difficult to think of God in the role of Creator. Then the added assault of chemotherapy and/or radiation destroys even more of your body's cells. At times you may feel your own body is the enemy.

It's important to remember that none of the treatments or medications would work if scientists had not discovered the miraculous healing and repairing capabilities of our bodies. We are not machines created by factory workers. God made us in His own image. That is why many studies and medical journal reports show the power of prayer in patient recovery from surgery and illness. Prayer calls on the Great Creator and the Great Physician to take part in the repair of your body, His *great* creation.

God's Love Letter to You

Dear_____, (fill in your name)
    It was I, God, who created you. I am the one who made the earth and created you to live on it. With my hands I stretched out the heavens. All the millions of stars are at my command (Isaiah 43:7; 45:12 NLT paraphrased).
Your Creator, God

Let's Pray

Prayerfully personalize Psalm 139:13–18 MSG.

My Creator . . .

Oh yes, You shaped me, _____, first inside, then out; you formed me, _____, in my mother's womb. I, _____, thank you, High God—you're breathtaking! Body and soul, I,

_____, am marvelously made! I, _____, worship in adoration—what a creation! You know me, _____, inside and out, you know every bone in my body; you know exactly how I, _____, was made, bit by bit, how I, _____, was sculpted from nothing into something. Like an open book, you watched me grow from conception to birth; all the stages of my life were spread out before you. The days of my life all prepared before I'd even lived one day. Your thoughts—how rare, how beautiful! God, I'll never comprehend them! I, _____, couldn't even begin to count them—any more than I, _____, could count the sand of the sea. Oh, let me rise in the morning and live always with you! Amen.

Lopsided

The surgeon had to remove so much tissue in the lumpectomy that my breast pointed east. —Carol

With reconstruction and having the other breast surgically lifted, they're pretty perky for forty-three. I like that! —Angel

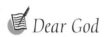 ## Dear God

Dear God,

The "sick," operated, and radiated breast is swollen, and I am lopsided. At Dr. West's recommendation I went to the shop at the BreastCare Center to find a new bra. Because of my frozen shoulder and the extra weight of the swollen breast, it was difficult finding a strap tolerable for my shoulders. The first one I took home, after trying on about fifty bras, had too much lace and irritated my radiated skin. They graciously allowed me to return it, and we continued searching for just the right one. By the time we were done, bras draped out of every drawer and cupboard, and the counter was elbow deep in different sizes, colors, shapes, fasten up the front, fasten down the back, zippers, clasps I could not reach around and hook . . . It was exhausting!

How grateful I was for Kay, the patient and kind shop owner. While she was as frustrated as I was, she didn't give up. It was nice finally to be even. What a relief to have the pain subside and not be lopsided anymore.

Equally Yours, Janet

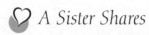 ## A Sister Shares

During the reconstruction process, I evidenced God's sense of humor, concern about the

smallest detail, and His living Word. I had decided to be about a C cup. Shortly after the permanent saline-implant surgery, I went shopping for new bras. The sales person pulled out her tape measure and wrapped it around—32D. "It can't be," I exclaimed. "I'm supposed to be a C!" That night my head spun with how to correct it. Could they take saline out of the implants? I needed to talk to my doctor. On and on until I said, "Lord, this is silly. Please let me just go to sleep."

Reading the Bible the next morning, I came to 1 Chronicles 28:20 NLT, which I had previously underlined. It starts out "Be strong and courageous. . . . Don't be afraid or discouraged by the size of the task." The words now had my attention. The passage continued—"for the LORD God, my God, is with you. He will not fail you or forsake you. He will see to it that all the work related to the Temple is finished correctly."

God responded to my little concerns in such a direct way. Laughing and crying, I thanked the Lord for His amazing love and care. My doctor's physician's assistant said saline could be removed, but she advised waiting. That was good advice, because I did end up being a C once I fully healed. I now had a great sense of confidence about the following surgeries—after all, God would see to it that all the work related to this temple would be finished correctly. —Grace Marestaing

Mentoring Moment

Shirley V. Galucki, MD, tells a cute story: "Some years ago one of my nieces, who has three brothers, was visiting her female cousins. All the girls were under the age of five. When it was time for their baths, the three girls went into the tub together. Suddenly my niece jumped out and ran to her mother. "Mom, I'm not the only one! They're just like me on the outside."[3]

Breast cancer changes the outside. This requires a sense of humor and patience. I have heard of women writing a message to the surgeon on their chest so he would remember the size they agreed on, only to find out his idea of B was really a C. Others had reconstruction done at different times, and one is tear shaped and one is round. Or the newly reconstructed breast is perky, but the natural breast is sagging. You may want to have repeated surgeries to correct all of this, or you might choose to adjust it with the correct-fitting bra and/or a prosthesis or insert like I did. Remember, it is important you feel comfortable with your decision.

- Weigh all your options.

- Talk to your doctor.

- Go through the "Peacekeeping Worksheet" on page 349.

- Pray about it.

- Ask God to help you adjust and live with the results.

Whether it was a partial, single, or double mastectomy; lumpectomy; reconstruction; or prosthesis, we each have a story to tell about getting the desired look. This was an interesting process for me. My left breast had always been bigger than my right, and now with the swelling from surgery it was quite noticeable. The BreastCare Center has a lovely shop, and the manager helped me find a bra with an insert pocket to put a pad in on the smaller right side to even out my clothed appearance. I still wear that bra with the insert.

Carol, with her breast "pointing east" after surgery, later had a reduction on the healthy breast to compensate for the unevenness. Angel had her remaining breast lifted to match the reconstructed breast. Most insurance companies cover symmetry surgery on the healthy breast. Talk to your doctor about your concerns, and don't give up until you have a look that suits you. Don't feel guilty pursuing it. You've been through a lot, and it's worth the effort to feel good about your appearance. Do what is necessary to achieve a sense of well-being, and then try to let it go and move on. As women we often are our own worst enemies. We think others are looking at our flaws. People aren't; believe me. They are too busy looking at their own.

God's Love Letter to You

Dear_____, (fill in your name)

If you decide for me, living a life of God-worship, it follows that you don't fuss about what's on the table at mealtimes or whether the clothes in your closet are in fashion. There is far more to your life than the food you put in your stomach, more to your outer appearance than the clothes you hang on your body. Look at the birds, free and unfettered, not tied down to a job description, careless in my care. And you count far more to me than birds. Has anyone by fussing in front of the mirror ever gotten taller by so much as an inch? All this time and money wasted on fashion— do you think it makes that much difference? Instead of looking at the fashions, walk out into the fields and look at the wildflowers. They never primp or shop, but have you ever seen color and design quite like it? If I, God, give such attention to the appearance of wildflowers—most of which are never even seen—don't you think I'll attend to you, take pride in you, do my best for

you? What I'm trying to do here is to get you to relax (Matthew 6:25–31 MSG paraphrased).
Your Equalizer, God

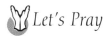 Let's Pray

Lord, You created us female, and we worry about our appearance. We are grateful for the many restoration possibilities, and we pray for courage and stamina through the process of putting ourselves back together again. It is taxing on our emotions and bodies, and we sigh and droop with the thought of going through any more. Don't let us give up or get discouraged, disgruntled, or disappointed with the outcome. Someday we will have brand-new, painless, perfect bodies when we join You. What a glorious day that will be, and we wait in anticipation. Until then, we ask for Your gracious hand of mercy as we restore the earthly temples You gave us. Thank You for making us women. Amen.

To Reconstruct or Not?

To love one's one-breasted body, to love one's body at all—this has been no easy matter for women. —Marilyn Yalom[4]

I had to accept that reconstruction was not going to be an "instant" process. With chemotherapy thrown into the mix, it would take well over a year to reach completion. This is not a project for the impatient. —Grace Marestaing

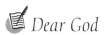 Dear God

Dear God,

Lord, with the family's and Your help, I chose a lumpectomy, which the surgeon called a partial mastectomy. So since we ruled out a complete mastectomy, reconstruction was not a decision I had to make. I do pray, dear Father, that through writing this book and interacting with other breast cancer sisters, You infuse my heart with compassion for those who are making this decision.

Compassionately Yours, Janet

♡ Two Sisters Share

When diagnosed with cancer in one breast, I opted to have only that one removed. I didn't see any reason at the time to remove the healthy one. I decided not to reconstruct, and my husband agreed. When I finished chemotherapy treatments, they scheduled a mammogram on the healthy breast. There was some question about the findings, and I agonized until the results were finally normal. It was just so scary. I could not imagine going through that every time I had a mammogram. I elected then to have my other breast removed and decided at that time to have reconstructive surgery. When they were injecting the saline into the expanders, I felt like breasts were growing under my armpits! —Darlene Gee

My decision was mastectomy. At this point I wasn't even thinking about reconstruction. During my planning meeting with my surgeon, one of the first things he said was, "I asked Ginny to meet with us because I'd like her to show you her reconstruction." Ginny was a patient-representative volunteer who works alongside the doctors as part of the support team. He did not say, "You should do reconstruction . . ." I will always be grateful for his gentle direction, because Ginny did show me her reconstruction, and I was amazed. She also explained that in my state, insurance is required to cover reconstruction and any necessary breast-symmetry procedures. Reconstruction was the next decision, along with consulting with the plastic and reconstructive surgeon who is part of the comprehensive team available at the BreastCare Center where I was so fortunate to be treated. —Grace Marestaing

☕ Mentoring Moment

Not experiencing this choice myself, I talked to women who had gone through the reconstruction decision process. What it all came down to was a very personal decision that each woman made for her own reasons, choosing the option that best fit her lifestyle. If you are married, be sure your husband accompanies you to the doctor appointments where your options will be discussed.

Often, the choice is to start reconstruction during the original mastectomy surgery, so you make reconstruction decisions before the initial surgery. Others opt to go back for a second or sometimes multiple surgeries. For some women, a prosthesis is the answer. "It's just unbelievable to see the change in women after they get fitted with the right prosthesis," said Mary La Fornara, certified breast fitter at Hoag Memorial Hospital Presbyterian Cancer Center in Newport Beach. "The shoulders are not droopy. The women stand up straighter. . . . They have a lot going on inside, but to the outside world, they're whole again."[5]

The reconstructive process includes many choices: What size? What shape? Free flap? Implants? Saline? Silicone? Nipples? No nipples? Colored (tattooed) nipples? Not tattooed? Darlene Gee said, "It didn't matter to my husband, and I hated wearing a bra, so I chose not to have nipples. I love the freedom of going braless and not even owning a bra! However, if I had to do it over again, I would choose a pear shape because now I have two grapefruits." One woman said she had her first reconstructed breast round but selected tear shape for her second one. Some women have the nipples formed but do not choose to have the areola color-tattooed. You see how personal these choices are, and there is no *one* right answer. Grace Marestaing helped her mom shop for a prosthesis, but when her own cancer occurred two years later, she opted for a complete reconstruction. Each woman did what was best for her, given her life circumstances and what made her feel complete.

Again, use the "Peacekeeping Worksheet" on page 349, looking at the options from all points of view. Talk to women who have had different types of surgeries and reconstruction and ask them to show you the results. This is very normal, and every woman I talked with said either she had someone do this for her or she has done it for someone else. That's another benefit of a support group, but your doctor also should be able to arrange for you to meet with someone who is willing to show you her reconstruction.

That helped Grace make her decision. Passing on to others what she learned from Ginny, Grace is a patient representative at the BreastCare Center and now mentors other women in the decision-making phase by letting them see her own reconstruction.

Pray hard for God to give you direction. After all, our bodies are gifts from Him. They are His temples, so it is only fitting that He has some say in what we do with them.

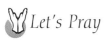 God's Love Letter to You

Dear_____, (fill in your name)
This is GOD speaking. I'll see to it that my Temple is rebuilt (Zechariah 1:16 MSG). Then you will know that I the LORD have rebuilt what was destroyed and have replanted what was desolate. I the LORD have spoken, and I will do it (Ezekiel 36:36 NIV paraphrased).
Your Temple Builder and Restorer, God

Let's Pray

Our Father, we are the clay; You are the potter. We are all the work of Your hand. We feel broken and want to glue the shattered pieces back together again to resemble the bodies You originally created. We are grateful for options and choices, but which one is best for each of us? You are the Creator of our temples, so we humbly seek Your guidance and direction. You knew before the cancer diagnosis that our bodies would go through this, and we are sure You have a creative plan. We want to work within it, so again we call on You, our dear Creator, to put us back on the Potter's wheel. Amen.

An Extreme Makeover!

I call breast cancer "my God makeover." —Grace Marestaing

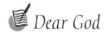 ## Dear God

Dear God,

Even though I didn't have reconstructive surgery, I feel like I have a new body. A better one at that. Those fifteen pounds shed and healthier eating habits have people saying I look better than before I was sick! After Dave's initial nervous weight gain with all the great food people brought us, he has lost right along with me, so it was a double blessing.

Father, I am so sorry it took cancer to get me in shape, but thank You for the blessing of a restored body here on earth with the promise of a perfect body when I join You in heaven.

Shapely Yours, Janet

 ## A Sister Shares

Three years, five surgeries, and chemotherapy later, I am very happy that my process of decision making took me down this path. In my journey with breast cancer, I lost about seventy pounds, I'm very pleased with my reconstruction, feel much more fit and confident about my appearance, and have a new lease on life in more than one way. —Grace Marestaing

 ## Mentoring Moment

My friend Grace Marestaing, my "Grace Abounds," is a petite, cute, black-haired, darling woman. Breast cancer not only resulted in her reaching her desired weight, but she got a complete made-to-order breast reconstruction, and her straight hair came back curly. I did not know Grace before, but I never would have imagined she didn't always look this way.

What You Should Know about Prosthesis

- Talk with your doctor about prosthetic options before surgery so you can make an informed decision.

- You can get more information on prosthesis through the American Cancer Society 1-800-227-2345.

- If you decide on a prosthesis, ask for a prescription for it.

- Check with your health insurance company to find out what and how much they cover. Plans typically cover a prosthesis every other year and two to three post-mastectomy bras every year.

- If you cannot afford a prosthesis, contact the Y-ME Prosthesis Bank at 800-221-2141 (English) or 800-986-9505 (Spanish).

- You usually can find a certified prosthesis fitter and retailer through the cancer center at a hospital near you. The fitter can help you find the right prosthesis.

- You may be able to wear a temporary prosthesis when you leave the hospital after mastectomy.

- Your first prosthesis fitting usually can be scheduled six weeks to eight weeks after surgery, when the swelling has subsided and scars have healed more.

- You are entitled to change your mind about reconstruction if you find later that a prosthesis isn't working for you.[6]

Reconstruction on the Rise

Most women who have undergone a mastectomy—and in some cases, lumpectomy patients—choose reconstruction over an external prosthesis, Orange County breast surgeons say. "There's a tremendous emotional, psychological, and rehabilitative value to reconstruction," said Dr. Ed Luce, president of the American Society of Plastic Surgeons. "Scars remind patients of the loss of the breast. Reconstruction restores their self-esteem. It says in an eloquent, nonverbal way that those who are giving care to the patient have absolute confidence in her ultimate recovery and survival."

Nationally, the number of breast reconstructions has increased 174 percent in a decade—from 29,607 in 1992 to 81,089 in 2001, according to the surgeons group. Most of these follow breast cancer surgery. The increase can be attributed partly to the Women's Health and Cancer Rights Act of 1998, which mandates health-insurance coverage for breast reconstruction and alteration of the other breast for symmetry in women who have had a mastectomy.[7]

Over lunch one day, she commented that breast cancer gave her a completely new body and a new life.

Darlene Gee laughingly tells the story of looking in the mirror after surgery and seeing what some would have taken for a concentration-camp survivor—a massive scar across her chest, bald head, pale and peaked complexion, and no eyebrows or eyelashes—but she thought her body looked so beautiful because now she was thin!

Grace Bell, on the other hand, said, "The most difficult time for me after my radical mastectomy was when the bandages were removed. I told the doctor, 'Just wait a minute.' I wasn't ready to face the reality of how my body now looked. The first few weeks back home were very hard. I felt like I had a rubber band around my chest, and I could hardly breathe."

If breast cancer negatively altered your body image, a makeover that makes you sad or mad, I hope you can find solace in knowing these bodies are only temporary. Some glorious day we will completely shed them for the new bodies Christ gives all those who believe in Him. However, until then:

- Pamper yourself.

- Bathe in luxurious bath salts.

- Slather the richest, most feminine lotion from head to toe.

- Get a pedicure and manicure.

- Treat yourself to a massage from someone trained in how to handle breast cancer.

- When your hair grows back, experiment with new hairstyles. In the meantime, use a wig to try a new 'do.

- Buy new makeup.

- Visit a makeup counter in the mall, and get tips on accentuating the positive and eliminating the negative.

- When you feel up to it, shop for a very feminine outfit or new underwear—or both.

My radiation center offered a "Look Good . . . Feel Better" lunch, sponsored by the American Cancer Society. It was a free makeover workshop led by a breast cancer survivor. What an interesting sight we were sitting around the table—some bald with no eyebrows or eyelashes, others sporting newly grown hair stubbles, others with wigs, and those of us with hair. They issued facial cloths to remove makeup, which revealed something we all had in common—pale, placid skin resulting from radiation and chemotherapy treatments.

Each of us received a box of makeup and skin-care samples donated from various cosmetic companies. They provided mirrors and went through steps of applying makeup, including how to draw in eyebrows and line our eyes to compensate for lost eyelashes. Everyone enjoyed restoring femininity to what can be a dehumanizing experience. Keep your ears open for a similar class, or call the American Cancer Society for one offered in your area.

God's Love Letter to You

Dear_____, (fill in your name)

Now, I, the Lord, am also the Spirit, and the Spirit of the Lord gives freedom. You have had the veil removed from your eyes so that you can be mirrors that brightly reflect the glory of the Lord. And as the Spirit of the Lord works within you, you become more and more like me and reflect my glory even more (2 Corinthians 3:17–18 NLT paraphrased).
Master of the Makeover, God

Let's Pray

Prayerfully personalize Psalm 34:4–6 NLT paraphrased.

I, _____, prayed to you, Lord, and you answered me, freeing me from all my fears. When I, _____, look to you for help, I will be radiant with joy; no shadow of shame will darken my face. I, _____, cried out to you, Lord, in my suffering, and you heard me. You set me free from all my fears. Amen.

What About Your Hair?

Kay was at the staff wives' retreat, and she talked from her heart about her cancer. She literally flipped her wig and exposed her bald head for us—it was so courageous of her. She is sexier than all get-out bald! Her vulnerability blew me away. —My friend Jane, speaking of Kay Warren

BUT THE HAIR ON HIS HEAD BEGAN TO GROW AGAIN AFTER IT HAD BEEN SHAVED. —JUDGES 16:22

Look Good . . .
Feel Better

The "Look Good . . . Feel Better" makeover program is sponsored by the American Cancer Society; The Cosmetic, Toiletry, and Fragrance Association (CTFA); and the National Cosmetology Association (NCA). It is a free, national program especially for women undergoing cancer treatment. They offer instruction, tips, suggestions, and advice on dealing with hair loss and skin, complexion, and nail changes. It includes complimentary cosmetic products donated by participating CTFA members and is demonstrated by volunteer cosmetology professionals. They do not promote or endorse any specific product or brand. For more information on the "Look Good . . . Feel Better" program and where one might be offered near you, call 1-800-395-LOOK, or call your local American Cancer Society office, or visit their Web site at www.lookgoodfeelbetter.org.

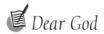 Dear God

Dear God,

I am sure You shook Your head during the family planning conference when my first question after hearing the course of treatment was, "Will I lose my hair?" They assured me I wouldn't. My hair truly is my favorite body gift from You. I know many women lose all their hair, and this can be a very sad and difficult time for them.

My left shoulder freezing up made it so difficult to fix my hair. I continue to pray, Lord, for a healing, but until that happens, doing my hair is painful. My frozen shoulder finally gave me permission to do what I have always wanted to do . . . cut my hair short. I love my new, quick hairdo. Much easier when I am traveling too. Dave is adjusting. Can you believe, God, that it took cancer for me to finally give myself more hours in my day from less primping and prepping of my hair? I consider this a real cancer blessing.

Your shorthaired girl, Janet

Two Sisters Share

Once I started chemo, I thought it best to quit playing bells at church every Tuesday, but since I was giving someone a ride to our rehearsals, I decided to keep going to church on that evening, so I joined the Tuesday night Bible study. The hair starts falling out in fourteen days so those girls planned an impromptu hat party. It was strange because the bell choir suddenly came into the Bible study. I thought it was someone's birthday, but I ended up with a wonderful selection of millinery! It was quite challenging to think about what to wear with each hat. My daily routine became—put on the face, the glasses, and then the hat! —Shirley

I knew with chemo that I would lose my hair. But I didn't think about losing *all* my hair, including eyebrows and eyelashes. Now I don't have to shave, shampoo, or pluck. That is too good to be true. A nice side effect. Imagine, some women spend hundreds of thousands of dollars in their lifetime for hair removal. I get mine free. No more bikini waxes.

One lady from church called and told me to go and order my wig right away as it only takes seven to nine days for my hair to fall out after the first treatment. So Mom and I went to a wig shop. Oh my, I couldn't believe it. It was like a candy store. Hundreds of wigs just waiting for me to try. You'd have to see it to believe it. The store itself was beautiful, a place you'd actually want to shop in. They were wonderful and treated me with such kindness. After over an hour of trying on all the styles, I selected two. —Linda M.

☕ Mentoring Moments

Worrying about our hair is a universal concern. When the late Peter Jennings made the television announcement that he had lung cancer, he chuckled as he admitted that he, too, asked, "Hey doc, am I going to lose my hair?" While I did not lose my hair, I definitely had to make hair care easier. In talking with women who had chemotherapy, they suggest researching wigs before your first chemo treatment. The average time it takes to lose your hair following the first chemo treatment is thirteen or fourteen days, so you want to be ready. Not everyone loses her hair, so talk to your doctor about the type of chemotherapy you are having and the expectation for hair loss.

Also, check with your doctor's office and the local American Cancer Society office to find out where they refer women to purchase wigs. You may discover a shop in your area offering free or low-cost wigs. Call your insurance company—or better yet, put that on the "Bless You! Here's Where I Need Help" form (page 374)—to see what they cover in this area.

This would be a good reason to attend a breast cancer support group, because those who have been through this can mentor you. When I went, I heard one name familiarly tossed around. Upon asking who this was, they all said, "Oh she is the best wig specialist in town. We all have gone to her, and she works her genius." Several ladies were wearing wigs that looked like their own hair. They also told stories about their husbands, hairdressers, or themselves shaving their heads. They advise that if your doctor said you would lose your hair, and you notice it starting to fall out, go ahead and help it along by shaving your head to avoid the uncomfortable feeling of not knowing when or where you'll find clumps of lost hair.

Getting a wig can provide an opportunity to try a new hair color or style, or you may prefer something as close to your current color and style as possible. Enjoy the freedom of doing what seems right for you. Maybe instead of wearing a wig, you prefer a pretty scarf or hat—even stocking hats are quite fashionable. There is a ministry at Saddleback Church called Crafts for Christ that knits and crochets caps for ladies who have lost their hair through chemotherapy. Then again, some women find wigs, scarves, and hats too hot and uncomfortable and just decide that bald is beautiful!

I have noticed that many women who lose their hair keep it short when it grows back. Like me, they find short hair easier to care for, saves time, and actually looks quite stylish. Darlene Gee kept her hair short and spiky, and it makes her look vivacious and chic. Others of you can't wait to grow it back to your waist! One woman shared that she asked the Lord to bring her brown hair back in salt-and-pepper gray, and that is exactly what she got! If you find your hair grows in totally gray, you might take comfort in Proverbs 16:31: "Gray hair is a crown of splendor; it is attained by a righteous life."

God's Love Letter to You

Dear_____, (fill in your name)

Every detail of your body and soul—even the hairs of your head!—is in my care; nothing of you will be lost (Luke 21:18 MSG). Are not two sparrows sold for a penny? Yet not one of them will fall to the ground apart from my, Your Father's, will. Even the very hairs of your head are all numbered. So don't be afraid; you are worth more than many sparrows (Matthew 10:29–31 paraphrased).
Your Caretaker and Hair Counter, God

Let's Pray

Dear Lord, our hair is our shining glory. Then along comes cancer and burns it all away, or we have no energy to deal with it, and with that goes much of our security and self-confidence. Our hair swept away in the garbage leaves us bare, naked, vulnerable, and scared. Let us remember You are our mantel, our refuge, and our security; our hair or our breasts do not define us. Inside, we are still the same women. Help us bravely and boldly withstand this latest assault. We are Your beautiful daughters. Amen.

Your Letter to God

Acknowledge the importance of how your body looks and your feelings about the new you. Do you have clarity as to the breast reconstruction that best suits your body, lifestyle, and season of life? Is your husband in agreement on the final decision? If you have reconstruction, can you mentor a cancer sister or give her helpful hints? Have you experienced the loss of hair? Write down your thoughts about your experience with body changes, hair, and breast cancer.

Dear God,   *Date:*

_____

_____

_____

CHAPTER FOURTEEN

Coping with the Private Issues

YOU ARE LIKE A PRIVATE GARDEN, MY TREASURE, MY BRIDE!
YOU ARE LIKE A SPRING THAT NO ONE ELSE
CAN DRINK FROM, A FOUNTAIN OF MY OWN.

—Song of Solomon 4:12 NLT

Good Girls Don't

About fifty people have looked at my breasts and commented on them. I do not even feel like they are mine any longer. —Nancy Tuttle[1]

We watched a videotape about the process [reconstruction with a tummy tuck] and then it was time for me to be examined again. I thought to myself, "How many people will see my birthday suit before we're through?" The doctor looked at my breasts as if he were a sculptor and I was the clay. —Brenda Ladun[2]

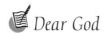 Dear God

Dear God,

As a young woman I worried my breasts were too small. After all, breasts make us feminine and sexy. Then giving birth to Kim, they were suddenly functional for nursing. That seemed so natural, even though there were those back then who thought breastfeeding was barbaric. My generation believed "good girls" don't expose their breasts for any reason, even nursing. Today new mothers unabashedly nurse in public. They stay modestly covered, but even when they don't, no one seems offended.

Still, Lord, I never have even shown cleavage. Now everyone is looking at my breasts! Every doctor, nurse, and technician has to see, touch, manipulate, tattoo, position, cut, stitch, measure, and radiate my breasts. Standard procedure is to bare my breasts. I don't think I will ever get used to it. The hardest was tattoo day. It just happened Frank was the radiation therapist assigned to do the tattooing. "Where is Mary Ann?" I asked. Oh, she was doing a CT scan on someone. I cried the entire time Frank measured and made those tiny black dots. Trying to put me at ease, he very professionally explained the reason behind the tattoos and why permanent is good for current treatment and also in the future we will know where I was radiated; but that did not help me deal with it any better.

Thank You, God, for Mary Ann's being present for most of my future treatments. They probably got the hint I was more comfortable with a woman. No offense to Frank—he was a great guy who made me laugh and had creative tips for our house remodeling. It's just that my husband is the only person I want seeing my breasts. Well, oh yes, the surgeon, the radiation doctor, the oncologist . . . OK, God, I get it. They are just doing their jobs. I need to get over it.

Bashfully Yours, Janet

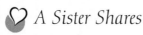 A Sister Shares

The night before I was to have my breast removed, I remember lying in the bathtub with candles and praise music on—sort of a memorial service to say good-bye to my breast, as

silly as it sounds. I began reflecting on the life cycle of the breast. When you're young, you can't wait to "bud" and are so proud when they sprout and grow and you get your first bra. Then later, if we are honest, we can use them in very discreet ways to attract a mate. Then our husband takes great delight in them, and later we use them for the ultimate tender act of breastfeeding and sustaining life for our babies. Life goes on, and they begin to sag and droop, but we still love them because they have served us well . . . then ultimately, they deceive you.
—Darlene Gee

 ## *Mentoring Moment*

Darlene called her above reflection "An Ode to the Breast." From the minute those little buds on our chests started growing, parents cautioned us to keep them covered. One day, without warning, our breasts started taking shape, and it was time for our first bra. Do you remember how awkward and embarrassing it was going to the bra department with your mom? My friends and I swap stories of standing outside the dressing room passing bras under the door for our daughters to try on, just like our moms did with us. And oh horrors if the woman store clerk wants to help us! Measuring tape? No way.

A word that seldom comes up in conversation, unless chatting with our girlfriends, is now the focus of discussion. What once was private and a sign of our femininity and sexuality is now public, scientific, and clinical. All these years of keeping our breasts under cover, and now they are on public display at every doctor appointment and talked about as objects. Our whole family is now talking breasts! *Our* breasts! We feel people nonchalantly glancing down at our breasts to see if they are still there or how surgery affected our appearance. Part of us wants to walk around with a big shield in front of our chests, with a sign that says, "Keep Away—Under Construction." How do we adjust?

Each of us will find our own way to adapt to this change. What helped me, and might help you, too, is to look at our breasts as a sick body part. Our breasts perform varied functions, and now we focus objectively on their body-part role. If left untreated, the rest of our body could die. Therefore, I was grateful for the men and women who fought down the sneers and jeers of their colleagues and friends to learn how to save lives from breast cancer. If you found other ways of coming to grips with the inevitable modesty and awkwardness of the initial focus on our breasts, please share that with other breast cancer sisters.

If we are open and willing to talk about breasts, more women might seek treatment earlier. It breaks my heart when a woman over forty tells me she has never had a mammogram, performed a self-breast exam, or had a clinical exam. Maybe she will be fine, but maybe she won't. Our openness in discussing this part of our bodies provides a comfort level for others and increases the awareness of the desperate need for a cure.

God's Love Letter to You

Dear_____, (fill in your name)

Your body is a unit, though it is made up of many parts; and though all its parts are many, they form one body. . . . And the parts that are unpresentable you treat with special modesty, while your presentable parts need no special treatment. But I, God, have combined the members of your body and have given greater honor to the parts that lacked it, so that there should be no division in your body, but all parts should have equal concern for each other. If one part suffers, every part suffers with it; if one part is honored, every part rejoices with it (1 Corinthians 12:12, 22–26 paraphrased). Honoring your body, God

Let's Pray

Lord, we know You love *every* part of us . . . including our breasts. You wrote about breasts in the Bible, and You gave them to us for both pleasure and function. Right now it seems one of our prized body parts has deceived us. We always felt the right to use our breasts the way we saw fit, and now others tell us what we can and cannot do with them. There is talk of even removing them from our body. In Ephesians 6:10–18, You remind us to daily put on the breastplate of righteousness and take up the shield of faith. Of course, that is the answer to our discomfort. We simply put on the armor of God every morning—ready to face the world full-breasted, partially breasted, one-breasted, or without breasts . . . it doesn't matter anymore when we are clothed in our protective armor. Thank You, Lord, for thinking of our every need. Amen.

How Will Breast Cancer Affect Your Marriage?

Between caring for Kay's basic needs, I sit quietly, think a lot, and thank God for my wife, and God's amazing invention of marriage. With all its ups and downs and "in sickness and health,"

I'm certain that marriage is God's primary tool to teach us unselfishness, sensitivity, sacrifice, and mature love. —Pastor Rick Warren

My husband said he didn't marry my breasts . . . so I decided to have them both removed. —Donnette[3]

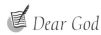
Dear God

Dear God,

You know how I worried about possibly having a complete mastectomy. Dave has always been a "breast man" and enjoyed my breasts just like the Scriptures say he is to do. I wondered, *What would we do if ever they did need to be removed? How would it affect our marriage relationship? Would Dave be devastated?* You, Lord, prompted me to stop worrying about it and just ask him. I will never forget his loving response: "We would work it out . . . we would just figure out something else." What reassurance that I was more important than my breasts. Dave loved me, not just my body.

A grateful wife, Janet

Two Sisters Share

My husband didn't handle the situation very well; he retired from USMC after twenty years of service the week before I received the cancer diagnosis. We had sold our home in California to move to Louisville, Kentucky, so he could work flying for UPS. Since my cancer was in stage four, I had to have a radical mastectomy immediately, followed by aggressive chemo and radiation. The doctors did not allow leaving California until after three chemo treatments, and then I continued treatments at my mother's in Pennsylvania. When completed, I joined my husband in Kentucky. He could not accept me the way I was. I tried to get him to counseling, but he didn't want to go that route and ended up divorcing me. I went to counseling for two years to help accept the losses in my life. I don't know what I would have done without a strong faith in God. From the moment of diagnosis I knew from within that God was with me, and I would beat cancer. [And she did!] —Karen

After being single for fifteen years, I began dating a very nice man, David, at Thanksgiving 1986. Just three months later, I found a lump in my breast while taking a shower. With my hands and body covered with soap, there it was—as plain as day! I had no doubt it was breast cancer. My attitude was, "Let's get this over with so I can get on with my life." I phoned my doctor the following day, and he scheduled a mammogram and a consultation with a surgeon for me right away. The surgeon confirmed my suspicions. I had breast cancer. He recommended a radical mastectomy.

Then it was time for me to tell David, and I knew that wouldn't be easy. I suggested to him that he go on with his life—to do his own thing—because I was unsure of what my future would be. His reply to me was, "I am as close to you as 99 is to 100. Case closed." What a comfort to know he supported me and would be with me as I faced breast cancer! I had a radical mastectomy in February. The surgery was successful, and there was no recommendation for chemotherapy or radiation. I was done with treatment! Best of all, David and I got married in April! —Martha

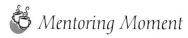 Mentoring Moment

As if talking about our breasts all the time is not embarrassing enough, we also have to consider how our surgery and treatment is going to affect others. For those of us who are married, the person most directly affected is our husband. I have heard a range of husbands' responses. Grace Marestaing tells me that sitting in patient conferences she sometimes hears a husband refer to his wife's breasts as "*my* breasts." Technically and spiritually, that is true: "The wife's body does not belong to her alone but also to her husband. In the same way, the husband's body does not belong to him alone but also to his wife" (1 Corinthians 7:4). The *New Living Translation* even goes so far as to say the husband and wife have authority over each other's body: "The wife gives authority over her body to her husband, and the husband also gives authority over his body to his wife." Some husbands might be inclined to interpret that verse to their own advantage; however, the same verse in *The Message* paraphrase says, "Marriage is not a place to 'stand up for your rights.' Marriage is a decision to serve the other, whether in bed or out."

Breast cancer is attacking younger and younger women, and some receive a positive diagnosis while engaged. The fiancé now must decide if he is going to honor the vows he will soon make to love his wife "for better or for worse, in sickness and in health." At the breast cancer support group I attended, one woman told the story of her boyfriend of two years suddenly proposing when she was diagnosed with breast cancer that required a bilateral mastectomy. She was surprised and elated! The group also talked about a fiancé recently honored on Oprah Winfrey's TV program for doing the same thing. These men are keepers!

Izzy was forty years old when she had one breast removed, and a nurse overheard her husband say to the doctor, "What am *I* going to do?" His concern was more for himself than for Izzy. On the other hand, Darlene Gee, who had a double mastectomy and reconstruction, says her husband makes her feel beautiful, and he loves her short hair!

Age often does not affect the husband's delight in his wife's breasts, and that is scriptural too. Proverbs 5:18–19 reads, "Enjoy the wife you married as a young man! Lovely as an angel, beautiful as a rose—don't ever quit taking delight in her body. Never take her love for granted!" (MSG). An elderly grandpa who still cherishes his wife's breasts may be devastated with the news she is going to lose them to cancer. He will need support and encouragement as much as a younger husband.

In a 2003 interview, the then-eighty-six-year-old actor Kirk Douglas discussed his depression after a stroke in 1996 that coincided with his wife, Anne, having a mastectomy. He said he is more in love with his wife now than when they married forty-nine years ago. Then he commented that they made love every night to give her confidence as she recovered from the mastectomy, and he plans to marry her again to celebrate their fiftieth anniversary, which I later read they did. I did the math; Kirk was seventy-nine years old when Anne had her mastectomy! I love that story.

Remember your body has suffered an assault, but his probably is still functioning pretty well. What can you do to help your husband? I know that is a tough question while you are justifiably preoccupied and probably overwhelmed just adjusting to your body changes. Quite often surgery, radiation, chemotherapy, and drugs affect your libido. The last thing on your mind is sex, and, honestly, you don't feel very sexy right now. There might be a season where it is not even appropriate to try having sexual relations. If you are like me, I was petrified of anything bumping or hitting my sore breast or frozen shoulder. You also may be nauseated and sick from chemotherapy or plain exhausted from radiation.

Our tenth wedding anniversary fell two days after radiation started—not very romantic. Well, actually, it was. There is a romantic bed-and-breakfast tucked away in Julian where we spent several previous anniversaries, which just happens to be days before Christmas, December 19. I prayed about it, and even though exhausted with radiation, the remodel, and the holidays, the Lord gave me a picture of rest and relaxation with my husband at this little hideaway. So on a hunch and a prayer, I called to see if they had a room available—they did. That was my confirmation we should go. My husband agreed. So packing a few candles and my sexiest nightgown, away we went. It became a very memorable experience for us. We made sure I had plenty of rest, and like Kirk Douglas, my husband made me and my sore breast feel very much loved.

If you have had a mastectomy and reconstruction, it is natural to feel a little hesitant and shy; but how about looking at your new situation with wedding-night anticipation? *What will this be like, and what can I do to make it a good experience?* Here are some ideas to get you started if you just aren't up to thinking of any right now. Then when you feel better, add things that are special to you and your husband.

- Keep the lights off or down low, and light candles.

- Wear your prettiest nightgown.

- If you are hesitant, wear two-piece nightwear and leave the top on.

- Spray on perfume (keep clear of your scars or radiation areas).

- Take a relaxing bubble bath, if medically allowed.

- Play a soft CD in the background.

- Let your husband know you are willing to give it your best effort.

- Allow your husband to give you a careful back rub to relax you.

- Ask someone to put fresh sheets on the bed.

- Try to spend your day on the couch or another bed in the house—not the same bed you sleep in with your husband, so you won't think of it as a "sick bed."

- If treatments and medication cause "feminine side effects," consult your oncologist.

- Make sure you are not rushed and have privacy.

- If feasible and you feel up to it, take a weekend getaway where there is not much to do but rest and be with each other. The beach, a river, the mountains—you choose.

📖 *God's Love Letter to You*

Dear_____, (fill in your name)

 Dress festively every morning. Don't skimp on colors and scarves. Relish your life with the spouse you love each and every day of your precarious life. Each day is my gift to you. It's all you get in exchange for the hard work of staying alive. Make the most of each one! (Ecclesiastes 9:8–9 MSG paraphrased).
Your Heavenly Husband, God

🙌 *Let's Pray*

Lord, we are fighting feelings of inadequacy and guilt that we brought this devastating disease into our marriage. Please help us and our husbands remember the vows we took to love and stand by each other in sickness and in health, in good times and in bad. Now it is time for our husbands and fiancés to do that, but there could be a time in the future where we will be the one standing by our man.

 We pray now more for them than ourselves . . . so often they just don't know what to do or say. Give us patience and extra measures of love. You picked them for us for such a time as this, and we know they can rally to the challenge. Give them confidence that we will be back . . . maybe better than before with a new sensitivity and awareness of how precious all aspects of life are—especially our marriages! We know You love us, Lord, and if our husbands should falter, You tell us You are a husband to the husbandless. We rest assured in being Your bride. Amen.

📝 *Your Letter to God*

How are you adjusting to the constant attention on your breasts? Are you married, engaged, or hoping to be? How is the man in your life responding to the changes in your body? If he is having difficulty, pray for him to embrace the role God gave him. Pray for patience while he adjusts and willingness to help with the transition in your physical relationship. If he is reacting in a way that encourages and supports you, thank God and pray for continued strength and courage for you both.

Dear God, _____ Date: _____

_____

_____

_____

_____

_____

_____

_____

_____

_____

_____

_____

_____

_____

_____

_____

_____

_____

_____

_____

_____

_____

_____

_____

CHAPTER FIFTEEN

Grieving the Losses

I AM BENT OVER AND RACKED WITH PAIN.
MY DAYS ARE FILLED WITH GRIEF.
A RAGING FEVER BURNS WITHIN ME,
AND MY HEALTH IS BROKEN.
I AM EXHAUSTED AND COMPLETELY CRUSHED.
MY GROANS COME FROM AN ANGUISHED HEART.
YOU KNOW WHAT I LONG FOR, LORD;
YOU HEAR MY EVERY SIGH.

—Psalm 38:6–9 NLT

The Grieving Process

JOB STOOD UP AND TORE HIS ROBE IN GRIEF. THEN HE SHAVED HIS HEAD AND FELL TO THE
GROUND BEFORE GOD. —JOB 1:20 NLT

*Some days you just "kick the wall," whisper to your inner-self softly with kind words—"It will
get better." —Martha*[1]

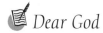 Dear God

Dear God,

When Dave and I went away for our eleventh anniversary, I cried the whole way up
the mountain to the cabin we rented. My mind traveled back to our tenth anniversary,
December 19, 2002, two days into radiation and not the way we had expected to celebrate
that milestone in our marriage. One year later I still grieved that loss. Ah, that is probably
what it is, grief—right? There has been a loss. Never again will life be as we knew it before
cancer. Things are literally BC—"before cancer" and AC—"after cancer." Just like Jesus's
life and death became a reference point for history, so breast cancer will be for our family
history. I don't like that. It makes me sad. What a helpless feeling being forced to live with
it whether I want to or not.

Two days after diagnosis Jane and I were on our way to Virginia to do a Woman to
Woman Mentoring training. The night before we left, I noticed on our itinerary we did
not have airplane seats together. I was so mad. I fired off an e-mail to the travel agent,
which of course was pointless because it was around midnight, and we left early the next
morning. Later I laughed and told Jane that God was probably protecting her from my
mood by having her sit behind me instead of next to me! On that same trip I called Dave,
and within minutes I was angry over some little thing. We hung up disgruntled, and then I
called back to apologize and cried on the phone for a half-hour. I still have angry moments,
but now with Your help I recognize the source and consciously choose not to let it overtake
my mind and mood.

My prayer is for this cancer experience eventually to be a slight catch in my breath—no
longer a raw and painful sob.

Grieving still, Janet

 A Sister Shares

I felt like I was in shock for weeks, but then there was the next emotion to deal with—
anger. I never got angry at God, but I did have unexplained anger at times. Little things
would bring feelings of rage. If I dropped something, it might make me really mad. I

later realized I wasn't mad at that particular event. I figured out this was part of the healing process. I would get mad about something so insignificant that it would make me shake my own head at myself. While I took my daily walk, I felt anger well up inside me. I had no particular reason to feel that way, but it was there. I knew I was angry I had cancer. I wasn't angry at anyone. I was just angry. Walking and praying and talking helped. I consulted with my friend Lisa Baggett about the anger. She had been a counselor and told me it was normal.

I finally asked the Lord to take the anger away. I had no room in my life for it. After all, I was trying to enjoy every day. Doug [her husband] supported me through that time when I was an argument waiting to happen. . . . He just knew I was working through the process of coming to grips with the fact that I had cancer. Sometimes even the things he said to try to help would lead me to tears. I wanted him to fix everything for me. But through the tears I came to a wonderful revelation. Jesus is perfect, but the rest of us sometimes say and do the wrong things. That's okay; we are human. But with the Lord's guidance, we can stay on track.
—Brenda Ladun[2]

Mentoring Moment

You may recognize the following steps in the grieving process because we all go through them at our own pace. Can you check off your journey?

The Steps of Grief

- ❑ *Shock* is our first reaction. The punch or sinking sensation in the pit of our stomachs—dizzying, nauseating, room spinning, unbelievable!

- ❑ *Denial* is a survival reaction until we get our bearings. "This can't be happening to me." We hold on to the possibility it's all a mistake and try ignoring it or maybe even postponing treatment.

- ❑ *Acknowledgment* replaces denial. Now we must face it head-on, and it hurts so bad and makes us so mad!

- ❑ *Anger* is often intense. Maybe we aren't angered easily, but now we are *angry*. Angry at ourselves, our genetics, the enemy cancer, and maybe even God.

- ❑ *Acceptance* and resignation is the eventual outcome of anger.

- ❑ *Sadness* seeps in as the dust settles on anger and acceptance, and the emotional and physical pain engulfs us.

- ❑ *Depression* is the deepest form of sadness and can become debilitating and dangerous if we don't take steps to move through it.

- ❑ *Joy* can be the aftermath of healthy grieving. With prayer, support, counsel, and our doctor's help, God says, "Weeping may remain for a night, but rejoicing comes in the morning" (Psalm 30:5).

We grieve for the loss of the bodies and lives we knew. Maybe we weren't always happy with them, but they were ours. Grieving is natural when pain, suffering, and loss plague our minds and hearts. Whether it's cancer cells, lymph nodes, lumpectomy, partial mastectomy, total mastectomy, chemotherapy, radiation, loss of hair, drug therapy, or killing good cells to get the bad ones, destruction and death of part of our bodies is necessary for our survival. Intellectually, we understand. But emotionally, we grieve. Even Christ, who died so we could live, grieved. On His journey to the cross, "He began to be filled with anguish and deep distress. He told them, 'My soul is crushed with grief to the point of death'" (Matthew 26:37–38 NLT).

While a sense of humor certainly is invaluable, we must not mask or bury hurt and anger by laughing them off. "Laughter can conceal a heavy heart; when the laughter ends, the grief remains" (Proverbs 14:13 NLT); but "Blessed are those who mourn, for they will be comforted" (Matthew 5:4). A buried emotion has energy. Eventually it rises to the surface and explodes. Job understood this when he said, "Even if I say, 'I'll put all this behind me, I'll look on the bright side and force a smile,' all these troubles would still be like grit in my gut" (Job 9:27–28 MSG).

We need to progressively transition through this grief process so we don't become bitter, cynical, discouraged, and lose hope. To accomplish this progression:

- Acknowledge where you are in the grieving process.

- Inform your family and friends so they don't take it personally.

- Allow yourself to experience each step in the process, and then move to the next.

- Pray that finally your mourning does turn to dancing again.

Eventually, although we never forget the cancer experience, we come to a place where the grieving turns to joy when we see how God will use our breast cancer for *His* good and glory.

📖 God's Love Letter to You

Dear_____, (fill in your name)
Go ahead and be angry. You do well to be angry—but don't use your
anger as fuel for revenge. And don't stay angry. Don't go to bed angry.
Don't give the Devil that kind of foothold in your life (Ephesians 4:26–
27 MSG). Don't be afraid, for I am with you. Do not be dismayed, for
I am your God. I will strengthen you. I will help you. I will uphold you
with my victorious right hand (Isaiah 41:10 NLT).
Restorer of Joy, God

🐰 Let's Pray

Prayerfully personalize Psalm 30:8–12 NLT.

Merciful God,

I,_____, cried out to you, O LORD. I,_____, begged
you for mercy, saying, "What will you gain if I,_____, die,
if I,_____, sink down into the grave? Can my dust praise
you from the grave? Can it tell the world of your faithfulness? Hear
me,_____, LORD, and have mercy on me,_____.
Help me,_____, O LORD. You have turned my mourning
into joyful dancing. You have taken away my clothes of mourning
and clothed me with joy, that I,_____, might sing praises
to you and not be silent. O LORD my God, I,_____, will
give you thanks forever! Amen.

Working through Sadness

WHY AM I DISCOURAGED? WHY SO SAD? —PSALM 42:5 NLT

A CHEERFUL HEART BRINGS A SMILE TO YOUR FACE; A SAD HEART
MAKES IT HARD TO GET THROUGH THE DAY.
—PROVERBS 15:13 MSG

📝 Dear God

Dear God,

In the beginning, I understood my tears came from a place
of shock, fear, pain, even denial, but why do I still cry? I cried

uncontrollably at odd times those first few weeks after diagnosis and surgery. That seemed normal. But a year later, waves of sadness rush over me when least expected. I used to be a very happy, optimistic, and passionate person. Now, I am often sad with a sense of woe and gloom. What's with that? I don't like it. When the sadness lifts, it is like a curtain going up on a sunny day. Speaking of which, if it is a cloudy, overcast day, my spirits match the weather. This is all such a new experience, and I am not sure how to adjust. Help! I need You big time with this one.

Sadly Yours, Janet

A Sister Shares

Because I didn't want to give in to my illness, I pushed myself every day. I continued walking five miles three times a week. I began to feel depressed and eventually confided in my doctor. He explained that depression was often common in cancer patients and prescribed an antidepressant. Slowly I began to feel better. The medication has improved the quality of my life dramatically. I realize now I should have been more honest about my fears and inner feelings early on. —Della

Mentoring Moment

Do you wake up in the morning crying over everything or maybe not even get out of bed? Or the day is going pretty well, and then the littlest thing turns your spirits from bright to sad? Do you cry out like the psalmist in Psalm 42:4, "My heart is breaking as I remember how it used to be?" (NLT). Is it any wonder we are sad, though? There are so very many changes going on in our bodies, physically, hormonally, emotionally, and spiritually. Sadness is in the realm of feelings we need to allow ourselves to experience and not stuff down or dance away from like they aren't there; but the key is to finding out what can pull us up out of the dumps.

It wasn't until I wrote this chapter that I actually identified the cause of my weepiness and emotionalism—a deep sadness. It helped finally to accept and verbalize that I was truly sad. Then I could talk to God and let Him know my fears and frustrations and ask for help finding happiness in the midst of the ugliness of this disease.

I find that depression departs when praise fills my heart. In my daily quiet time I write in a "Prayer-and-Praise Journal" like I give you on page 378. For years I have done this, and for years it has sustained me. It is so important to go back and write the answers to prayer requests so we can see the miracle of God at work.

Exercise is also a form of mental therapy and release for me. A walk in the fresh air or a trip to the gym, and I am refreshed and ready to take on the world. So it was tough when I didn't even feel like taking a walk, not to mention going to the gym. Grace Marestaing told me about the first day she decided to reinstate her daily walk; she put on her tennis shoes, stretched, and headed out the door for her usual five-to-ten-mile hike. Laughingly she recalls, "I made it to my neighbor's driveway and had to turn around and come home." Now that could make you sad! But the next day she made it a little farther, and that made her happy; and a little farther the next day, until on her second breast cancer anniversary she did a three-day Walk for the Cure. Now, that really made her happy!

Return as soon as possible to doing things you enjoy, but take baby steps. For example, if you are a musician, start by playing some favorite CDs and then move up to playing your musical instrument or singing. Are you a gardener? Start out watering the garden, then progress to planting new flowers. Call an upbeat friend, chat for a while, and then invite her over. Are you tired? Take a nap. Just close your eyes and be restored.

Here again is where a mentor or someone who has experienced breast cancer and its ensuing emotions can come to your side and comfort and encourage you like no one else can. Listen to what Grace says about helping someone with this emotional process:

> The process of dealing with the reality is just that—a process. It covers the gamut of emotions, but I've found they don't all happen at the same time. The mind tends to compartmentalize and deal with what it can, and each person reacts to the news differently. As an example, while I was very calm and cognitive in the initial stages—getting the information, making choices of treatment with my doctors, and so forth—I found myself dealing with the sadness and more emotional side at the year anniversary of my diagnosis. As volunteers at the BreastCare Center, we make sure each woman has heard all the information, and we help them deal with one step at a time. We can acknowledge their sadness and assure them their emotions are normal. We are there to catch some of that from the perspective of a person who has been there.

In dealing with our emotions, we have to consider the step we are at in our journeys. Experience the sadness, but know what and how to replace that sadness with a much more comfortable feeling—gladness.

Sad Is Not Bad
by Margaret Blackstone

If you are going through this frustrating period now, the best things you can do for yourself are to rely on those you trust, get plenty of rest, and keep yourself occupied with positive activities, including meditation or other means of relaxation that allow you to keep your mind free of fear or panic. Try to think of this as a door being opened, not closed. Of course, you'll have periods of grief for the "old you," but sad is not bad. Sad is what you go through as you grieve that some things in your life will change, and you may not have a lot of control over how they change. For your sake and your health's sake, try to approach this new chapter in life as a challenge, not as a defeat.[3]

God's Love Letter to You

Dear_____, (fill in your name)

When you give birth, you have a hard time, there's no getting around it. But when the baby is born, there is joy in the birth. This new life in the world wipes out memory of the pain. The sadness you have right now is similar to that pain, but the coming joy is also similar. When I, the Lord, see you again, you'll be full of joy, and it will be a joy no one can rob from you. You'll no longer be so full of questions (John 16:21–23 MSG paraphrased).
Delighting in you, God

Let's Pray

Prayerfully personalize Psalm 119:25–29 MSG.

I, _____, am feeling terrible—I couldn't feel worse! Get me on my feet again. You promised, remember? When I, _____, told my story, you responded; train me well in your deep wisdom. Help me, _____, understand these things inside and out, so I, _____, can ponder your miracle-wonders. My sad life's dilapidated, a falling-down barn; build me, _____, up again by your Word. Barricade the road that goes Nowhere; grace me, _____, with your clear revelation. Amen.

It's All Over, so Why Are You Depressed?

After my last procedure for reconstruction, I felt like I was on a mountaintop all alone. This was it. I'd made it, but now what? No more procedures to schedule, no next phase to look forward to. It was a strange feeling. I thought I'd be jumping up and down, because it was over. But I guess I was like a person who's been trapped in a dark cave for a long time. I came out, and the sun was too bright. I had to adjust. —Brenda Ladun[4]

I felt the sadness and more emotional side at the year anniversary of my diagnosis. —Grace Marestaing

The patient is tearful and crying constantly. She also appears to be depressed. —Excerpts from a medical record

Dear God

Dear God,

I remember Liz at the radiation center warning me there could be a huge letdown at the end of radiation. She said she experienced it, and I probably would too. I questioned, "How could that be? Won't I be so glad to have this all over and behind me?" As I approached those last intensive "boost" days of radiation, where the radiation beams focus in on the cancer area, Liz's words replayed in my head. *Would I feel a letdown? Would depression really hit me hard?*

Lord, maybe subconsciously I planned for this, or You protected me by having plenty to do those last days of radiation and following. There were writing deadlines and speaking engagements to fulfill. I never could have made those early trips without my Jane. Her help and getting right back into things allowed me to bypass any deep depression, although there was the lingering sadness.

Gratefully Yours, Janet

Two Sisters Share

Friends and family think it is "over" when you finally have that last chemo treatment. They forget it is still in your system for another month or so. You feel like you have lost everything—your hair, eyebrows, eyelashes, breast, strength—in general, you feel lousy! Everyone wants to celebrate with you, and you are *still grieving* for what you have been through. I cried every day for three weeks after my final treatment. Then one morning I woke up, and the Lord had removed it. I realized those days of crying were actually cathartic. —Darlene Gee

As of now my surgeon doesn't want to see me again for two months. My radiologist doesn't want to see me again for three months. My medical oncologist doesn't want to see me again ever! If it weren't for the support group, I'd be *having withdrawal symptoms*—now, there is no other reason for me to be in the hospital or the breast center. I almost miss the doctors and nurses who have taken such good care of me! —Heather

Mentoring Moment

The last treatment. You longed and prayed for this day. Hard to imagine depression at this point, isn't it? But it happens. There is a huge, sudden letdown. For months now the focus has been on you. Family and friends did things for you, took you places, asked how you are, and brought you meals. Doctors, nurses, and technicians focused on *you*. If you had radiation, it provided a place to go daily for maybe thirty-five to thirty-seven days or even longer, where everyone wanted to know how you felt and fussed over you. Were you eating enough? Drinking liquids? Maintaining your weight? Here, have a snack.

During chemotherapy, doctors and nurses attended to your needs, and you got to know other patients and enjoy their company and conversation during treatments. Then one day, you're done. Just like that, the doctors and nurses wish you well and then turn their attention to new patients. You may never see your fellow chemo friends again unless you make an effort to get together or run into each other in the doctor's waiting room. During those "sick times," everyone tried to help you feel better. While it is not the way we prefer to get attention, nevertheless, we had it.

Perhaps our families and friends have "had it" too! They reach a giving limit. In a crisis, people often do heroic things, like lift a car off a person. We were in a crisis mode. Those around us gathered up all their adrenaline and energy, maybe even put their own lives on hold, to help us weather the storm. We needed them; they managed to be there. However, as the crisis passes and we move into recovery, or the reality of no recovery, their energy wanes. Not meaning to be callous or uncaring, they are tired. This has been an emotional turmoil for them too.

Going from the center of attention—"it's all about you"—to everyone getting back to their normal activities now that you can function somewhat on your own can be quite a shock. And you feel so strange about it. The worst is over, so you think, *What is wrong with me?* Or maybe the doctors said full recovery is not in your future, and you still so desperately need support—where did everybody go?

Just like Liz counseled, don't beat yourself up over this, and don't be too hard on everyone else. If you prepare, hopefully, it won't catch you by surprise. As you see on your calendar the approaching end of your surgeries and treatments, try to plan things to occupy your time and mind that make you feel useful again:

- Resume an activity you put on hold.

- Start taking small walks, building up to longer ones.

- Pamper yourself with a massage or pedicure.

- Put all your pictures in an album.

- Volunteer to serve for an hour or two at your children's school or the church office.

- Start back to work a couple of hours a day as you build up to going back full time.

- Ask if there is work you could do from home if you are not up to going into the office.

- Read the book that has been sitting on your shelf for so long.

- Start a project you have always wanted to do.

- If you are not up to doing a project yet, have fun making a project-idea folder.

- If possible, plan a relaxing trip with friends or family—cruises are very relaxing.

- If you have not already, now might be the time to join a breast cancer support group.

Don't overdo. That is another extreme that will put you right back in bed. Know your limits. Talk to your doctor about what is appropriate, and then gradually add normal activities back into your day. Our minds are such an important part of the healing process. As much as possible, think on what is pleasant. Your body responds to your mind. In this order, remember to:

- Spend time with God

- Rest

- Eat nutritious foods

- Exercise

- Have some alone time

- Start a task or job

Nancy Tuttle wrote she always planned a wonderful trip during breaks in her treatments. "It is important to have something to look forward to. During the first break we took an eleven-day Hawaiian cruise. During the next break we went on a cruise to Greece and Turkey. On our last trip we went to Israel—what a blessing!"[5]

Shirley writes, "I took on small-term projects, like knitting an afghan, building a dollhouse for our granddaughter, and taking short trips. Also e-mails were nice, but the cards, flowers, and letters were great, and I have a 'big C' scrapbook that I put together—interspersed with the e-mails." Linda M. volunteered to write to those serving overseas in the military.

I did not take antidepressant medication, although my radiation oncologist did suggest it. However, many women are helped by it as well as counseling.

📖 God's Love Letter to You

Dear_____, (fill in your name)

Do not be anxious about anything, but in everything, by prayer and petition, with thanksgiving, present your requests to me, God, and My peace which transcends all understanding, will guard your hearts and your minds in Christ Jesus. Finally, whatever is true, whatever is noble, whatever is right, whatever is pure, whatever is lovely, whatever is admirable—if anything is excellent or praiseworthy—think about such things (Philippians 4:6–8 paraphrased).
Rejoicing over you, God

🙏 Let's Pray

Prayerfully personalize Psalm 42:5 MSG.

Merciful and loving Lord, please lift my spirits . . .

Why am I, _____, down in the dumps? Why am I, _____, crying the blues? If I fix my eyes on God—soon I'll be praising again. He puts a smile on my face. He's my, _____'s, God. Amen.

Feeling Guilty

God makes no two flowers or snowflakes or women alike. —Anne Ortlund

There may be a letdown or guilt at feeling sad or depressed about something in light of the fact you survived breast cancer and you are alive. —Grace Marestaing

🖋 Dear God

Dear God,

Part of my struggle with being sad is feeling like I don't deserve to be sad. My cancer and treatment was so less invasive than many other women's experience. I still have my breasts, and I didn't lose my hair. I don't feel justified grieving. My frozen shoulder seems mild in comparison to what others endure. Many women have it so much worse than I, Lord; I grieve for them too. I am so very grateful my cancer is curable and required less radical treatment, but I need help not comparing myself with someone else. I cannot measure my grief and sadness on a scale according to how bad things are. Lord, let my guilt turn to gratefulness. Guilt does not come from You. Please forgive me.

Not guilty, Janet

Two Sisters Share

Not every lesion is cancerous! I have learned *not to compare myself* with any other woman who I know has had or will have breast cancer. There are too many variables. —Darlene M.

I thought I let my family and friends down by being afflicted with this disease. I imposed upon myself the same expectation I had imposed upon my mom. My mother's breast cancer diagnosis was in 1984. She had a mastectomy, recovered well, and is still cancer free. In spite of that, I was totally unprepared for the news I had a malignant tumor. My mom had always been the pillar of strength in my eyes. Because my mom had gone through the same experience and it didn't seem to bother her, I thought I should have been able to do the same.

Through my experience, I saw my mom differently. I began to understand that her motives and the way she portrayed herself as being able to handle everything was her way of protecting me from the burdens of the realities and troubles of life. I realize now she is a real person also. —Brenda N.

 ## Mentoring Moment

Guilt is yet another phase of grieving. It can happen at any stage of the journey. Maybe like Brenda N., you feel guilty that your family has to deal with this disease or you aren't measuring up to how you think someone else dealt with it. Perhaps like me, you feel guilty bringing it into your family heritage, or still being sad a year or two later, or not feeling justified being sad when you had a less invasive surgery. A fellow chemo patient dies, and you feel guilty you lived.

Comparing is never a good idea. Only negative things result from it. The Bible warns us: "We will not compare ourselves with each other as if one of us were better and another worse. We have far more interesting things to do with our lives. Each of us is an original" (Galatians 5:26 MSG).

God's Love Letter to You

Dear_____, *(fill in your name)*
    Make a careful exploration of who you are and the work you have

been given, and then sink yourself into that. Don't be impressed with yourself. Don't compare yourself with others. Each of you must take responsibility for doing the creative best you can with your own life (Galatians 6:4–5 MSG).
Freeing you of guilt, God

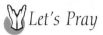

Let's Pray

Father, we know the voice in our heads telling us we are undeserving or filling us with doubt is not You. Help us cast out any negative thinking that causes us to worry or makes us feel unworthy. You tell us we are worthy in Your sight. You made each of us individual and unique, and we are on our own earthly journeys. There is comfort in that, Lord. Please keep our ears listening to Your still, small voice. Amen.

Where Were Those You Expected to Be There?

QUICK, GOD, I NEED YOUR HELPING HAND! . . .
ALL THE FRIENDS I DEPENDED ON GONE. —PSALM 12:1 MSG

AND YOU, MY SO-CALLED FRIENDS, ARE NO BETTER—THERE'S NOTHING TO YOU! ONE LOOK
AT A HARD SCENE AND YOU SHRINK IN FEAR. —JOB 6:21 MSG

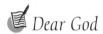

Dear God

Dear God,

Where, oh where, were those who made so many promises? The ones who said, "I'll be there the morning of surgery" or "I'll take you to radiation, and we can have lunch" or "I'll come by and keep you company," but then didn't. Then there was the person I thought You put in my life because she, too, had experienced breast cancer, but instead of mentoring and comforting me, she made it seem like a piece of cake, and why didn't I do the same?

Of course, so many went above and beyond, but I couldn't help but wonder what happened to the others. Did they forget about me? Did their own lives get so crazy, they couldn't fit me in? Was it just too painful to be around me going through this?

Let me prayerfully continue to love them, Father. Please remove any bad feelings or resentment in my heart. Help me speak the truth in love as I let them know I missed their presence or was disappointed they didn't follow through. If I can do this, it might help them not hurt the next person.

Regretfully Yours, Janet

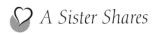 *A Sister Shares*

Yesterday I spent a good part of the day at the BreastCare Center with a friend who started neoadjuvant chemo [chemo before surgery to reduce the size of the tumor]. She was starting chemo that day. I already had two students not coming to their lesson, moved another couple of them, and was able to stay with her through the five hours. I had a real sense of an assignment from the Lord, and was glad to be there because she was by herself. She just hugged me and cried when she saw me. —Grace Marestaing

 Mentoring Moment

Grace and I had several discussions together lamenting the sadness and disappointment when people let us down. However, Grace did not allow that to let her become bitter. Instead, she uses it as a reminder and impetus to be there for others as she volunteers one day a week at the BreastCare Center and steps into the void others experience in their journeys. Just today, I read of a high-school senior graduating this month after having cancer in her sophomore year. She had won a contest by sending in her diary entries during this scary and tear-filled time of her young life. One of the things the article noted was her comment about the "friends" who never came to visit.

So many women going through a crisis tell me the people they expected to be there weren't, and the ones they least expected were! It makes us sad, and maybe mad, to think we might have fair-weather friends and/or family members. We need to pray for them because they missed the blessing of loving someone more then themselves.

But how about those who came through who barely knew us? Maybe someone at work who occasionally says "hi" came to visit you *every week*. Or the church acquaintance who arranged meals through the church! While the disappointment is real with those who let us down, I find shifting the focus to the ones that went out of their way to help replaces the sadness with gladness. Perhaps a new relationship will come out of their acts of kindness and mercy toward us.

📖 God's Love Letter to You

Dear_____, (fill in your name)

    Be merciful, just as I, your Father, am merciful. Do not judge, and you will not be judged. Do not condemn, and you will not be condemned. Forgive, and you will be forgiven (Luke 6:36–37 paraphrased).
Your Forgiver, God

🐰 Let's Pray

Merciful Savior, thank You for forgiving us our many sins. You never condemned us or made us feel guilty. Lord, help us remember we do not earn or deserve mercy; You grant it unconditionally, never taking it back. Help us mercifully forgive those who disappoint us, and keep our minds focused on the many ways others came forward with acts of mercy and kindness toward us. You are a merciful and forgiving God, filled with grace and love. Let us go and do likewise. In Your gracious name we pray. Amen.

✍ Your Letter to God

Write about where you are in the grieving process. Ask God to give you wisdom and discernment as to what would help relieve any bouts of anger, sadness, or depression. Write the names of those who disappointed you, and write "Forgiven" next to their names. Start another praise list of those who were there for you. Is it longer? Ask God to help you make the transition from "It's all about me" to "It isn't all about me anymore."

Dear God,   *Date:* _____

_____

_____

_____

_____

_____

_____

_____

Chapter Sixteen

Restoring the Joy!

Hallelujah!
Thank God! Pray to him by name!
Tell everyone you meet what he has done!
Sing him songs, belt out hymns,
translate his wonders into music!
Honor his holy name with Hallelujahs,
you who seek God. Live a happy life!
Keep your eyes open for God, watch for his works;
be alert for signs of his presence.

—*Psalm 105:1–4 MSG*

It Feels Good to Be Happy!

A HAPPY HEART MAKES THE FACE CHEERFUL, BUT HEARTACHE CRUSHES THE SPIRIT.
—PROVERBS 15:13

I'M HAPPY FROM THE INSIDE OUT, AND FROM THE OUTSIDE IN, I'M FIRMLY FORMED.
—PSALM 16:9 MSG

A diagnosis of cancer can, like Pastor Rick says, make you better or bitter. You have a choice. I am definitely better and happier than I have ever been. Cancer is an incredible clarifier of what's important in life. —Darlene Gee

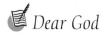 Dear God

Dear God,

In spite of all the sadness, happiness prevailed. The tears did fall, but then the smile returned. People always tell me how much they enjoy my smile. You gifted me with a childlike joy and enthusiasm, and often friends surprise me with something special just to hear me shriek with excitement. My shrieks were pretty weak for a while, but I do believe they have returned. Many joyous outbursts come from the insight of realizing things that only You could have done!

How happy it made me experiencing my best friend, Jane, care for me so lovingly as we traveled on our speaking events. It allowed her to shine as she stepped in when my energy waned. I watched the Woman to Woman Mentoring Team not miss a beat through any of my illness. They all rose to the challenge—not just carrying on but excelling beyond me. It is with a great deal of pride and gratitude that I decrease, so they may increase. I am not sure that would have happened had I not been so ill.

My dear Grace Abounds is probably the biggest blessing of my cancer. Meeting Grace and establishing what will be a lifelong relationship makes my heart smile. I can't imagine life without Grace. Yet had we both not had breast cancer, we never might have met. And I can't forget "RawSome Robyn" teaching me how to change my diet. I love shopping now at the health-food stores, and You know how I really used to dread grocery shopping. I am so happy with the way we eat and the restored pleasure in preparing food for Dave and me.

Lord, even though the sad times still happen, they are fewer and fewer. And when they come, I know they will not linger.

Happy and smiling, Janet

Two Sisters Share

There are lots of negatives about suffering cancer, but we also have some positives. Cancer can't overcome our spirit or shatter our hope. Cancer can't destroy our friendships or take away sweet memories. Cancer can't take away our soul or disrupt our eternal life. Bitterness began to sour my very soul . . . bitterness, disbelief—hate had been simmering so long with my pain. The timing of this event in my life was such a sacrifice. It was not a make-believe situation, but maybe it put me in touch with how life really is. Maybe it was a loving type of sacrifice on my part. . . .

You step outside on a cold, still morning and take a panoramic view of all the surroundings. God had covered the landscape with frost and ice. We took a fifty-minute drive to see God's wonderland of beauty. His was the making of such a beautiful, happy day. Happiness is like a butterfly. . . . When you chase it, it is just out of your reach, but if you will sit down quietly, the butterfly will often light right upon you. —Martha[1]

I have been in the work force since I was seventeen. I always wanted to have some time off and someone to do the cooking and cleaning. Not to mention I hate shaving my legs and having to do my hair. Now I have no hair anywhere to worry about! God gives us what we want, just not always the way we want it. In the midst of all this I actually am experiencing days I even forget I have cancer. The back pain has become a part of everyday life, and I pay particular attention to my limitations and don't even try and overdo them. Life is so good. —Linda M.

 ## Mentoring Moment

You may have read the title of this section and thought to yourself, *Happy? What do I have to be happy about?* Perhaps you wondered if I had truly lost it. None of us is ecstatic or delighted to have breast cancer. If we could choose, I think most would say please pass me by with this character-building experience. But since it did happen, the focus now changes to how can we see good in this? Solomon, the wisest man (except Jesus) who ever lived, said, "When times are good, be happy; but when times are bad, consider: God has made the one as well as the other" (Ecclesiastes 7:14).

Author Gary Smalley talks about finding the pearl in every situation, and that has become the motto at our house when something goes wrong. In the midst of the fear, pain, and sadness of breast cancer, there is *nothing* funny about it. You may have to really search to find something to be happy about. But it will happen, and it usually comes with gratitude. Happiness is really a choice. My pastor often says you have to act yourself into a feeling, and sometimes that is what it takes to get us out of a down mood. Sit down quietly, close your eyes, then read a few passages from your Bible—God will meet you there. He will restore that sometimes-elusive happiness. "God will let you laugh again; you'll raise the roof with shouts of joy" (Job 8:21 MSG).

God's Love Letter to You

Dear_____, (fill in your name)

I, the LORD your God, have arrived to live among you. I am a mighty savior. I will rejoice over you with great gladness. My love will calm all your fears. I will exult over you by singing a happy song (Zephaniah 3:17 NLT paraphrased).
Restorer of Happiness, God

Let's Pray

Prayerfully personalize Psalms 86:3–5 NLT and 119:71, 111 MSG.

Restorer of my joy, please . . .

Be merciful, O LORD, for I, _____, am calling on you constantly. Give me, _____, happiness, O LORD, for my life depends on you. O LORD, You are so good, so ready to forgive, so full of unfailing love for all who ask your aid. My troubles turned out all for the best—they forced me, _____, to learn from your textbook. . . . I, _____ _____, inherited your book on living; it's mine forever—what a gift! And how happy it makes me! Amen.

A Transforming Blessing

For me, breast cancer was a transforming life experience—physically, personally, and spiritually. I would not change what I have gained from my battle. Strange to say—but it has been a gift in my life. —Grace Marestaing

Cancer has given me time to study the Bible and the desire to develop a closer relationship with God. —Nancy Tuttle[2]

All the tears of pain passed, and I knew in that moment that having cancer would change my life and become such a blessing to me. A rare gift and privilege for me to carry. —Linda M.

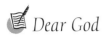 Dear God

Dear God,

I am different now . . . in a good way. I have a new depth. I am more aware of others and their needs. While I still want to do my best, I can stop when it's time to rest, take a break, or go to bed. I have a hunger to help women stop wasting their lives in overwhelming worry. The price of lost moments is too high. Skidding up to death's door and facing my mortality, I know if You were to take me home today, I have made a difference in the world. I did not just take up space on earth but fulfilled Your plan and call on my life. Every woman should be able to say that . . . it is within her reach.

I often wonder, though, if it doesn't take a brush with death or tragedy to get our attention. I speak boldly now. Some are uncomfortable, but You said they would be. I feel a new depth of spiritual awareness. My vision is clear . . . my path is straight . . . my hope does not falter . . . my confidence is in You Lord, and I will live to Your glory. And so I say as many others before and after me, thank You for my breast cancer.

Gratefully Yours, Janet

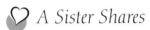 A Sister Shares

My breast cancer was a blessing in disguise. In 1999, the year after my breast cancer surgery, I quit work to care for our grandson Michael. My husband, Earl, was already retired. In May 2002 Earl received the diagnosis of lung cancer. He had surgery on June 3. All during this time God kept speaking to my heart and showing me in His Word, "Do not be afraid." I thought everything would be OK. I had claimed Psalm 41:3 "The LORD will sustain him on his sickbed and restore him from his bed of illness."

On June 15 Earl died. God did "restore" Earl—to heaven. By quitting work because of my breast cancer, God allowed me to have extra quality time with Earl, making special memories. The Sunday after Earl's funeral services as I sat down in the pew at church, God "spoke" to my heart and said, "This is the time I was telling you not to be afraid." Our Father God has indeed done more than I could ever imagine to provide for me, His grateful daughter! —Linda Taylor

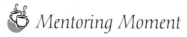 ## Mentoring Moment

Suffering transforms us. Our character goes to new depths—never reached had our lives gone merrily along. I am always telling God I am enough of a character without more suffering. Suffering reveals new realms for understanding others, ourselves, and most important, God. I think every one of us journeying through breast cancer would say we now have a new, deeper level of warm, heartfelt compassion for the sick and weak—especially those suffering from any kind of cancer. Now we see through His eyes the things that break His heart, and our hearts break.

Many women referred to breast cancer as a blessing and gift and thanked God for it. That does not mean they enjoyed breast cancer or are glad it happened; however, most women said this experience changed their lives for the better. I know how hard that might be for you even to think of right now. It was tough for me too. As I went through treatments, most of my prayers were, "Help, Lord!" or "Protect me, Lord!" or "I am so sad, Lord" or "It hurts so bad, Lord!" My "Thank You, Lords" were more for getting me through a tough time or making a decision. However, now on the other side of the intensity, I realize everything God was doing in my life that probably never would have happened had I not been forced into the throes of breast cancer—up close and personal.

Don't worry if it is too soon to think positively about your breast cancer. Tuck these thoughts in your mind and heart, and when the time is right, reread this area and journal. Or perhaps you can say, "Lord, this would not have been my choice, but thank You for the ways You are using it to mold and make me into a godlier woman."

I pray as you move from grief to acceptance of this new life, you can look back like so many have and see you are not the woman you were before breast cancer. Not just the physical changes but also the internal transforming changes. Can the loss become a gain? We have to make a choice. We can't go back.

God's Love Letter to You

Dear_____, (fill in your name)

My thoughts are completely different from yours, and my ways are far beyond anything you could imagine. For just as the heavens are higher than the earth, so are my ways higher than your ways and my thoughts higher than your thoughts. I send out my word, and it always produces fruit. It will accomplish all I want it to, and it will prosper everywhere I send it. You will live in joy and peace. The mountains and hills will burst into song, and the trees of the field will clap their hands! (Isaiah 55:8–9, 11–12 NLT paraphrased).

Transformer of Lives, God

Let's Pray

Prayerfully personalize Psalm 18:20–24 MSG.

Precious heavenly Father, I am so grateful that . . .

You, GOD made my, _____'s, life complete when I placed all the pieces before you. When I, _____, got my act to-gether, you gave me a fresh start. Now I, _____, am alert to your ways; I don't take you for granted. Every day I review the ways you work; I try not to miss a trick. I, _____, feel put back together, and I'm watching my step. GOD, You rewrote the text of my, _____'s, life when I opened the book of my heart to your eyes. Amen.

You Can Rejoice in the Trials

I still praise God every day for His wonderful love and mercy. After all, every day is a gift, and nothing comes into our lives that He's not in control of. —Edna

I am praying for a physical healing, but I am enjoying the journey of spiritual healing along the way. —Nancy Tuttle[3]

As for myself and Emily [teenage daughter], we refuse to crawl into a hole and let this kick our butts. We intend to enjoy every day we have and take full advantage of the kindness bestowed on us. —Linda M.

Dear God

Dear God,

We all squirm in our seats and laugh nervously when the pastor starts talking about trials being good for us and growing our spiritual maturity. When I hear a message like that and everything is going great in my life, I tend to say, "Thank You,

Lord, and please let it last." However, during a crisis like breast cancer, this type of message actually is a comfort and brings joy instead of being uncomfortable. I know something big is going to happen in my spirit. I wish it could be another way . . . that I would just grow and blossom for You without ever having to endure a hardship . . . but Your Son, Jesus, endured the cross, showing me that would be impossible. Jesus had to sacrifice, and I will have to do the same.

After much prayer I realize that giving in to breast cancer gives Satan a foothold on my mind and ministry, and I will fight that happening to the very end. Therefore, Lord, with Your help I can be glad and give thanks in good times and in bad . . . that takes a lot of prayer and a lot of faith, but I am ready for both! You never said it would be easy, but You also never told us to give up or give in . . . so today I choose to rejoice and be joyful in all circumstances. Lord, I only can do that with Your strong arm holding me up.

Joyfully Yours, Janet

A Sister Shares

Many friends sympathized with me, but my husband and I are quick to tell them not to feel sorry for us because we feel truly blessed. Through our difficult trials and my having breast cancer, I have learned . . .

- To lean on God and surrender the situation to Him because I can do nothing on my own.

- To trust God because He is always there for me and will not lead me to something unless He provides a way for me to get through it.

- That just as God supplied the Israelites with their daily bread from heaven (see Exodus 16:4), He provides for me on a daily basis. When we face difficult situations, God sends the strength and nourishment to face what comes our way, not all at once, but day by day.

- That because of the difficult situations I've been through, I am able to help others by offering words of comfort and encouragement. —Lisha

Mentoring Moment

Looking back at our lives, we usually see blessings emerge from hardships. We are actually glad for the experience, difficult as it was at the time. When first faced with breast cancer, I could hardly imagine finding anything to rejoice and be happy about. This was what I had dreaded all my life, and now here it was right in my lap . . . or should I say, chest. Once I worked through the stages of treatment and grief, I could clearly see the blessings. One of them was being able to write this book for you. My reward comes when you have *Dear God, They Say It's Cancer* in your hands and are pouring your heart out to the Lord. So with great happiness and anticipation, I write to you every day until it is finished.

Writing down what you have to be thankful for—all the blessings you continue to see through this breast cancer adventure—may just put that smile back on your face too! After "Your Letter to God," at the end of this chapter, there is a page titled, "I Am So Happy Because . . ." It is a place for you to linger awhile and literally count your blessings. If you have trouble getting started, how about beginning with gratitude for *today's* gift of life. I am sure about halfway down the page your heart will start to sing, and you, too, will say, "I can rejoice in my trials." Then enjoy the poem "Gratitude," which my Grace Abounds wrote in the midst of her breast cancer trial.

God's Love Letter to You

Dear_____, (fill in your name)

Dear sister, whenever trouble comes your way, let it be an opportunity for joy. For when your faith is tested, your endurance has a chance to grow. So let it grow, for when your endurance is fully developed, you will be strong in character and ready for anything. If you need wisdom—if you want to know what I, God, want you to do—ask me, and I will gladly tell you. I will not resent your asking. But when you ask me, be sure that you really expect me to answer, for a doubtful mind is as unsettled as a wave of the sea that is driven and tossed by the wind (James 1:2–6 NLT paraphrased).
Growing you, God

Let's Pray

Prayerfully personalize with me Romans 5:3–5 NLT.

God of joy, light, and blessings, we lift up Your holy name in prayer . . .

We, _____ and Janet, can rejoice, too, when we, _____ and Janet, run into problems and trials, for we, _____ and

Janet, know that they are good for us—they help us learn to endure. And endurance develops strength of character in us, and character strengthens our confident expectation of salvation. And this expectation will not disappoint us. For we, _____ and Janet, know how dearly God loves us, because he has given us the Holy Spirit to fill our hearts with his love. Amen.

Your Letter to God

Where are you right now on the happiness scale? If low, ask God to remind you of something that puts a smile on your face, restores joy, and shows you the light and rainbow at the end of the tunnel. Start writing. If happy, write down everything that makes you happy. On dark days, come back and read what you wrote today. Have you had difficulty rejoicing in this trial? Do the hardships far outweigh the blessings at this point? I am so sorry, and I totally understand, and so does God. Pray for comfort the world cannot give. Let God wrap His arms around your heart and cheer you up. As blessings begin to unveil, and they will, write them down so you won't ever forget God's faithfulness through all generations.

Dear God,
                                                                    Date:

_____

_____

_____

_____

_____

_____

_____

_____

_____

_____

_____

_____

Gratitude
by Grace Marestaing

Gratitude—
What is your shape and color?
What is the woof and warp of your substance?
What is it about your contours that calls us close
when sometimes we would rather look away?
What is it in your expression that turns a key
and cracks the door of hope—
revealing further in, the gifts our hearts desire?

Gratitude—
When we withhold you,
when we fail to respond to your prompting,
we are trapped.
We lock ourselves away from the wisdom
and the healing we so need.
So this day, intent refreshed, renewed
we have a little clearer view of who you are.
We come to sing your songs to the simple and profound.
We sing with grateful heart for birds and trees,
for laughter, chocolate shakes,
the smell of fresh-baked bread;
for the beauty and provision of each day;
for wind and rain, for storms and calm.
How can we not express the dearness of the heroes
of our lives—
those whom we love, who love us back,
who walk along and stand beside.
The heroes, too who help us fight—
the warriors in whose skills we put our trust,
the ones whose care helps us survive.

Gratitude—
In speaking you we know you best.
You are the journey of heart-felt thanks.
Without you perception's marred;
we miss the joy,
the world is less.

© GMM. 2003

I Am So Happy Because . . .

Many Things to Be Grateful for   I Have Seen Many Blessings

- _____   - _____
- _____   - _____
- _____   - _____
- _____   - _____
- _____   - _____
- _____   - _____
- _____   - _____
- _____   - _____
- _____   - _____
- _____   - _____
- _____   - _____
- _____   - _____
- _____   - _____
- _____   - _____
- _____   - _____
- _____   - _____
- _____   - _____
- _____   - _____
- _____   - _____
- _____   - _____

Chapter Seventeen

Discovering a New Focus and Purpose

I'm not saying that I have this all together, that I have it made. But I am well on my way, reaching out for Christ, who has so wondrously reached out for me. Friends, don't get me wrong: By no means do I count myself an expert in all of this, but I've got my eye on the goal, where God is beckoning us onward—to Jesus.
I'm off and running, and I'm not turning back.
So let's keep focused on that goal, those of us who want everything God has for us. If any of you have something else in mind, something less than total commitment, God will clear your blurred vision—you'll see it yet! Now that we're on the right track, let's stay on it. Stick with me, friends. Keep track of those you see running this same course, headed for this same goal.

—*Philippians 3:12–17 MSG*

Changing Focus

Cancer was a wake-up call that enabled me to focus on what is truly important to me. Our Lord is so good. —Anita

Cancer has made me a better person because I now focus on the truly important things in this life and look forward to eternity with Him. —Edna

Breast cancer was a message to change. It provided the opportunity to experience a precious wilderness time with God. In spite of the nausea and weakness, I felt sheltered by His wings and covered by other's prayers. —Lynn

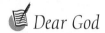 Dear God

Dear God,

You constantly reprioritize and refocus my life. The tragic murder of Daddy when I was ten embedded in my soul the precious fragility of life. Only You know the numbers of our days. Early on I understood bad things happen to good people; live ready to die. Sadly, You watched me struggle through rebellious backsliding years, trying to outrun You. How unprepared I was to die had You taken me then. Thank You for sparing and bringing me back into the fold. The prodigal daughter returned, giving her entire life to You.

Initially, I was confused with the cancer diagnosis! "No, not now, God," I railed. "Not just when I finally understand my purpose and passion in life is serving You. Would You bring me down in the middle of it?" Ah, but Your Son, Jesus, only had a ministry for three years. He did what He came to do. He didn't finish all the work on earth, but He did fulfill His purpose—to die for our sins. Lord, please help me know and fully accomplish my purpose. Don't let me waste a precious moment. Every day has new meaning. With Your help I will do only things that enhance my life and the kingdom.

Constantly, I ask for direction. How do You want me to use these restored days? It would be foolish to spend them mad or angry. No time for stress or overwhelmed feelings. No spending precious earthly time wasting the potential You gave me. Lord, give me a message to speak boldly. Synchronize my focus with Your plan and purpose for my life.

Purposely Yours, Janet

A Sister Shares

God,

Cancer has made me aware that my time on earth is temporary. I don't want to waste my days with meaningless activities. I want to choose to spend my time doing things that will help me to grow more Christ-like. God, I give You my time.

Your child, Nancy[1]

 Mentoring Moments

Have you heard it said, God never wastes a hurt? His plans are for good and not for harm. Even in the worst circumstances God's plan is still to bring out the best. Maybe someone comes to know the Lord during our cancer. Maybe it is a fine-tuning of our own hearts and depth of compassion.

The one thing breast cancer universally brings is a brush with our mortality. In our youth, we anticipated the luxury of years to make an impact on the world. We often wasted precious moments on meaningless activities. Breast cancer causes us to acknowledge that earthly life is not forever. For many, the light goes on to do whatever we can with our remaining years, no matter how few or many. They will be the exact days God planned for us, and our job is to maximize the gift of every moment.

We come to grips with our life's goals and accomplishments. Are they in line with the legacy we want to leave? If so, then we rest in that fact and continue. However, if we have spun our wheels, dragging through a worried, exhausted, overwhelmed, and tired life, we now ask ourselves the question, "Why? Why continue living like this?" Then comes the next question, "What needs changing so I can live a balanced life with time for my family, Bible study, ministry, quiet time with God, hobbies, recreation, and fun—yes, *fun!*?" Perhaps it means cutting back hours at work, taking an early retirement, or downsizing so household duties or your schedule are not so draining. As you pray, let God reveal to your heart His focus for your life during and after breast cancer.

More Sisters Share How Their Focus Changed

Returned to Work with New Vigor

It was during her second journey down the road to cancer recovery that Margaret Kelly began to take inventory of what was important in her life. "I love the people I work with," she says. "To just decide to give up my career because I had cancer would be letting cancer win." At the end of a nine-month sabbatical, Margaret returned to RE/MAX [her real-estate job] with new vigor for life and work.[2]

Left Work to Focus on Grandson

I now regard time differently; my focus has changed. I quit teaching and daily watch my grandson. I now have time to pour my love into him while his single mom works. The lack of freedom frustrates me, but viewing life in the light of eternity, there is no better use of each minute than investing in the life of a child. —Lynn

Don't Sweat the Small Stuff

Breast cancer is just another illness. I learned to accept that life is about living each moment. It is important to cherish those who love us and whom we love, accept others and ourselves, forgive differences, and recognize that no one or anything is perfect. I have to remind myself continually to "not sweat the small stuff." —Brenda N.

Intentional Space and Margin

This process of breast cancer has made me intentional about leaving space and margins in my life . . . time for quiet, walking, exercise, precious relationships with friends and family, enjoying new friendships, and fun. I no longer say yes just because there is an empty space on my schedule. I'm more careful about how many things I take on. I'm more likely to ask for help. —Grace Marestaing

Saddleback Church Breast Cancer Support Group Comments

- Little things don't bother me.
- Cancer helped put everything into perspective.
- Cancer is a great clarifier of life.
- Everything on earth is temporary.
- I value every new day.
- I allow more "me" time.
- I don't spend time being frustrated. I have a completely new outlook.

📖 God's Love Letter to You

Dear_____, (fill in your name)

    If you are humble, I will lead you in what is right and teach you my ways. If you keep my covenant and obey my decrees I, the Lord, will lead you with unfailing love and faithfulness (Psalm 25:9–10 NLT paraphrased).

Your Refocus, God

🙏 Let's Pray

Prayerfully personalize Psalm 40:1–3 NLT.

I, _____, waited patiently for you, LORD, to help me, and you turned to me, _____, and heard my cry. You lifted me, _____, out of the pit of despair, out of the mud and the mire. You set my feet on solid ground and steadied me as I, _____, walked along. You gave me, _____, a new song to sing, a hymn of praise to you, God. Many will see what you have done and be astounded. They will put their trust in the LORD. Amen.

Finding Purpose in Your Breast Cancer

Living on purpose is the path to peace. —Rick Warren[3]

I had the assurance of His love for me, and somewhere in this chaos I knew there was a greater purpose. —Grace Marestaing

Don't box God into only one way of responding to your prayers for healing or into having only one "purpose" for your suffering. —Kay Marshall Strom[4]

✒️ Dear God

Dear God,

    Initially, I went about this cancer journey like a dreaded job I had to do. That's the driver personality in me, I guess. Look at the goal— get well fast—then move on to the next assignment. Gradually, I realize a cancer-beating goal is never completely finished. This job never ends. I always will be surviving breast cancer and continuously looking over my shoulder to see if it has returned, again demanding attention.

Purpose for me used to mean accomplishments—getting an A, giving a well-received talk, making a delicious dinner, finding just the right outfit. It all had to be perfect—the best. Even as I prayed and sought the purpose in my cancer, I was looking for it to be tangible—writing the book I longed for, sharing my breast cancer to encourage others, helping people understand the need for good nutrition for better quality life—doing, doing, doing.

But, of course, none of those are Your primary purpose for my life, are they? Cancer is helping me evaluate through Your eyes the fleeting, temporary satisfaction and glory of accomplishments—of doing. Like a drug—one leads to a craving for another. Feelings of satisfaction so short-lived that I search out the next big hurdle or task to overcome, conquer, and claim. I am going through withdrawal of not finding purpose in my own worth and seeking it instead in Your worth. Gradually, being replaces doing.

As my mind and heart emerge from the prideful fog, I more clearly see Your purpose for me is to become more like You. I receive my "Well done, good and faithful servant" when I display the fruit of the Holy Spirit: love, joy, peace, patience, kindness, goodness, faithfulness, gentleness, and self-control. Help me know what that looks like, Lord. Humble me. Break me. Mold me. Use me for Your purpose.

Seeking Your purpose-driven life, Janet

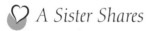 A Sister Shares

My life underwent internal changes. Accomplishments and actions energized me before; often relationships suffered. With breast cancer, I felt helpless to *do* anything; and dependent on others' help, I felt inadequate and useless at times. Slowly my motivations began to change. I had unlimited time to visit and interact with family and friends who stopped by to visit and assist. My parents and I restored our relationship and realized how much we loved and cherished each other. I could ramble on and on about other issues that were dealt with and resolved. Having experienced the "worst," cancer, I experience less fear and more peace. I know God will shelter and help me through anything. I know He has numbered my days just like each one of His children's, and I am content to rest in that. —Lynn

Mentoring Moment

My pastor, Rick Warren, wrote the bestseller *The Purpose Driven Life*. That book is breaking all records for sales! Translated into many languages, it has a fit for every segment of humanity. Why is it so popular? Because everyone is searching for purpose in life. Why in the world are we here? We all need to know we are not accidents and that things don't just randomly happen to us. The first words on Day One of Pastor Rick's book are:

> It's not about you. The purpose of your life is far greater than your own personal fulfillment, your peace of mind, or even your happiness. It's far greater than your family, your career, or even your wildest dreams and ambitions. If you want to know why you were placed on this planet, you must begin with God. You were born *by* his purpose and *for* his purpose.
>
> The search for the purpose of life has puzzled people for thousands of years. That's because we typically begin at the wrong starting point—ourselves. We ask self-centered questions like What do *I* want to be? What should *I* do with *my* life? What are *my* goals, *my* ambitions, *my* dreams for *my* future? But focusing on ourselves will never reveal our life's purpose. The Bible says, "It is God who directs the lives of his creatures; everyone's life is in his power."
>
> Contrary to what many popular books, movies, and seminars tell you, you won't discover your life's meaning by looking within yourself. You've probably tried that already. You didn't create yourself, so there is no way you can tell yourself what you were created for![5]

On Day Three, Pastor Rick asks the question, "What drives your life?" Guilt? Resentment? Anger? Fear? Materialism? Need for approval? He says all these and other forces can drive our lives, but they "all lead to the same dead end: unused potential, unnecessary stress, and an unfulfilled life." He then outlines five great benefits of living a purpose-driven life. Knowing your purpose . . .

1. Gives meaning to your life

2. Simplifies your life

3. Focuses your life

4. Motivates your life

5. Prepares you for eternity[6]

If you have not read Pastor Rick's book, I highly recommend you pick it up. Or better yet, when someone asks you the inevitable question, "What do you need?" or "What can I get you?" tell him or her to buy you *The Purpose Driven Life*. If you have already read it, reread it looking for God's purpose and plan for your life with breast cancer added to the mix.

Right now it may be unthinkable to consider God has a master purpose and plan for your breast cancer. Can you accept that He will bring good and purpose out of it? God is God, and we are not! That means we will never fully understand everything this side of heaven. Bad things do happen to good people—they did in biblical days and throughout history. The purpose often comes when we learn what God wants us to do as Christians who are encountering a hardship. Do we look for ways to glorify God in and through our crisis? What a challenge that is, and one you may not feel up to at this point . . . don't worry about it. Stay prayerful, and when God sees that you are ready, He will reveal His perfect purpose and plan to you.

God's Love Letter to You

Dear_____, (fill in your name)
    My purpose is to give life in all its fullness (John 10:10 NLT).
Jesus Christ, your Lord and Savior

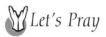

Let's Pray

Prayerfully personalize with me Colossians 1:15–17 MSG.

Our loving Lord and Father of our Savior, Jesus Christ . . .

We, _____ and Janet, look at this Son and see the God who cannot be seen. We, _____ and Janet, look at this Son and see God's original purpose in everything created. For everything, absolutely everything, above and below, visible and invisible, rank after rank after rank of angels—everything got started in him and finds its purpose in him. He was there before any of it came into existence and holds it all together right up to this moment. Amen.

How Does God Want to Use Your Breast Cancer?

Breast cancer changed my life dramatically. I lost my husband, home, employment, financial security, and part of my body. I will probably be alone the rest of my life because I am not willing to risk more loss. My focus has been changed to finding why God saved me, what is my purpose for being here? What do I have to offer as a servant of God? —Karen

THE LORD HAS A REASON FOR EVERYTHING HE DOES. —PROVERBS 16:4 CEV

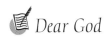

Dear God

Dear God,

How are you going to use my breast cancer to further Your kingdom work? I know you have a plan and purpose for me, and I want to work within that. Lord, let me not fight it. Help me know what to say and when to say it. How can I help others be more at ease with their breast cancer? How will You use it in my speaking? My writing? My relationships? Lord, for sure this very book is all part of Your master plan and a powerful use of my cancer. I will be obedient. I will go where You say and write what You say. Stay present in my mind and heart; let my words be Your words.

Obediently Yours, Janet

 ## A Sister Shares

Today I gave my testimony for the third year at Christian Outreach Week. I'm sure it blessed others, but not as much as it blessed me. This year Randy asked to speak with me on how my cancer brought him back to the Lord. God does answer prayers in mysterious ways, and does work everything for good to those who believe, and does answer a mother's most fervent prayer for the soul of her beloved son. During Randy's portion of our talk, I felt so much love! Randy previously asked me how to get the head knowledge of Christ into his heart. Well, I saw that happening as he talked emotionally about how my cancer affected his life, while looking at me with so much love in his eyes. He was surprised so many mothers heard his message as one of "The Prodigal Son," which gave them hope for their wayward children. A girlfriend approached me and said, "Randy will be a great man of God." What a *grand purpose* for my cancer. —Nancy Tuttle[7]

 ## Mentoring Moment

Once we accept there is a purpose, the next step is to stay in tune with God as to what, where, and how He will use our breast cancer to further His kingdom work. It will be different for each of us and fit our personalities, talents, gifts, and environments. He will fulfill His purpose and plan in our lives if we let Him.

In the "Sanity Tools," appendix B, you'll find My Breast Cancer Purpose and Plan. It is a place for you to brainstorm and pray for God to reveal how He plans to use your breast cancer.

God's Love Letter to You

Dear_____, *(fill in your name)*

Give yourselves to me, God. Surrender your whole being to me to be used for righteous purposes (Romans 6:13 TEV).
I will use you, God

Let's Pray

Prayerfully personalize Psalm 119:137–46 MSG.

Father, you are a purposeful God . . . your promise has been tested through and through, and I, your servant _____, love it dearly. . . . Your righteousness is eternally right, your revelation is the only truth. Even though troubles came down on me hard, your commands always gave me delight. The way you tell me, _____, to live is always right; help me understand it so I, _____, can live to the fullest. I, _____, call out at the top of my lungs, "GOD! Answer! I'll do whatever you say." I called to you, "Save me so I, _____, can carry out all your instructions." Amen.

Talking about Your Breast Cancer on Purpose

You just don't realize the impact of someone choosing to use their public position for a really personal thing. —Martha Maynard, president of the San Antonio affiliate of the Susan G. Komen Breast Cancer Foundation

In the past Nancy suffered from breast cancer and I had my cancer surgeries. We found that through our open disclosures, we were able to raise public awareness. We were happy that as a result many more people underwent testing. —The late president Ronald Reagan, announcing that he had Alzheimer's

I COULD WRITE A BOOK FULL OF THE DETAILS OF YOUR GREATNESS. —PSALM 145:6 MSG

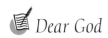 ## Dear God

Dear God,

Growing up, *breast cancer* was a hush-hush term. Probably because no one publicly wanted to say, "breast." I am amazed how many women never mention their breast cancer. You know I don't want my breast cancer wasted. I feel my speaking platform to large numbers of women is an important reason You allowed me to experience this. What can I say to help them? A message of hope and faith. Please help me present it in a way that draws attention to You, not me. This won't be easy. It means reliving breast cancer over and over, but to You be the glory. Let me know how little or how much to say. Give me words that aren't prideful or martyr sounding. Help me focus on You and all those who shared in my pain and recuperation. Grant me encouraging, compassionate words and listening ears to absorb others' stories. Remind me to pray for them. Thank You for all those who prayed for me after hearing my story. Let it be Your story told through me.

Your storyteller, Janet

 ## Three Sisters Share

Leslie Mouton, thirty-six at the time, an anchorwoman for KSAT-TV and a Christian, used her public role to educate viewers on her private battle in a three-part series. The first night she still had hair; viewers saw her lying on an operating table as her voice narrated. The second report showed Leslie crying during her first chemotherapy treatment. But the third night she went before the cameras without her wig. "This is my reality," she told viewers. "I'm bald." As some hinted that she might have done this as a ratings ploy, she said, "No, this was God's time line."[8]

Brenda Ladun, a young mother with three children under six and an anchorwoman for ABC 33/40 in Birmingham, told the world about her breast cancer. "I decided soon after I was diagnosed that I had to share this news with others. *If I felt this good,* I thought to myself, *and I had cancer growing inside of me, I have to warn others. There were other mothers, sisters, and daughters out there with a killer growing inside of them . . . and they didn't even know it.*" She wrote and taped an announcement for the day of surgery and it aired on the six o'clock news while she was still in a 13-hour surgery. After the announcement, her coanchor said that instead of sending flowers, please make donations to the Susan G. Komen Breast Cancer Foundation and that ABC 33/40 was providing free mammograms in Brenda's honor through a local hospital. The next Saturday more than a hundred women got free mammograms. "Do I regret going public? I wondered if I would. I didn't know how people would react. But I've received only more blessings from sharing my diagnosis with viewers. . . . James Spann, our meteorologist, is highly respected and well known as a Christian in our community. I told him I was going public with the news, and he said, 'This is your mission.' And it remains my mission, to warn people about cancer and ease the blow in some small way."[9]

Dr. Carolyn Kaelin, a breast cancer specialist, teacher at Harvard Medical School, and mother of two young children, was in her forties when she self-diagnosed breast cancer. Dr. Kaelin bravely and kindly allowed an interview with Diane Sawyer on national TV during *Good Morning America.* During the interview Dr. Kaelin pointed out that in-between diagnosis and her own surgery, it seemed so surreal to be sitting next to her own patients, knowing she would soon be a patient herself. Chemotherapy was an eyeopener, giving her new insight and allowing her to walk in the footsteps of her patients. She said, "The fatigue levels you. Food tastes like tinfoil for ten days after a treatment." Humbly, with a big smile on her face, she shared, "I learned lessons of humanity through the painful process and the sleepless, longest night of waiting between the biopsy and the diagnosis."

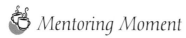 Mentoring Moment

These women chose television to go public with their breast cancer. They demystified breast cancer and came alongside every viewer with breast cancer and said, "It's OK to be bald. Don't feel you need to hide your illness, but at the same time life can and will go on for you."

We don't have to be a TV anchorwoman or a famous doctor or a president's wife to go public. When and if we are willing to talk openly about our breast cancer, God will put women in our paths who need to hear our encouraging and frank words. If you want to talk about your breast cancer, do it. If you don't, that's OK too. Don't feel guilty either way.

Understandably, you may not want to talk much in the beginning while still wrapping your arms around this whole experience of having breast cancer, or you might not be able to stop talking about it. We all have different styles and personalities. Some talk through everything; others internalize and process. Some can't find the words; others fear being misunderstood, so they hold it all inside. My prayer is for this book to be a safe place for you to talk to God. No judgment, only love. Talking is healing. If you have a safe friend, start there. God may eventually want to use you to help someone else, so talking about your breast cancer lets others know you are available.

Be prepared that talking about your breast cancer could take you one step further, as Heather discovered. "When you've shown your breast to a total stranger in the restroom of a restaurant, there's nothing sacred," Heather said, explaining how it can help a woman determine whether to have a mastectomy or lumpectomy. Grace Marestaing, who had a double mastectomy and reconstruction, does the same on the days she volunteers at the BreastCare Center.

Going public requires openness, vulnerability, and possibly literal nakedness to help another woman make a decision that will be with her for the rest of her life. For practice, speak first about comfortable things in surroundings that won't embarrass you or others. Support groups are a safe place because everyone is in similar circumstances. Nothing you say there is too personal or gruesome, because they have experienced it too.

Men may be uncomfortable with the topic of breast cancer in a couple's group, although I see more and more men open to the discussion. It is important we don't talk about our illness to get attention or put the focus on us. Instead, we speak in a way that lets others know how they can help or that we are willing to help them.

📖 God's Love Letter to You

Dear_____, (fill in your name)

Following the directions and doing the things that I, GOD, commanded Moses for Israel will make you successful. Courage! Take charge! Don't be timid; don't hold back (1 Chronicles 22:13 MSG paraphrased). Your Source of Courage, God

🙌 Let's Pray

Prayerfully personalize Daniel 10:16–18.

Heavenly Father . . .

Then one who looked like a man touched my, _____'s lips, and I, _____, opened my mouth and began to speak. I, _____, said to the one standing before me, "I am overcome with anguish because of the vision, my lord, and I, _____, am helpless. How can I, _____, your servant, talk with you, my lord? My strength is gone and I, _____, can hardly breathe." Again the one who looked like a man touched me and gave me strength. Amen.

A New Boldness

As a nurse, God definitely uses me when I talk with my patients facing potentially life-threatening situations. I know what it's like and can share my faith and what works for me. —Darlene M.

I START TALKING ABOUT YOU, GOD, TELLING WHAT I KNOW, AND QUICKLY RUN OUT OF WORDS. —PSALM 40:5 MSG

I WILL PRAISE THE LORD AT ALL TIMES. I WILL CONSTANTLY SPEAK HIS PRAISES. I WILL BOAST ONLY IN THE LORD; LET ALL WHO ARE DISCOURAGED TAKE HEART. COME, LET US TELL OF THE LORD'S GREATNESS; LET US EXALT HIS NAME TOGETHER. —PSALM 34:1–3 NLT

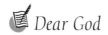 ## Dear God

Dear God,

There is a new sense of urgency. People are dying every day without eternal salvation. I can speak to what it feels like to be OK with dying. Of course, I would rather stay here with my family longer, but I rest in the assurance that when my time comes—and it will—I am ready to go. Many people today are not.

Not too surprising . . . breast cancer made me bolder than usual. You know I've not been afraid to ask anyone if he or she is a Christian, but now it seemed I had to know. Some people in the medical profession were just so matter-of-fact about their work. I am pretty resilient, but many others aren't. Could I soften them for the next patient? Remember all the prayers asking for wisdom of what to say to whom? "Lord, give me 'a word' for them," my heart repeatedly pleaded.

I particularly remember the woman administering dye for the lymph-node mapping. She was nice but reserved. Trying to adjust to dye shooting through my veins, I struck up a conversation. Most people ask me what I do. Often, they are not ready for my answer, "I'm a Christian author and speaker." That brings a variety of responses. At best, they ask what I write and speak about. My explanation about writing the Woman to Woman Mentoring resources and my passion of helping women get closer to God and each other is sometimes a conversation stopper, but other times it leads them to ask, "What do you mean by 'Christian author'?" Others talk about their own faith or lack of it. In this case, the woman was a Christian, but her husband wasn't. I told her about the book *Power of a Praying Wife* and encouraged her to get it. She said she would.

Boldly Yours, Janet

♡ *A Sister Shares*

While volunteering at the BreastCare Center, if a patient I'm working with knows the Lord, the spiritual link is made and I reinforce my experience with breast cancer as a person of faith and the comfort I received from the Lord. But one thing I say to all patients I work with is they will be on my personal prayer list. I have never had any person reject that offer. —Grace Marestaing

Mentoring Moments

The evangelist Bill Bright once said, "Although I have shared Christ personally with many thousands of people through the years, I am a rather reserved person and I do not always find it easy to witness. But I have made this my practice, and I urge you to do the same: assume that whenever you are alone with another person for more than a few moments, you are there by divine appointment to explain to that person the love and forgiveness he can know through faith in Jesus Christ."[10]

Perhaps you accepted Christ for the first time while reading and journaling in this book. That is good news to share with everyone. When someone asks how you are feeling, how about answering, "I am so blessed because I have eternal life and Jesus Christ as my Savior. It couldn't get much better than that. Right now I am experiencing difficult times, but I am so glad Jesus is there to comfort me. Do you know Him too?"

Or maybe you're a longtime Christian. Sometimes familiarity brings complacency. Now is the time to put your faith on the line. Others will look to see if you truly believe what you profess. Try not to miss witnessing occasions. Does your doctor, nurse, technician, or fellow patient know the Lord? Maybe God's plan and purpose is for you to introduce that person to the great Healer and Physician, Jesus Christ. Staying strong is tough—even for a Christian, but our call is to live out our faith.

You still may be seeking and wondering about accepting Christ. You've been journaling and praying throughout this book, but you're still unsure. Your boldness might take the form of asking questions of Christians whom God puts in your path. Ask for help understanding where God is when you are sick. Find those who can assure you He is right beside you, sharing the pain.

📖 God's Love Letter to You

Dear_____, (fill in your name)

    Always be prepared to give an answer to everyone who asks you to give the reason for the hope that you have. But do this with gentleness and respect (1 Peter 3:15). You will receive power when the Holy Spirit comes on you; and you will be my witnesses . . . to the ends of the earth (Acts 1:8).

Your Boldness Provider, God

🙌 Let's Pray

Prayerfully personalize Psalm 138:2–3.

I, _____, will praise your name for your love and your faithfulness, for you have exalted above all things your name and your word. When I, _____, called, you answered me; you made me bold and stouthearted. Amen.

✒ Your Letter to God

Is your life focus and purpose changing? Have you asked God how He wants to use your breast cancer, or is it too painful right now? Let God know how hard this is but how freeing it will be to find a purpose in the pain and a way to use it for His glory. Are you struggling with how much to say when and where? Sit awhile and listen to His quiet, gentle answers. Have you considered God might use your breast cancer to help others know Him? Ask for bold courage and a revelation of when and what to speak. If you seized opportunities, journal the experience.

Dear God, _____   *Date:* _____

_____

_____

_____

_____

_____

_____

CHAPTER EIGHTEEN

Living with Breast Cancer

I'M PROUD TO PRAISE GOD,
PROUD TO PRAISE GOD.
FEARLESS NOW, I TRUST IN GOD;
WHAT CAN MERE MORTALS DO TO ME?
GOD, YOU DID EVERYTHING YOU PROMISED,
AND I'M THANKING YOU WITH ALL MY HEART.
YOU PULLED ME FROM THE BRINK OF DEATH,
MY FEET FROM THE CLIFF-EDGE OF DOOM.
NOW I STROLL AT LEISURE WITH GOD
IN THE SUNLIT FIELDS OF LIFE.

—Psalm 56:10–13 MSG

How to Let Others Know You're Not Back Yet

Emily secured a date for homecoming. I have to take her shopping at the mall to find a dress. I will ask Grandma to come along as I get tired after about an hour and have to park myself with the "older" generation while she shops. There is nothing like having to wait for someone to take you somewhere to run a small errand. Even though your loved ones don't mind, it can still be frustrating. —Linda M.

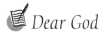 Dear God

Dear God,

I find myself repeatedly telling friends and family, "You know, I may look like I'm back, but I'm not. I don't have energy, memory, or endurance. I still need your help. It makes me feel bad to ask you, but my energy cup is often empty." You know I want to look good and not look sick. I want quickly to resume my normal activities, but I find there are new limits to my endurance. My family and friends have limits, too, and I am sure they are tired of me being sick and helpless. They are also fearful, and fear is draining. They want the old mom, wife, friend, and ministry worker back in action because it tells them I'm OK. I think sometimes they need that reassurance more than I do.

Still, trying to make a comeback too soon could ruin all the good work You did in healing me. I search for the right words. Sometimes, feeling so overwhelmed, I burst out crying; then they "get it." I don't want to push it to that point or come across as a martyr either. Lord, I don't want anyone thinking I am dragging this out to get attention or help. Believe me, I would rather do things myself. You know that about me. I guess they do too. Oh Lord, this is a struggle. I don't like being hysterical. Give me the words and timing to convey how much I value their help and still need it.

I'll be back, Janet

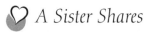 A Sister Shares

I need to say some thank-yous to you who continually supported my family by sending food. We so enjoyed it, and when I have a treatment, you can pretty much count out the other two [her husband and daughter, Emily] cooking or cleaning. It waits for at least seven days to get normal again. So the food really helps them out, and they enjoy the surprise goodies you send our way! I firmly believe that once you become a mom, there is no being ill allowed. No matter how sick you become, you still have to take care of your "babies." —Linda M.

☕ *Mentoring Moments*

As I conversed with fellow patients in the radiation-center waiting room, I discovered a common complaint you probably also experienced. Once past the immediate crisis of diagnosis and surgery, family and friends often are ready for you to get back to "normal" again—not your new normal but your old normal. Cancer treatment involves a series of events that drag on week after week, and people have to return to their daily activities, and they want you to do the same. They might put things on hold during those first crucial weeks, but they reach their limit. Always a trusted few hang in until the very end, but even they often need reminding that while you might look good on the outside, healing is still taking place on the inside.

Feelings of guilt arise because you, too, think you should be "up and at it" again sooner than your body is ready. Talk to your doctors about this, and ask what is realistic for your stage of recovery. Then objectively present the doctor's explanation and terms to those around you. Hearing this from your doctor may help them receive and internalize it better. Don't be afraid to say something like this: "Hey, gang, nobody wants to be back to normal faster than I do, but I'm not there yet. With your continued help, it will come. Please hang in with me a little longer. I promise not to abuse your graciousness. I love you and appreciate all you have done and look forward to returning to my activities as soon as possible. With Christ as my strength, and you as my earthly support, I will be back soon."

That might be a little flowery for you, but personalize it to something those close to you will appreciate and understand. I had to sit my husband and children down on more than one occasion and lovingly remind them, "Remember, I'm not back yet." The important thing is not trying to meet others' expectations of when you should be "back." Even your doctors will tell you everyone is different. They can only give averages or what usually happens. No one but God and you know your timetable; and remember, you have a new definition of *normal*.

A number of the ladies who sent in stories for this book, like me, went through cancer treatment during Christmas. The one common thread I saw was we all commented on what a great Christmas it was because it was simple and quiet. Linda M. said, "We had a quiet

Christmas, which was extremely wonderful—didn't have to do a lot of running around and not a lot of expectations." Bonnie said, "It was the quietest and least festive Christmas we have ever had, but yet very poignant." I found the same thing. Making it simple made it more enjoyable.

Ask others to pray for your family to adjust to the changes in you and the household. Linda M. had an e-mail force of prayer warriors, and she delighted in seeing the answered prayers: "My husband and daughter have now become a team. The two of them have really surprised me. I suggested they make some of the decisions themselves. It is such a relief to see the two of them developing into adults together. Someone was really devoting prayer time to this one!"

God's Love Letter to You

Dear_____, (fill in your name)
Put away all falsehood and "tell your neighbor the truth" because we belong to each other (Ephesians 4:25 NLT).
Helping you with your comeback, God

Let's Pray

Prayerfully personalize with me Colossians 1:11–12 MSG.

Lord Jesus . . .

We, _____ and Janet, pray that we'll have the strength to stick it out over the long haul—not the grim strength of gritting our teeth but the glory-strength God gives. It is strength that endures the unendurable and spills over into joy, thanking the Father who makes us, _____ and Janet, strong enough to take part in everything bright and beautiful that he has for us. Amen.

You Need an Outlet

Radiation made me nauseous . . . during this time I did research on our family tree. —Grace Bell

Breast cancer was a message to change. It provided the opportunity to experience a precious wilderness time with God. I read a book about intercessory prayer and learned how much God covets our prayers and acts on them. This was my entrance to intercessory prayer. I am now on the prayer team for my church. —Lynn

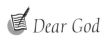 *Dear God*

Dear God,

You know how busy I always keep myself with doing "purposeful" things. Writing, speaking, and ministry fill my days and nights. Those still are so important, but strangely, cancer has awakened a desire to try something I have never done before. Please help me know what that might be and how it could help my recovery both physically and mentally.

Searchingly Yours, Janet

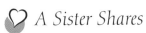 *A Sister Shares*

The New Year brought my last three chemo treatments and a nomination by my Girl Scout leader peers for the honor of carrying the Olympic torch in the 1996 Torch Relay as a community hero. . . . I was worried about my stamina, which was not good. The torch was coming through Knoxville in late June. Hopefully by then, my cancer experience would be behind me. The day of the run a motorcyclist came ahead and turned a knob at the bottom of my torch. He handed it back to me. "Enjoy your moment!" Claresse Hobbs approached me. We touched our torches high. She hugged me, and it was all mine . . . I proudly represented Girl Scouts and breast cancer survivors. . . . I watched as Mohammed Ali took my flame and lit the caldron to open the Atlanta games. I listened as Celine Dion sang the song specifically written for the Olympics. One sentence held me. "There's nothing ordinary in the living of each day." I savored my moment. I am grateful to be alive. I traveled a great distance that year. It was a year of extremes, good and bad. I no longer take life for granted. I don't sweat the small stuff. I don't know what the future holds for me, but I do know there was a rainbow at the end of my tunnel. —Bonnie[1]

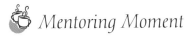 *Mentoring Moment*

Like Bonnie and me, are you at a point where venturing into something new sounds exciting? Is there something you always wanted to do but never took the time before? Now, with a new definition of *time,* you are thinking to yourself, *Why not give it a try?* The BreastCare Center has a Center for Wellness, which provides a newsletter and catalog of activities and programs designed for healing the total body. Everything from drumming—yes, beating on a drum—to creative art classes—to the Laughter Club. I am not artistic or creative, but my "Grace Abounds" was teaching a creative art course, so I thought, *Why not? I'll support Grace.* I actually learned how to make a gift book! It was fun and different.

Grace also bought an annual pass to Disneyland, which is near her home so she can go there for daily walks. She said it is entertaining and she feels safe walking there at night. Grace knows the exact miles around Frontier Land, Fantasy Land, and all the other lands. What a novel idea! The night I visited the Saddleback Church Breast Cancer Support Group, Darlene Gee had a bag full of pictures she took while on a two-week mission trip to Africa with our church just a little over three years after her last mastectomy surgery. Her eyes glowed, and her face was radiant as she kept us laughing and crying with stories from the trip. She also has hiked the Grand Canyon since her surgery!

I read in a magazine about a woman who found emotional healing from baking cakes. She said, "During difficult times, we all do different things to help us heal. I found that in my own life, during my darkest, worst days, my therapy was to bake. I've always found that [crises are] a great opportunity to learn something new—there's great growth in that. . . . I think if you get out of yourself, you're able to view yourself in a different light and view your strengths. You've got to move out of the position and activate the creative part that's in yourself. And I think if you dip into those talents, you've got them for life."[2]

My husband and I joke that my recovery entailed revamping our entire kitchen! I took great delight in learning about juicing and eating raw and organic, which meant I researched and bought a juicer, smoothie maker, high-speed blender, food processor, toaster oven that dehydrates, special containers for ripening and keeping raw fruits and veggies—just for starters. We no longer used a microwave, so I also bought stainless steel pots and pans and two sets of dishes that were ovenproof for heating up leftovers in the toaster oven. Our kids say, "Mom, every time we come, you have a new set of dishes!" I thought to myself, *Why not?* Who knows how many more sets of dishes I will enjoy in my lifetime?

Next, I had fun researching and comparative shopping in health-food stores that carried organic foods. This was quite a project as I read labels and learned my way around. Now instead of dreading shopping, it is exciting and fun. I can hardly wait to try a new healthy recipe or a different way of food preparation.

Karen mentioned she took a psychology class during her difficult chemo treatments. Do you enjoy or would you like to learn gardening? cooking? sewing? playing an instrument? writing poetry? traveling? exercising? quilting? photography? making memory books? taking computer classes? painting? researching the family tree? Fill in the blank _____ _____, and like the Nike commercial, now is the time to "Just do it!"

📖 *God's Love Letter to You:*

Dear_____, (fill in your name)

You should use whatever gift you have received from me to serve others, faithfully administering my grace in its various forms. If you speak, do it as one speaking my very words. If you serve, do it with the strength I, God, provide, so that in all things I may be praised through my Son, Jesus Christ. To him be the glory and the power for ever and ever (1 Peter 4:10–11 paraphrased).
Creative Gift Giver, God

🙏 *Let's Pray*

Father, we are tired of being sick and having our lives revolve around breast cancer. Awaken in us a desire to do something new . . . maybe something we have never considered before or a project we thought would be a luxury. Please free us from any guilt or concern that this might be "wasting time." Remind us that our earthly time is but a moment, that we should do today the things You put on our hearts and not wait until tomorrow . . . for tomorrow might never come. Thank You for the gift of ideas and creativity that no amount of cutting, radiating, or chemo drugs can ever take from us . . . Your Spirit prevails in our hearts. We love You, Lord. Amen.

It Could Come Back

I am living with cancer, not dying from cancer. —Angel

I struggle with the fear of the cancer returning and wondering if the strong support system will be there again if that happens. —Cindy

My cancer has returned, and I have been undergoing lots of tests and some very aggressive treatments. The chemo I'm taking is a very strong mix of some of the newest medicines, and it makes me very sick, but it is working. My tumors are shrinking! —Edna

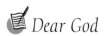 *Dear God*

Dear God,

The word *recurrence* must be part of my vocabulary. I don't want it to be . . . I don't want to think about it, but it always hangs over my head. Every time someone asks if I am OK, I respond that the doctors say I should have 100 percent recovery, but I truly feel only as safe as my last mammogram or doctor appointment. Even awaiting another six-month mammogram next week, I know there is always a chance breast cancer could return. There are too many stories of recurrence to ignore that possibility. How would the family deal with that? Would everybody be there for me again or be burned out on breast cancer and not able to deal with it anymore? Oh Lord, I cannot imagine how lonely that would be. It was so hard the first time; it must be devastating to relive it. In many ways cancer is like living with a time bomb. You don't know if it is defused or if it's ticking away, ready to catch you off guard and blow your life apart again . . . maybe this time actually taking you to a place of no return. I have to admit these thoughts go through my mind at random times.

Lord, I must put my complete faith and trust in You. I will do everything the doctors tell me to do when they tell me to do it . . . no playing games with this . . . and I pray You continue to protect me and restore me to complete health. However, if there should be a recurrence, I also pray my family and friends would rally back around me, and You would give the doctors the same wisdom and insight You did the first time. Let them catch it early again—breast cancer will not win the battle for my life.

Confidently Yours, Janet

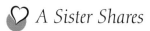 *A Sister Shares*

Hello, my faithful prayer warriors! Most of you heard I had an MRI, bone scan, and CT scan that said my breast cancer had spread to my thoracic spine, after nine and a half years! After waiting an agonizing two weeks, we got the news that the PET scan was negative, which means there is no cancer in any of my body—even the bones! Our prayers were answered, praise God! Therefore, we are singing, dancing, and thanking the Lord for His loving kindness. Love, Sue

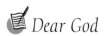 *Mentoring Moment*

This was a very difficult section to write, and yet I knew I must. There are so many of you living the fear of recurrence right now, and some of the ladies who shared with you in this book have also experienced the much feared and dreaded recurrence:

- Sue escaped, praise the Lord.

- Angel has had recurrences in her neck, hip, lungs, and brain, all from her original breast cancer site. The good news is, they have found no new sites of origin, and so far they have been able to combat each new tumor that rears its ugly head. However, she will have chemotherapy every three weeks for the rest of her life and never ignore a new pain, ache, or lump.

- Linda M.'s breast cancer first identified itself in her bones. As doctors traced the site of origin to her breast, she awaits a double mastectomy.

- Edna's breast cancer returned.

- Della recovered fully from her recurrence.

- Heather had a new site in her other breast and had a double mastectomy two days ago.

- Nancy Tuttle's recurrence ended a seven-year battle with breast cancer.

- Leslie's recurrence took her life while I was writing this book.

A recent study found that only 63 percent of women were getting annual mammograms five years after breast cancer surgery. Speculated reasons—complacency after the initial scare, but more likely, fear of a recurrence. Please don't let yourself fall into this statistic. A recurrence detected early enough can have a good outcome. Yes, it's scary, but don't let fear stop you from taking care of your future health.

There is a fine line between unnecessary worry and following up about every little pain. Angel said her first indication of the brain tumors was a ringing in her ears, which her doctors attributed to the medication she was on, but she relentlessly pursued a brain scan, which showed, indeed, she did have two brain tumors. Later she had pain in her hip, and the doctor wanted to give her a cane and pain medication, but again her insistence that she have a bone scan revealed a tumor in her hip.

I asked Angel if she was surprised at the recurrence of her breast cancer, and her response was, "Total shock." She had not lived life looking for it to happen again and did not expect it after having the positive lymph nodes removed during her original surgery. In fact, the news that her cancer had returned sent her into a complete nervous breakdown. Angel warns that it is so important to select a doctor who is responsive to your questions and requests and includes you in the course of treatment. You must be an active participant in this battle. If a doctor tells you he will be in charge and you will only do what he says, pursue with him your desire to participate in your treatments. It would be much easier to sit back and let the doctors take care of everything, but remember, as gifted as they are, they are human just like you and I. And no one . . . absolutely no one . . . knows your body better than God and you.

God's Love Letter to You

Dear_____, (fill in your name)

Oh, how sweet the light of day, and how wonderful to live in the sunshine! Even if you live a long time, don't take a single day for granted. Take delight in each light-filled hour, remembering that there will also be many dark days but most of it is just smoke. You who are young, make the most of your youth. Relish your youthful vigor. Follow the impulses of your heart. If something looks good to you, pursue it. But know also that not just anything goes; you have to answer to me for every last bit of it (Ecclesiastes 11:7–9 MSG paraphrased).
Always with you, God

Let's Pray

Prayerfully personalize with me Romans 8:38–39 NLT.

Dearest Lord Jesus . . .

We, _____ and Janet, are convinced that nothing can ever separate us from your love. Death can't, and life can't. The angels can't, and the demons can't. Our, _____ ____'s and Janet's, fears for today, our worries about tomorrow, and even the powers of hell can't keep your love away. Whether we are high above the sky or in the deepest ocean, nothing in all creation will ever be able to separate us from the love of God that is revealed in You, Christ Jesus our Lord. Amen.

Eliminating Stress

The doctor ordered me a wheelchair so I can do some strutting since I can't walk for long periods of time. With my new, blue, trusty chair I won't worry about tiring out. I'll just worry about the person pushing me tiring out. I was kind of embarrassed to ask for it, but it will enable me to go further now. —Linda M.

I had a very active, high-stress lifestyle because I thought I was invincible. Cancer is something that happened to other people. It couldn't happen to me. —Margaret Kelly[3]

I am tired of feeling stressed about things I have no control over. —Nancy Tuttle[4]

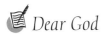 ## Dear God

Dear God,

I read so many studies that prove how damaging stress is to our bodies. It hits us at our weakest points. I don't know if stress had anything to do with my breast cancer, but I do know my whole body would benefit from a more relaxed and less worried lifestyle. Being the Type A, productive person You made me, I know this is not going to be easy. Please point out when I am worrying unnecessarily, and help me learn techniques to eliminate stressful thinking. My mind is so active that it often gets me into trouble.

As I begin to feel better, there are glimpses of the old "doer" Janet returning. I need balance. I want to do all You want me to do and learn not to worry about the rest. This will be a stretch, but I know with Your help I can do it! Thank You, Lord, for pointing out that this could make a huge difference in regaining my health and staying healthy, as well as model to my children and friends how not to get caught up in the world's idea of a productive life.

Cool and calmly Yours, Janet

 ## A Sister Shares

There were actually some positives during my breast cancer journey. One is that life becomes very simple and focused; you don't have to make up excuses if you want or need to take a nap. It becomes very easy to say no to the things you don't really want to do.

However, as one regains wellness, life's schedules and obligations start pressing in again. I went from working twelve-to-fourteen-hour days, sometimes seven days a week, to an entirely different kind of pace. This took some learning. I remember a day when I felt pretty bad but thought I could "push through" the day's responsibilities. But there was another plan at work. My phone started ringing that morning, and for completely different reasons and circumstances all of the students scheduled for that day called to say they were not going to make their lessons. It was like they had gotten together in agreement, which I knew they hadn't—it was weird. I had a sense of my Holy Time Manager at work clearing my calendar and saying, "Today you need to listen to your body; be still and rest—and it's OK if you do." —Grace Marestaing

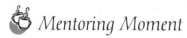 *Mentoring Moment*

Often, God will intervene like He did with Grace to point out we are pushing ourselves to the stressful breaking point and need to set boundaries. Or like Linda M., we must swallow our pride and admit we need assistance—even a wheelchair if necessary. Where do you carry your stress and how does it manifest itself in your life?

- ❏ Headaches?
- ❏ Stomachaches?
- ❏ Irritability?
- ❏ Nervousness?
- ❏ Sleeplessness?
- ❏ Backaches?
- ❏ Neck aches?
- ❏ Asthma flareups?
- ❏ Diarrhea?
- ❏ Exhaustion?
- ❏ High blood pressure?

It seems the more high-tech and convenience oriented our world becomes, the more stress filled our lives are. There is so much noise. Fax machines and phones ringing, e-mail in-boxes filling, TVs and radios blaring, kitchen appliances whirring, cars racing, cell phones singing, answering machines recording, computers talking, people yelling, music playing in stores, gyms, and restaurants—a world of bombarding sounds. And everything seems so urgent because people can reach us as much as we want to let them. This is not healthy, and America's health statistics speak to that. No one questions that stress has a negative impact on our health. As we move into menopause, we must consider our heart health as well as our breast health. Stress is not good for either.

After you identify your stress points, start looking for what stimulates them. Then one by one eliminate the causes. For example, I have trained myself not to react to things that do not need my immediate attention, and even some that do will just have to wait for a more convenient time. In taking a sabbatical to write this book, I had to let others take care of many things, which means they didn't always turn out the way I would like. When that happens, I consciously shift my focus to how glad I am they took care of it and let them deal with the results. Many have shined by my giving them the gift of *responsibility* and *authority*.

There have been those, like the friends of Job, who somehow feel they need to set my life straight, but I can *choose* not to react. I find blessed assurance in knowing I am doing just what God wants me to do, and I don't have time to receive or respond to their critical comments. Wow, that alone just reduced my stress level tremendously.

You, too, will find many have their opinions about what you should or should not do, and while well-meaning, they may cause your stress level to increase as you feel a knot in your stomach or pounding in your head. Don't go there. Stop at the first sign of stress. Pray and ask God to remove the stressful thought from your mind. Release it and don't go back. Every time the thought comes to your head, let it go again. Take deep, soothing breaths, and then slowly let them out . . . until your pulse is back to normal, the stress signs are gone, and there are no wrinkles on your forehead.

I realize many of you cannot isolate yourselves completely from stress. You may have young children who need attention, or you are self-supporting and have to get back to work. However, you still need to do the following:

- Let others help.

- Lower your expectations of them and you.

- Find some time each day to be alone with God.

- Practice some of the things we have talked about to bring calm to your spirit.

- Agree not to stress over the small stuff, and then remember . . . hey, in the big picture of life, it's all small stuff anyway.

You may need accountability in this—I do. My natural way of reacting and responding often comes into play, and it is my husband or best friend, Jane, who both remind me to let it go. We can make a change. It will make a difference. Our very lives depend on it.

📖 *God's Love Letter to You*

Dear_____,(fill in your name)

Humble yourselves under my mighty power, and in my good time, I will honor you. Give all your worries and cares to me, God, for I care about what happens to you. Be careful! Watch out for attacks from the Devil, your great enemy. He prowls around like a roaring lion, looking for some victim to devour. Take a firm stand against him, and be strong in your faith. Remember that your Christian brothers and sisters all over the world are going through the same kind of suffering you are. I, God, kindly called you to my eternal glory by means of my Son, Jesus Christ. After you have suffered a little while, he will restore, support, and strengthen you, and he will place you on a firm foundation (1 Peter 5:6–10 NLT paraphrased).

Your Stress Buster, God

🐰 *Let's Pray*

Prayerfully personalize Psalm 27:3–8 MSG.

Oh Lord, when I, _____, feel stressed, I come to you . . .

When besieged, I'm calm as a baby. Every one of us needs to pray; when the dam bursts, we'll be on high ground, untouched. I,_____, am asking you, GOD, for one thing, only one thing: to live with you in your house my whole life long. I, _____, will contemplate your beauty; I'll study at your feet. That's the only quiet, secure place in a noisy world. The perfect getaway, far from the buzz of traffic. Hold me, _____, head and shoulders above all who try to pull me down. I'm headed for your place to offer anthems that will raise the roof! Already I, _____, am singing God-songs; I'm making music to GOD. Listen, GOD, I'm calling at the top of my lungs: "Be good to me! Answer me!" When my heart whispered, "Seek God," my whole being replied, "I, _____, am seeking him!" Amen.

Releasing Fear

As a believer in Jesus Christ, I knew He had become a man and paid the debt for my sins by dying on the cross, that He had risen from the grave, and that I was assured of eternal life in heaven. So whether I lived or died, it was going to be OK. This helped me release much of my fear. —Nancy Tuttle[5]

THE LORD IS MY LIGHT AND MY SALVATION—SO WHY SHOULD
I BE AFRAID? THE LORD PROTECTS ME FROM DANGER—
SO WHY SHOULD I TREMBLE? —PSALM 27:1 NLT

A HEART AT PEACE GIVES LIFE TO THE BODY. —PROVERBS 14:30

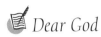 Dear God

Dear God,

The majority of time I am calm and at peace. I think most of my fear or nervousness comes from not liking the unknown. What damage will the radiation do? What will be the long-term effects? Will they decide ten years down the road that radiation was not such a good idea after all like they did with hormone replacement therapy (HRT)? How will we pay all the bills? Will this affect Kim? How will I adjust to the "new me"? What will I forget to do? Did I turn everything off? Blow out all the candles? Did I pay the bills with the right amount? It scares me when I look the next day at something I wrote and see transposed numbers or names.

What it sounds like, Lord, is my biggest fear is failure. Oh, now, that is scary! I am afraid I might do something wrong through my forgetfulness or maybe even fail at getting well and back to my old self. I know You do not want us living in fear and trembling. Lord, teach me to rest in You. To cast out the source of fear that would make me ineffective . . . paralyzed . . . compromised—knowing You want me effective . . . active . . . stopping at nothing in the life and ministry You gave me.

Fearfully Yours, Janet

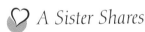 A Sister Shares

From the treatment options presented, I chose a complete mastectomy with seven months of chemotherapy. There wasn't time to think, feel, or assess anything. I couldn't even think about reconstruction; I just had to get through the treatments. It wasn't until months after the treatment was completed that I realized just how betrayed I felt. I was both angry and afraid. My left breast was gone, and my entire body image was destroyed. I had a very difficult time communicating just what I was thinking or feeling. I was extremely angry, yet there was no one to blame. There was no real explanation. My thoughts and feelings did not make any sense to me or anyone. I turned inward and isolated myself from my supporting family and friends. It took a lot of soul searching before I discovered my fears and anger were rooted in the loss of my independence and control. I felt like a failure.

It has been a long road of dealing and healing. I have learned to share my fears and to cry with those who love me. I have learned to have compassion for myself and to allow myself weaknesses and failures. I had to come to accept and understand that bad things happen to good people before I could let go of my anger. The Word of God reminds us not to worry about anything, but in everything to give praise and thanks to God. Why fret about the unpleasant things in our lives? We can't change anything by worrying. We don't have to be perfect to be acceptable. I still get anxious whenever its time for a checkup, but I have confidence I can face anything the future holds. I know I am not alone. My faith in God is strong, and my family is there for me. —Brenda N.

Mentoring Moment

What is it you fear? I know there has to be something—maybe actually there are multitudes of things. Don't chastise yourself or beat yourself up over your fears. Breast cancer is scary. Every time we say we had or have breast cancer, it brings that nagging fear back into our hearts. Writing this book and immersing myself in the topic 24/7 for months has demystified breast cancer, removed the stigma, and destroyed my fears. Yes, I encountered unnerving scenarios during my research—women who were terminal or had a recurrence— even sadly, some died or had already died, and I only know them by their memoirs. But those same months I also immersed myself in the Lord. I have searched and read the Scriptures and prayed nonstop that He would write with me and through me. I have asked others to support my writing through prayer. I encountered distractions too numerous to mention trying to discourage me, but Christ has spurred me on, and He will you too. There is no fear, no obstacle, no pain, no doubt, no worry, and no disappointment too big for our Lord. My prayer is that as you journal and write your own letters to God, you, too, will feel released from your fears.

God's Love Letter to You

Dear _____, *(fill in your name)*
    Can you add a single hour to your life by worrying? Since you cannot do this very little thing, why do you worry about the rest (Luke 12:25–26 paraphrased)?
Your Fear Buster, God

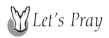 ## Let's Pray

Lord, you tell us in the Bible that Your perfect love casts out fear. We know You love us and we should not be afraid, but You are perfect, and we are not, and so we still fear. Help us put our faith in You and trust the plans You have for us. We don't want to waste a minute living anxiously. We cannot do this alone, but with Your help all things are possible. Amen.

Your Letter to God

Have you had to tell your family the hard truth that you are not back yet? How did that feel? Talk to God about something that would fulfill your heart's desire and be an appropriate adventure or experience. Ask for discernment to know when to follow up on a new ache or pain. Pray for removal of stress and fears. It is helpful to write down all the fears lurking in your mind—yes, *all* of them. Tell God you don't want to have ownership of them any longer, and ask Him to give you courage and confidence not to take them back.

Dear God,   *Date:*

Chapter Nineteen

Relying on God

I call to God; God will help me. At dusk,
dawn, and noon I sigh deep sighs—he hears,
he rescues. My life is well and whole,
secure in the middle of danger.

—*Psalm 55:16–18 MSG*

Can You Hear Him Now?

At the time, I knew no one who had breast cancer, so I shared my feelings and pains with my doctors, but mostly I talked with God. —Grace Bell

WE HEARD THE VOICE OUT OF HEAVEN WITH OUR VERY OWN EARS. —2 PETER 1:18 MSG

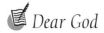 Dear God

Dear God,

You often speak to me through others. Like the day I was struggling with writing, and Grace e-mailed a scripture she prayed for me: "He who began a good work in you will carry it on to completion" (Philippians 1:6). Just the words You knew I needed to spur me on as I wearied. Another time she sent, "And do not forget to do good and to share with others, for with such sacrifices God is pleased" (Hebrews 13:16).

When it seemed my frozen shoulder and arm would not let me write another word, Grace e-mailed, "Love you, friend . . . keep writing, we will be like the guys that held up Moses's arms during the battle." Thank You, God, for speaking through Grace as Your encouraging voice to me and for showing me Your face.

Your listening servant, Janet

A Sister Shares

Standing in the shower with the warm water flowing over me, I began crying. I was drowning in pain emotionally and physically. It was more than I could bear. I felt so weak and small. I was of no use to anyone, and it just didn't seem there was any reason to fight this disease. I felt hope slipping quickly away. I am not one to ask God for something that might not be His will, but I prayed and begged between sobs that if there was any way He could spare me from this, please do so.

With my head against the shower wall, eyes closed, sobbing, I realized I was not alone. There was someone else praying a prayer like that also, asking His Father to save Him from an awful end. *He was now praying for me, with me.* A great calmness came over me, realizing it was Jesus. The painful tears passed, and I knew having cancer would change my life and become a blessing. A rare gift and privilege for me to carry. I went from despair to reconcilement, remembering God's promise that He would not give me more than I could handle—even cancer and all that comes with it. It brought such comfort. I was able to surrender all the worry, fear, anxiety, and pain. I knew I would be OK. I knew I could handle all of it. —Linda M.

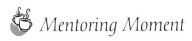 *Mentoring Moment*

Throughout this book I have given examples of God's revelations in the midst of my breast cancer journey. People long to hear God's voice or for His presence to be visible. They're looking for a burning-bush experience, but often God is not that dramatic. Instead, He takes *ordinary* life experiences and makes them *extraordinary*. Our job is not to let them pass by as coincidences.

I find the best way to hear God is to have meaningful time with Him daily. Psalm 37:4–7 in *The Message* reminds us to, "Keep company with GOD, get in on the best. Open up before GOD, keep nothing back; he'll do whatever needs to be done: He'll validate your life in the clear light of day and stamp you with approval at high noon. Quiet down before GOD, be prayerful before him." I always have my quiet-time bag ready with:

- My Bible

- Journal

- Highlighter

- Candle

- Lighter

- Pen and pencil

- Kleenex

- You could add your *Dear God, They Say It's Cancer* book.

Your quiet time with God might be the perfect time to read a section in this book and write "Your Letter to God," or just be still and listen.

God's Love Letter to You

Dear_____, (fill in your name)
Trust me, GOD, from the bottom of your heart; don't try to figure out everything on your own. Listen for my voice in everything you do, everywhere you go; I'm the one who will keep you on track. Don't assume that you know it all. Run to me (Proverbs 3:5–7 MSG paraphrased).
The Still, Small Voice, God

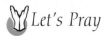 Let's Pray

Lord, You care enough to listen to our pleas and speak into our hearts. The intrusive din often drowns out Your soft and gentle whisper. Is it You waking us in the night wanting to talk? We long to be receptive to Your voice speaking through other people, circumstances, experiences, praise music, the Bible . . . Give us alone time and moments every day when all we hear is You. Still our minds and thoughts. Speak in ways we understand. Resting now in the sounds of stillness . . . wind chimes singing . . . birds chirping . . . children laughing . . . dogs barking . . . sounds of life. Amen.

God Always Answers Prayer

Our prayers are heard and answered. Sometimes not the way we expected, but answers eventually come. —Linda M.

> THE LORD HAS HEARD MY CRYING. THE LORD HAS HEARD MY PLEA;
> THE LORD WILL ANSWER MY PRAYER. —PSALM 6:8–9 NLT

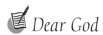 Dear God

Dear God,

I have felt the power of prayer throughout this difficult journey. There were times when I knew someone was praying for me and later learned they were. It was such a comfort knowing others, some whom I will never meet, were going before You on my behalf, even when I couldn't. Often women come up after a speaking engagement to say they have been praying for me. Just a couple of weeks ago after a Woman to Woman Mentoring Training in Baton Rouge, Louisiana, a woman took me aside and asked if she could pray for me right on the spot! Oh, I love that, Lord.

Please help me be sensitive to others' need for prayer. Remind me the best thing I can do for a physically or emotionally hurting woman is pray for her. Thank You for the many answered prayers.

Prayerfully Yours, Janet

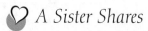 A Sister Shares

Mom and I are pure proof that prayers do work! We certainly didn't recover on our own. We have a lot of help and prayer. God has showed me "Ask and you shall receive" really happens. Because so many asked on my behalf, wonderful things happened in my life. I changed and I expect some of you changed also. It's no lie: prayer works. Is it just one religion? Well, there are at least six different religions praying for me. That is something to be said for prayer. I believe all of your prayers are answered. Now when I pray, I feel you praying for me as well. Sometimes I get this warm flush (besides the hot flashes) and know someone is out there saying a prayer for me. It brings much comfort, and I never feel alone and lost. Thank you for your never ceasing prayers for my family. —Linda M.

A Husband Shares

Most people of faith understand that while every prayer is heard, not every prayer is answered—at least not in the way we would like it to be. And that was the case with the many, many prayers and good wishes that were sent out on behalf of my beautiful wife, Marilyn "Tule" Dillow. I can hardly bear to write these words. But Tule died last week, at our home, as I held her hand, after a short, hard fight with advanced breast cancer. But Tule didn't fight her battle alone. And for that I want to extend my heartfelt thanks. Last fall, with Tule's permission, I wrote a column about her battle with breast cancer, the purpose being to encourage women and the people who love them to make sure they have regular and frequent breast exams. In that column I noted that neither Tule nor I was trying to elicit any sympathy. After all, every day people face tragedies and tribulations, and ours were not more inherently important or noteworthy than anyone else's. Nevertheless, afterward we were deluged with a constant flow of prayers and good wishes from readers, most of them people we didn't even know. Tule was amazed, and touched, by the kindness of strangers. It filled her heart and lightened her burden—and for that I will be forever grateful. —Gordon Dillow, reporter for the *Orange County Register*[1]

Mentoring Moment

Often women are shy about making prayer requests for themselves, but God does not want us to suffer in silence. Jesus says, "I tell you that if two of you on earth agree about anything you ask for, it will be done for you by my Father in heaven" (Matthew 18:19). There are so many verses reminding us to pray faithfully and sing praises when God answers, like David, "I'm singing at the top of my lungs, I'm so full of answered prayers" (Psalm 13:6 MSG).

However, God does not always answer prayer the way we think He should. He looks at the overall global picture, and *our* plans are not always *His* plans. An answer that we don't like is still an answer. Just like when kids ask for something and their parents say no. It wasn't the answer the kids wanted, but it was an answer. Looking at the greater good for their child, the parents may withhold what the child is asking for. God often does the same with us. We praise God if healing comes. But can we praise Him if healing doesn't happen? Being a follower of Christ *does not mean* we get a clean bill of health. It *does mean* Christ will be strong in us whether or not we have health.

Don't be bashful when people say they are praying for you or ask how they can pray for you. Thank them for their thoughtfulness, and tell them specifically where you need prayer. From the very first suspicion, we told people about the possibility it might be cancer because we knew the *best* way others could help was through prayer. That is the best way for you too. Then listen and look for His answers, and be sure to record them in the "Prayer-and-Praise Journal" on page 377. You will have an ongoing, encouraging record of the many ways God responded to your requests.

God's Love Letter to You

Dear_____, (fill in your name)
This is God, your God, speaking to you. Call for help when you're in trouble—I'll help you, and you'll honor me (Psalm 50:7, 15 MSG). Until now you have not asked for anything in my name. Ask and you will receive, and your joy will be complete (John 16:24).
Waiting for your prayers, God

Let's Pray

Prayerfully personalize Psalm 40:6–8 MSG.

Oh, precious Lord, I cast all my fears before You and I am listening and looking for Your answers. Help me to accept what I don't always understand . . .

You've opened my ears so I, _____, can listen. So I answered, "I'm coming. I, _____, read in your letter what you wrote about me, And I'm coming to the party you're throwing for me." That's when God's Word entered my life, became part of my very being. Amen.

Drawing Close to God

I grew closer to God through this valley by completely surrendering to His plan for my life.
—Linda Taylor

God's promise to be with me in the darkness of surgery kept my heart at peace as I faced each new surgery. —Grace Marestaing

THE LORD IS CLOSE TO THE BROKENHEARTED; HE RESCUES THOSE WHO ARE CRUSHED IN SPIRIT. THE RIGHTEOUS FACE MANY TROUBLES, BUT THE LORD RESCUES THEM FROM EACH AND EVERY ONE.
—PSALM 34:18–19 NLT

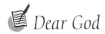 Dear God

Dear God,

I thought I was close to You before, but it was nothing like now. I am so aware of You in every aspect of my life. Throughout the day, I find myself talking to You, asking, which way to go? What to do with my time? What to say to a friend? What to write? It's as if during breast cancer You drew my heart into Yours in an unimaginable way. I felt broken many times in my life, but You must have felt I needed a deeper, more intense breaking to truly know You. There was still too much of me—it needs to be just about You.

Thank You for continuing to break me in all the right places. I want my heart to beat with Yours . . . and, yes, break with Yours. Continue to do with me what You must.

Sacredly Yours, Janet

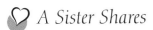 A Sister Shares

In April 2002 I heard the dreaded words, "Cancer again in the same breast." I was so nervous. I just *knew* it would be terminal this time. I wasn't afraid of dying, but I was fearful of a long, drawn-out illness. My surgeon recommended a radical mastectomy, and I chose reconstruction too. Thankfully, this time chemotherapy and radiation would not be necessary!

I recovered fully from the surgeries and now enjoy a full and busy life. Having cancer has taught me a lot about patience, and I now have more compassion for cancer patients and their problems. I value time with family and friends. I enjoy my church and have a closer relationship with God. I really appreciate life!
—Della

🍵 *Mentoring Moment*

Often we question, "Where is God in a crisis?" The answer—He is going through it with us. This world is not as good as it gets; it's just a dress rehearsal for the *real* life Christians will spend in eternity with Christ. The Lord says, "I have told you these things, so that in Me you may have [perfect] peace and confidence. In the world you have tribulation and trials and distress and frustration; but be of good cheer [take courage; be confident, certain, undaunted]! For I have overcome the world. [I have deprived it of power to harm you and have conquered it for you]" (John 16:33 AMP).

After the shock and fear of the dreaded diagnosis, many found it exciting watching evidences of God at every step. If it has been difficult for you to get close to God during your breast cancer, again I recommend seeking a spiritual mentor. As you draw closer to God in your crisis—and you will—and grow stronger spiritually—and you will—God is going to put someone in your life for you to mentor by teaching what you've been taught—and you will—right?

📖 *God's Love Letter to You*

Dear_____, *(fill in your name)*

Dear friend, do not be surprised at the painful trial you are suffering, as though something strange were happening to you. But rejoice that you participate in the sufferings of Christ, so that you may be overjoyed when his glory is revealed (1 Peter 4:12–13).
Suffering with you, God

🙌 *Let's Pray*

Prayerfully personalize with me Hebrews 10:22–23.

Lord, we ask You to lean in and hear our prayer. We come together praying . . .

Let us, _____ and Janet, draw near to you with a sincere heart in full assurance of faith, having our hearts sprinkled to cleanse us from a guilty conscience and having our bodies washed with pure water. Let us hold unswervingly to the hope we, _____ and Janet, profess, for You who promised are faithful. Amen.

Breast Cancer Tests Our Faith

I consider this gift of cancer a true testimony of faith. Of believing in the unknown. Of believing in a cure. God has showed me what true trust is: letting go of what bothers me most and believing He will take care of my family and me. Anyone with an illness or having lost someone needs to hold on to faith, hope, and trust. —Linda M.

*I put all my trust in God. He has given me a reason to fight this cancer.
—Angel*

*God taught me to trust Him in a way I'd never done before, and the
most important lesson—live one day at a time. —Grace Bell*

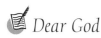 ## Dear God

Dear God,

I never trusted You more than during breast cancer . . . every
decision, risk, life-threatening or life-changing event . . . I take them all
to You and trust I am in Your will. With faith I can look at each new day
with renewed hope and courage. I must trust that even though I don't
like how the plan is going, You are OK with it! You are my hope.

I cannot imagine women going through this experience without
You . . . Oh how lonely and desolate they must feel. Please bring
others into their lives to pray for them and offer the hand of hope
only faith can afford. It is easy to follow where You lead when
everything is going right, but the true test of faith comes when it
isn't. I do believe. I do trust. I am Yours 100 percent!

Faithfully Yours, Janet

 ## A Sister Shares

I remember the night before my surgery when I didn't know if I was
going to live or die. I was struggling and pleading with God, telling
Him there could be no good in my children's not having a mother.
That simply could not be part of His plan for them. I was willing to
let the Lord take control of everything except my children, and, of
course, I had no peace. I got a phone call that night from an awesome,
godly friend who had lost her mother to breast cancer when she was
fourteen—my daughter was fourteen at the time. She shared that
although it was devastating and tragic, she would not be the person
she is today if she hadn't suffered that loss. I felt like God was telling
me to *trust* Him. I was able to pray a simple prayer telling God that
although I didn't understand the plans He has for me and probably
never would this side of eternity, I was surrendering my children to
Him, knowing He loves them even more than I do. It wasn't until

then that I could experience God's perfect peace, comfort, and strength, and finally relax in His arms. —Darlene Gee

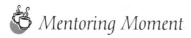 *Mentoring Moment*

Breast cancer can threaten our belief system as well as that of our families and friends. *What is God all about? I thought that being a Christian sheltered me from catastrophe.* Well, we only have to look at the life of Jesus or martyred missionaries to see that being a Christian does not eliminate pain and suffering. God never says we won't endure the same hardships as everybody else. What He does say is He will provide us with enduring *strength*, discerning *wisdom*, and sustaining *courage*. Trust takes time to develop.

We each seek doctors who share our treatment goals and vision for our future and replace doctors who gave up or were only willing to "manage" our illness instead of "fight" it. When it's time for surgery or treatments, and the anesthesia or chemo drips through our veins or radiation penetrates our bodies, we surrender complete trust in these human doctors. If we trust *imperfect* doctors with our lives, how much more should we trust a *perfect* God? He may choose to do "surgery" even without our signed approval or understanding, and we may never figure out His purpose this side of heaven; yet He still tells us to trust and obey. Can we do that yet? Can we have that kind of faith?

If you are seeking to know more about God or are a new Christian, know that developing trust and faith in God takes time, just like it did with your doctors. You had to meet with doctors, talk to them, watch their actions and reactions, and sense their sincere desire to do everything humanly possible for your best care. You will need to do those same things in developing your faith in God. For now, put your faith in His Word, the Bible, and look for ways God is evident in your life. Seek out those who know the Lord, and ask them to share how they have seen God real and alive in their lives.

We may not always like or agree with what God has planned for us, but because we know He has our best interest in mind, we trust Him. Some have called this "blind faith," but actually, it's just the opposite. He tells us, "You will seek me and find me" (Jeremiah 29:13). There are no coincidences in a believer's life—only God-incidences.

📖 *God's Love Letter to You*

*Dear*_____, *(fill in your name)*

Trust in me, the LORD, and do good. Then you will live safely in the land and prosper. Take delight in me, and I will give you your heart's desires. Commit everything you do to me. Trust me, and I will help you. Be still in my presence, and wait patiently for me to act (Psalm 37:3–5, 7 NLT paraphrased).

I AM Trustworthy, God

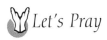 *Let's Pray*

Prayerfully personalize Psalm 56:3–4 MSG.

Our Lord and Father, we have complete faith and trust in You even though we do not completely understand why You are asking us to show it by going through breast cancer . . .

When I, _____, get really afraid I come to you in trust. I'm proud to praise God; fearless now, I, _____, trust in God. What can mere mortals do? Amen.

There Are "Angels" All Around

With the power of prayers from family and friends, God sent an angel to bring good news. The nurse called to say, "Your margins are free and clear!" —Gloria

GOD'S ANGEL SETS UP A CIRCLE OF PROTECTION AROUND US WHILE WE PRAY. —PSALM 34:7 MSG

PRAISE THE LORD, YOU ANGELS OF HIS, YOU MIGHTY CREATURES WHO CARRY OUT HIS PLANS, LISTENING FOR EACH OF HIS COMMANDS. YES, PRAISE THE LORD, YOU ARMIES OF ANGELS WHO SERVE HIM AND DO HIS WILL! —PSALM 103:20–21 NLT

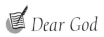 *Dear God*

Dear God,

I have felt lifted in the arms of angels throughout this breast cancer journey. Especially as I flounder around with my "Tamoxifen brain." So many stupid things I do, drop, forget . . . I feel angels there protecting me from harm or doing harm. Sometimes when I am tired or it is difficult to see while driving . . . like the time taking Kim to the airport early in the morning when I felt faint . . . it is as if angels did the driving. I am confident I will get home safely. Lord, I know someday those same angels are going to lift me up into Your presence, but for now, thank You for the many times they protect me and the many earthly angels You graciously put into my life.

Angelically Yours, Janet

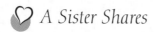 A Sister Shares

I remember looking at the doctor and saying, "You mean I will be on chemo for the rest of my life?" He said, "Yes." I made it out of his office and into the chemo room *before* breaking down. It takes between two to three hours to receive my treatment, and Mom and I cried the entire time. Toward the end, my favorite nurse came in to sit with us, and she brought me to a calmer state. I am sure that nurses who administer chemo must be angels. —Linda M.

Mentoring Moment

Grace Marestaing, my "Grace Abounds," is one of my angels. God placed her in my life with just the right combination of strength and quietness through the most devastating experience of my life. As I have shared, Grace always knows a scripture that will lift me up before she even knows what she is lifting me up out of!

There were so many "angels" God used to restore me during my weakest times. Shortly after surgery the kitchen cabinets needed emptying for our remodel, which was going on with or without me! Like an angel, my friend Cathy appeared at the front door with boxes and spent two days emptying every corner of my kitchen. She also promised not to give away any of my secrets, although she still talks about all the cans of tuna! When it was time to put everything back, radiation was taking its toll. My daughter Michelle was home for Christmas and lined all the new kitchen cabinets. Another friend, Lorna, called to say she had found the perfect Christmas fire screen to put in front of our remodeled fireplace. She later tackled a major upholstery project in our living room. My dear Jane and her husband wrapped all my grandchildren's Christmas presents, and Jane organized a food brigade that brought meals for two months.

I found great comfort in my "angels"—both earthly and heavenly—and I hope you do too. Of course, we can't see the heavenly ones, but we do see the earthly results. Someone offers assistance in areas where we need help. A check arrives in the mail to pay a medical bill. Brenda N. remembers during her mastectomy her teens were still very dependent on her for basic needs. Brenda says, "One day a lady came over, took my teenage son out to the garage, and showed him how to iron his own shirts, telling him that Mom could not do that anymore! What an earthly *angel* that woman was."

Look for the "angels" God puts in your life . . . they are there. Some you see; some work behind the scenes. Then one day you can be an angel to someone in need.

God's Love Letter to You

Dear_____, *(fill in your name)*

    Yes, because I, GOD, am your refuge, the High God of your very own home, evil can't get close

to you, harm can't get through the door. I order my angels to guard you wherever you go. If you stumble, they'll catch you; their job is to keep you from falling. If you'll hold on to me for dear life, I'll get you out of any trouble. I'll give you the best of care if you'll only get to know and trust me. Call me and I'll answer, be at your side in bad times; I'll rescue you, then throw you a party. I'll give you a long life, give you a long drink of salvation! (Psalm 91:9–12, 14–16 MSG paraphrased).
Your Guardian Refuge, God

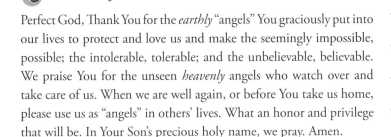 Let's Pray

Perfect God, Thank You for the *earthly* "angels" You graciously put into our lives to protect and love us and make the seemingly impossible, possible; the intolerable, tolerable; and the unbelievable, believable. We praise You for the unseen *heavenly* angels who watch over and take care of us. When we are well again, or before You take us home, please use us as "angels" in others' lives. What an honor and privilege that will be. In Your Son's precious holy name, we pray. Amen.

Our Hope Is in God

The miserable have no other medicine but only hope: I've hope to live and am prepared to die. —William Shakespeare[2]

Hope is never ill when faith is well.[3]

Several conversations in the last few days have reminded me where I came from with cancer to where I am today and the hope that I hold dear to me. —Linda M.

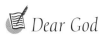 Dear God

Dear God,

Breast cancer brought a new awareness to every song we sing in church. And oh how many there are that talk about our only hope being in You. "My hope is in You Lord, my trust is in You Lord, my life is in You Lord . . . in You, it's in You." How many times we sing words like that and think, *Sure, I believe that,* but down deep we still place our hope in ourselves—our abilities, our strengths, and our efforts.

Breast cancer awakened in me the real truth that without You in my life, every day is hopeless . . . lacking meaning and purpose . . . just another day to mark off the calendar. Life is hectic, frantic, crazy, and futile without the hope that whether I live or die, it is all gain. So I live each day You give me, filled to the brim with the hope that I am walking the path You want for me and grateful that all the curves in the road and the valleys and gullies and cliffs and turns and switchbacks will eventually, in Your timing, end up at the foot of Your throne. Lord, keep me always ready to share my Source of hope.

Hopefully Yours, Janet

 ## A Sister Shares

God is our hope and promise. He is in control, and He does perform miracles. We are part of His family, and He does love us. Even when we are in serious trouble, we do not need to be afraid, but just trust Him. He is concerned about our daily needs, as well as our problems. He can see the big picture and knows what is best for us. We need to rest in Him, obey Him, and seek His will daily through prayer and reading the Scriptures. God looks at our hearts. Our problems can bring us closer to God and heal our hearts so we can reflect His light and love to others. I am waiting with patience for a new, healthy body, whether it be here on earth or in heaven with Jesus. Do you have that same hope? —Nancy Tuttle[4]

 ## Mentoring Moment

Nancy Tuttle wrote these words even as her cancer progressed to eventually end her earthly life and usher her into the presence of God. Her sustaining hope allowed others to see Jesus in her—including her son, Randall, who accepted Christ as his personal Savior as a result of watching his mom's faith and hope in the midst of her breast cancer. Hope is oxygen to our souls. We cannot live without it.

Never let anyone say your condition is *hopeless*. Even when Nancy was terminal, she was not hopeless, because her hope was not in the doctors or the length of this life. She knew that something bigger and better was waiting for her. And God is in the business of miracle making. We never know when a tumor will miraculously disappear. Or the test biopsy is positive, but the surgical biopsy is negative. On my eighteen-month check up they found suspicious calcium deposits again on the mammogram and scheduled me for a surgical biopsy. The morning of surgery they could not locate the area. It was gone. My family and friends witnessed a miracle.

There is nothing for sure except God. The Bible cautions us to stay prayerful and hopeful.

> Don't put your confidence in powerful people; there is no help for you there. When their breathing stops, they return to the earth and in a moment all their plans come

to an end. But happy are those who have the God of Israel as their helper, whose hope is in the LORD their God. He is the one who made heaven and earth, the sea, and everything in them. He is the one who keeps every promise forever. (Psalm 146:3–6 NLT)

Here are some ways to maintain life-sustaining hope when things *seem* hopeless:

- Don't keep company with "gloom and doom" people.

- Instruct doctors to tell you the truth but to stay hopeful in the way they treat and talk to you.

- Ask your family and friends to join you in hopeful discussions and thinking.

- Think how the negative can turn into a positive.

- Ask everyone you know to pray *expectantly* and *hopefully* for you.

📖 God's Love Letter to You

Dear_____, (fill in your name)

Always continue to fear me, the LORD. For surely you have a future ahead of you; your hope will not be disappointed. My child, listen and be wise. Keep your heart on the right course (Proverbs 23:17–19 NLT paraphrased). Your Wellspring of Hope, God

🙏 Let's Pray

Prayerfully personalize with me Romans 5:1–5.

Therefore, since we, _____ and Janet, have been justified through faith, we have peace with God through our Lord Jesus Christ, through whom we have gained access by faith into this grace in which we now stand. And we, _____ and Janet, rejoice in the hope of the glory of God. Not only so, but we also rejoice in our sufferings, because we, _____ and Janet, know that suffering produces perseverance; perseverance, character; and character, hope. And hope does not disappoint us, because God has poured out his love into our hearts by the Holy Spirit, whom he has given us. Amen.

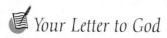 Your Letter to God

Have you seen God do the extraordinary in the ordinary? Is it difficult asking for personal prayers? Ask God to remove the stumbling blocks. If you asked for prayers, thank God for all who prayed for you. Where are you in your faith journey? Can you acknowledge that your only true and lasting hope is in God? Have you seen any transforming blessings? Ask for peace, confidence, and hope that can only come from complete surrender to Him.

Dear God,   *Date:*

CHAPTER TWENTY
Making a Difference

JABEZ CRIED OUT TO THE GOD OF ISRAEL,
"OH, THAT YOU WOULD BLESS ME AND ENLARGE MY TERRITORY!
LET YOUR HAND BE WITH ME, AND KEEP ME FROM HARM
SO THAT I WILL BE FREE FROM PAIN." AND GOD GRANTED HIS REQUEST.

—1 Chronicles 4:10

It Just Takes One Woman

It was almost a relief. I thought, "It's done. I've had it, and now I've had it again." —Renee

HE'S LOOKING FOR . . . JUST ONE GOD-READY WOMAN. —PSALM 53:2 MSG

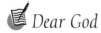

Dear God

Dear God,

So many times I cried out to You not to be the one in eight women who collides with breast cancer, but You knew I would be the one. All those years of silently petitioning came to the culminating pinnacle—it was me! What a relief; the decision was made. I must have sounded so selfish praying for it not to be me because that meant it would be another woman. Oh Lord, forgive me those prideful, selfish thoughts and prayers. I know you were saying, "Why not you, Janet? Why shouldn't it be you?" Back then Your words fell on fearful ears.

Thank You for changing my heart. I know what it means to give up your life for your friends, as You were the One who gave up Your life for mine. You were the One who spared me. If it works that way with breast cancer, Lord, I sincerely pray, "Let me be the one who carries the breast cancer cross for all the women You put into my path. Don't let it be them. Lord, protect these women. Use me to make a difference. Let it be me."

Willingly Yours, Janet

A Sister Shares

Throughout all of this it has been my strategy to keep my illness out in the open, making it an easy topic of conversation. It is good therapy for me, while in many cases it is inspiration or motivation for others. At least one friend who called for a mammogram appointment when she heard my story has been through a fine-needle aspiration that came up negative, thank goodness, but what if it hadn't? —Heather

Mentoring Moment

Those of us who carry the breast cancer burden feel a sense of responsibility to educate other women. Even as I wrote this book, the statistics have gone from one in eight to one in seven women who will get breast cancer. There is an old saying that misery likes company, but we don't want *this kind* of company. We would not wish this on anyone, and so we must encourage and nudge our friends to get their mammograms regularly and have an annual physical—putting it on our calendars to remind all those women near and dear to us. Does that seem a little smothering and intrusive? They won't mind if it saves their lives.

While praying the other morning, the Lord put on my heart that my best friend, Jane, had forgotten her mammogram appointment. Periodically I had asked if she rescheduled—she hadn't. That morning I e-mailed her and said, "Call for your mammogram appointment. Let me know the time and date; I will help you remember it." Much to her surprise, she got an appointment the next morning. Everything was fine, but my call let her know I cared about her. It was also a reminder that it is not OK to be lax about our health.

The license-plate holder on my car reads Mammograms Save Lives! A neighbor commented that seeing this was a reminder to make her annual mammogram appointment. Early breast cancer detection saves lives.

- I am one of those lives.

- I will never forget it.

- I will never let anyone else forget it.

You can make a difference. It may seem like you are only one woman, but if each one of us works in our spheres of influence, we will touch the world one woman at a time. Then they, too, can pass on the preventative-care message . . . woman to woman to woman to woman . . .

God's Love Letter to You

*Dear*_____, *(fill in your name)*
The first command is to love me, the Lord your God, with all your heart and with all your soul and with all your mind and with all your strength. The second is this: Love your neighbor as yourself. There is no commandment greater than these (Mark 12:30–31 paraphrased). My Son was "The One," God

Let's Pray

Prayerfully personalize with me 1 John 3:23–24 MSG.

God, You told us, _____ and Janet, to love each other, in line with the original command. As we keep your commands, we,

_____ and Janet, live deeply and surely in you, and you live in us. And this is how we experience your deep and abiding presence in us: by the Spirit you gave us. In Your Son's name we pray. Amen.

Breast Cancer Sisters

Fourteen years later it seems I can hardly go anywhere without encountering a person that either has had or knows someone who has been afflicted with breast cancer. —Brenda N.

Karen was a perfect stranger before I had cancer. Now I feel like she's a sister. —Brenda Ladun[2]

We are all incredibly touched by my mother's journey. . . . It has definitely made us all aware and sympathetic—and a part of this group of people who have, in a way, survived what breast cancer does to a family. —David Arquette[3]

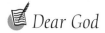 ## Dear God

Dear God,

Help me always remember every breast cancer woman is my sister, regardless of her position or stage in life, no matter how young or old, famous or unknown, rich or poor. This is a sisterhood not of our choosing. But I would imagine that if I introduced myself as a fellow breast cancer survivor to Olivia Newton-John, her face would light up, she would give me a hug, and there would be an instant bond of recognition. Breast cancer does that.

In Your eyes we are all the same . . . You don't have a caste system for rating one person more important than the next, and I am sure You want us to look at one another the same way. It is such a shame when it takes something like breast cancer to bring us to this ultimate awareness. I don't have to be a famous movie star or political figure to make a difference. If I can influence those You put in my presence, I will do my best to help them realize the importance of treating their bodies well, supporting the work of finding a cure for breast cancer, and knowing You, Lord, as their personal Savior. Breast cancer certainly levels the playing field. Anything is possible . . . maybe even meeting Olivia Newton-John!

Making a difference, Janet

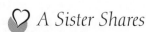 ## A Sister Shares

I wonder how I am still here and others are not. I realize I must have some kind of message I am supposed to deliver, a task, a mission, or something left for me here. And now that some time has passed, and I have learned to live with my condition, I can talk more freely without totally breaking up about my feelings and emotions. Did you ever notice after you buy a new car how many people have that same kind of car? Cancer is like that. You come to realize just how many other people share your illness. —Linda M.

 Mentoring Moment

What do Nancy Reagan, Olivia Newton-John, Betty Ford, Suzanne Somers, Peggy Fleming, Janet Thompson, Kay Warren, Grace Marestaing, and you all have in common? You guessed it—breast cancer—along with all the women who shared their stories in this book. Many of those women I may never see face to face, but one day while looking at Olivia Newton-John's picture in an advertisement for breakfast cereal, I noticed it said she was a breast cancer survivor and advocate. Immediately I knew Olivia and I were sisters!

What do David Arquette, Randal Niles, Kim Mancini, Nicole Kidman, Emily Morphis, Oliver Wolfson, and your children all have in common? You guessed it—their moms had breast cancer. My daughter, Kim Mancini, often tells me about acquaintances of hers whose mom had breast cancer. How does that topic come up? Because, just like with us, once breast cancer touches their lives, it becomes a focal point. Immediately they have a connection just as we do with other breast cancer survivors. They are the surviving family, and our breast cancer had a significant impact on their lives too—it gives them a common bond. They can reach out to help and comfort one another in ways no one else can.

Have you noticed yourself suddenly drawn to other women who have had breast cancer? Women who talk the same language—shunts, HRT, DCIS, implants, wigs, tattoos, chemo stories, radiation burn, shaving your head, hair coming back gray, stubble, prosthesis, reconstruction that doesn't mean you are remodeling your house, frozen shoulder that didn't get stuck in the freezer, and stage two or three—not a Broadway show. It is amazing how our language shifts so easily to calmly talking about things that previously would have horrified us. As I talked with many of the women in this book, through tears and laughter, we were quickly tracking with each other. No explanations needed . . . just nodding heads and reaffirming, "Uh-huh . . . I know what you mean." We didn't waste words talking about the neighborhoods we live in, or what career we had or have, or certainly not our economic status, unless it was to talk about insurance and the bills we all accrued.

We all can pray for and comfort one another and use whatever platforms God gives us to spread the awareness of breast cancer, whether it's in your children's classroom or playground, your workplace or neighborhood, among friends and family, in the boardroom, on stage or the movie screen, in the political arena, with written words, or with a book like this. Whatever you do, you can make a difference if you try!

God's Love Letter to You

Dear_____, (fill in your name)

Don't get tired of doing what is good. Don't get discouraged and give up, for you will reap a harvest of blessing at the appropriate time. Whenever you have the opportunity, you should do good to everyone, especially to your Christian brothers and sisters (Galatians 6:9–10 NLT paraphrased).

Your Father, God

Let's Pray

Lord, we had no desire to claim this sisterhood, but we want to reach out to each other as only breast cancer sisters can. Help us not let cultural, economic, or personal differences stand in our way. Please bring down the strongholds, break the barriers, help us unite not only in the breast cancer walks and runs, but also on the streets and sidewalks of everyday life. It's a lonely journey, and many of us just need a friend . . . a sister . . . who understands. Give us hearts to love and courage to reach out even in our own pain. Let us remember that in Christ, as well as breast cancer, we are all one family in the Lord. Amen.

Giving Back

I will have chemo every three weeks for the rest of my life. After my treatments I head over to the Kids Konnected office, which supports children whose parents have cancer. —Angel

That support system was there for me, and I wanted to give back. —Grace Marestaing

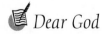 Dear God

Dear God,

I cannot go through this breast cancer experience without it making a difference in not only my life but also the lives of others. I know this book is part of that purpose, but then what? How can I continue giving back? Grace and many other former breast cancer survivors volunteer at the BreastCare Center; Liz volunteered at the radiation center; Angel goes to the Kids Konnected office and volunteers after her chemo treatments; Darlene M. uses her job as a nurse to encourage others; Sue and Dianne faithfully lead the Saddleback Breast Cancer Support Group and give much of their personal time helping the women who attend; Darlene Gee continues attending the support group to offer encouragement and wisdom from her experience; Lynn is involved in intercessory prayer at her church; Nancy Tuttle left her inspirational letters and writings to encourage us; Leslie Furth allowed her husband to chronicle in the newspaper her entire journey, even to the end.

My heart is open and ready. I will bend my ear close to hear. Somehow I feel the journey has just begun!

Expectantly waiting for my next assignment, Janet

A Sister Shares

The BreastCare Center & Oncology Center of Orange County includes trained and informed volunteers as part of the medical team. That support system was there for me, and I wanted to give back. Being a patient-representative volunteer is some of the most rewarding work I have ever done. We participate as an extra pair of ears in patient planning meetings with the surgeons, making sure the patient hears the necessary information; but mostly we are there for support. We match patients with a volunteer who is of similar age and has experienced the same procedures, and then we track with them through the process. They have our phone numbers, and we make ourselves available at any time. We also circulate through the chemotherapy room, bringing water, juice, crackers, or tea—or just sitting, chatting, and encouraging the patients. As one of the nurses said, "We can say things to the patients, but when you say the same thing, it is different. It carries more weight."

I can't tell you what a blessing it is to my life; it's the highlight of my week. Some have asked if I find it depressing. On the contrary, I feel a great sense of purpose there. As I walk in the door, I pray God's compassion and comfort will come through me to the patients.
—Grace Marestaing

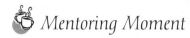 *Mentoring Moment*

As you journeyed through this book, are you feeling stronger emotionally, spiritually, and hopefully physically? Are you wondering how you might pass on all the love and help shown to you? Maybe it will be in the area of breast cancer; but then again, it might be somewhere else. Perhaps people brought you those all-important meals, and you could now take meals to shut-ins or the ill. How about reading to the hospitalized? Leslie Furth found that comforting as her eyesight failed.

Maybe, for you, it would be too uncomfortable to help as Grace does, but you could offer encouragement by phone to newly diagnosed women. As I mentioned earlier, Saddleback Church has a ministry called Crafts for Christ, and they knit or crochet "chemo caps" for women going through chemotherapy. Each cap has a gift card attached with John 3:16 and a personal note from the crafter. Perhaps that's a ministry you could start or suggest at your church. You could learn to knit or crochet if that is not already a talent of yours. These are just a few ideas. Maybe you aren't quite up to helping others yet, but give it some thought because it could be a huge step in your recovery. Healing happens while helping others.

God's Love Letter to You

Dear_____, (fill in your name)

Do for others what you would like them to do for you (Matthew 7:12 NLT). If anyone gives you even a cup of water in my name because you belong to Jesus, I assure you, that person will be rewarded (Mark 9:41 NLT paraphrased).
Filling up your cup, God

Let's Pray

Precious Lord, we come today having progressed through our journeys to the point we feel You might be ready to use us to make an impacting difference in the world. We are open and receptive. We wait with joyful anticipation the revelation of what that difference might be. No task is too small or insignificant when it comes to helping someone else. How will You use us to refresh and renew someone else's spirit as others have done for us? You tell us that even in our weakness Your strength prevails. We pray You will receive the glory and honor for all we do, and we come before You in such gratitude for all that others have done for us. We strive to serve You and give back. Amen.

Finding a Cure

You have to create possibilities that don't exist yet. —Dr. Robert Langer[4]

YES. GOD IS AROUND; GOD TURNS LIFE AROUND.
—PSALM 14:7 MSG

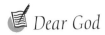 Dear God

Dear God,

Why are so many of us, especially in Orange County, San Francisco, and New York, getting breast cancer? Theories flourish about stress, environment, food additives . . . but no proven, concrete prevention or cure. Lord, I pray even as I write, that You are granting a light-bulb experience to a researcher working on a cure. Father, continue the national publicity. Let the rising incidence of breast cancer alarm those who have the knowledge and means to help. Don't make it touch each household before people become concerned about what's happening. I know when people do not follow Your ways, disaster happens. There are many things in the world today not pleasing to You, and I am sure You want our attention. Lord, let breast cancer get the world's attention.

For those of us with platforms, give us opportunities to talk about our breast cancer. The more breast cancer becomes a topic of conversation and concern, the better chance we have of finding a cure. As Dr. Bob Arnot says, any other disease moving as fast as breast cancer and affecting so many would qualify as an epidemic! Lord, bring awareness. Cause the public to care. Help us find a cure. Heal our land and bodies.

Pleadingly Yours, Janet

A Sister Shares

I consider this gift of cancer a true testimony of faith. Of believing in the unknown. Of believing in a cure. One day there will be a cure. I believe *all* of your prayers receive answers. I also believe that as a breast cancer patient, I will be part of the cure. My child and your children may never have to worry about cancer. Did you know that once the genetic code is broken, inoculation will be the treatment for cancer just like many other diseases? Imagine that . . . now that would be a miracle. It's a miracle that I will live longer than a cancer patient diagnosed ten years ago. Keep praying! —Linda M.

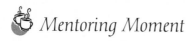

Mentoring Moment

Movie actor David Arquette's mother, Marti, died from breast cancer. David and his actor siblings, as well as his actress wife, Courtney Cox, have all participated in fund-raising events to support breast cancer research. David remarks, "It's so beautiful to see people come out and support their loved ones or run for someone they've lost. We're so moved. With all the tragedy that comes from breast cancer, you also get such an awareness of the good in people, how they come together to support each other."[5]

Women are not the only victims of breast cancer. Did you know that? It is rare and accounts for less than 1 percent of male cancers, but men do get breast cancer, and their treatment options are the same as ours. Rod Roddy, the announcer on *The Price Is Right* TV program who invited audiences to "Come on down!" died from colon and breast cancer. He had his left breast removed.

Admittedly, I looked at breast cancer from a safe distance until I was on the inside looking out. Suddenly I had a keen awareness of how far medicine has come, but I also had concern at how far we still have to go. My daughter's words in the hospital, *"Next year you and I will walk together, Mom,"* echoed in my mind as Grace prepared for a three-day Susan G. Komen Foundation Race for the Cure. Grace was two years cancer free as I approached my one-year surgery anniversary. I was not up to walking three days with Grace and was in another state speaking during our local one-day race. However, I could participate both financially and prayerfully.

We can help in many ways. Here are a few suggestions:

- Buy breast cancer postage stamps. They cost more, but the extra money goes to breast cancer research. Shirley Neal, who shared in this book, proudly tells everyone that her doctor founded the breast cancer stamp and encourages them to buy the stamps.

- Many organizations have fund-raiser programs. For example, I held a fund-raiser Tupperware party. A percentage of the proceeds went to the charity of my choice, which was the Center for Wellness Foundation, affiliated with the BreastCare Center. Pampered Chef also does fund raisers, as well as a Help Whip Cancer Promotion in May to raise funds and awareness for the importance of early detection of breast cancer. Each May I book a Pampered Chef show with my daughter Kim who is a consultant.

- In addition to sponsoring the two-day Avon Walk for Breast Cancer, Avon sells breast cancer promotional items, and a significant portion of the purchase price is retuned to the breast cancer cause. The necklace I am wearing on page 381 is from Avon.

- Brighton produces a breast cancer bracelet every October, and I now own three to mark each year I have been cancer free.

- Talking openly about your breast cancer helps raise awareness. Betty Ford was diagnosed with breast cancer in 1974, and she was open and honest about her surgery and recovery. My pastor, Rick Warren, announced from the podium that his wife, Kay, had breast cancer and encouraged all the women in the congregation to get mammograms. About five hundred women did just that, and several diagnoses resulted because Rick and Kay went public.

- Frequent and support businesses that sponsor breast cancer research.

- Include the research and the researchers often in your prayers. These are the "quiet heroes" Dianne Hales so beautifully describes: "The superstars of research are the new drugs, techniques, and treatments that emerge to save lives or make them more livable. But the people behind these successes tend to remain in the shadows, often by choice. Most of us do not know their names, recognize their faces, or ask for their autographs. Yet, without their dogged persistence (often over decades), intellectual brilliance, and burning passion to find answers, many new discoveries would never see the light."[6]

- Pray for fellow breast cancer sisters God puts in your path.

- Pray for doctors, nurses, technicians, and volunteers devoting their lives to saving ours.

Actively participating in the fight against breast cancer instills in us a sense of empowerment. Instinctively, we fend off a threatening foe and engage others to help. So harness those same survival energies and resources into attacking this public enemy to women—breast cancer!

📖 God's Love Letter to You

Dear _____, *(fill in your name)*

If my people, my God-defined people, respond by humbling themselves, praying, seeking my presence, and turning their backs on their wicked lives, I'll be there ready for you: I'll listen from heaven, forgive their sins, and restore their land to health. From now on I'm alert day and night to the prayers offered at this place (2 Chronicles 7:14–15 MSG paraphrased).
Fighting for you, God

🙌 Let's Pray

Prayerfully personalize Psalm 5:2–3.

Oh, precious God, in Jesus's name I pray . . .

Listen to my, _____'s, cry for help, my King and my God, for to you I, _____, pray. In the morning, O LORD, you hear my voice; in the morning I, _____, lay my requests before you and wait in expectation. Amen.

✍️ Your Letter to God

Have you been feeling guilty about asking, "Why not someone else instead of me?" Thank God today that you are important to Him. The God of the universe cares about you, regardless of your state in life, and He wants to use you to make a difference. Has God been tugging? Maybe asking you to use a special gift or area He knows would be perfect to help others? Ask God to give you some ideas of how and when you might give back. How can you help further the search for the cure?

Dear God, _____ *Date:* _____

_____

_____

_____

_____

_____

Chapter Twenty-One

Praying Expectantly

I CRY OUT TO THE LORD;
I PLEAD FOR THE LORD'S MERCY.
I POUR OUT MY COMPLAINTS BEFORE HIM
AND TELL HIM ALL MY TROUBLES.
FOR I AM OVERWHELMED,
AND YOU ALONE KNOW THE WAY I SHOULD TURN.
THEN I PRAY TO YOU, O LORD.
I SAY, "YOU ARE MY PLACE OF REFUGE.
YOU ARE ALL I REALLY WANT IN LIFE."

—Psalm 142:1–3, 5 NLT

Pray God's Word

Philippians 4:19, which says, "My God will meet all your needs according to his glorious riches in Christ Jesus" was the password to my computer as a reminder that God knew me, He knew where I was, and He knew what I needed—and I needed His help daily, sometimes hourly.
—Grace Marestaing

ALL YOU SAINTS! SING YOUR HEARTS OUT TO GOD! THANK HIM TO HIS FACE!
—PSALM 30:4 MSG

LET MY CRY COME RIGHT INTO YOUR PRESENCE, GOD; PROVIDE ME WITH THE INSIGHT THAT COMES ONLY FROM YOUR WORD. GIVE MY REQUEST YOUR PERSONAL ATTENTION, RESCUE ME ON THE TERMS OF YOUR PROMISE. —PSALM 119:169–170 MSG

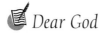 Dear God

Dear God,

You still make bodies the same as Adam and Eve's—all our parts and organs exactly the same as theirs were! You haven't changed a thing. What has changed is everything we put into our bodies and subject them to daily. Similarly, the Bible has never changed; it is the same today as yesterday and will be the same tomorrow, no matter how the world turns. Your Word is timeless. That helps put everything into perspective and drives home the relevancy of the Bible, written thousands of years ago yet still so completely and totally applicable to my body and life today.

Thank You for writing the Bible for me—not just for religious scholars or students of the Bible—so I can prayerfully claim all Your Words for my life. What an awesome, thoughtful, loving God You are, and Your words transcend all generations. That is a message I must get out. Please give me the hope in my heart and the words in my mouth to help others personally apply the Scriptures in the good times and the not so good. Your Word prevails, Lord, forever and ever . . . Amen.

Personalizing Your Word, Janet

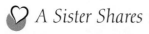 A Sister Shares

The verse that came to mind when the doctor told me the diagnosis was breast cancer is Job 23:10: "But he knows the way that I take; when he has tested me, I will come forth as gold." I can't begin to tell you the comfort I have derived from the truth in that verse . . . just remembering that the God of the universe *knows* where I am today, what I'm facing, what is behind me, and what is ahead . . . and that in His wisdom He allowed my situation . . . where is there much room for fear or anxiety? It holds me. —Kay Warren

 Mentoring Moment

Isn't it incredible to know that God made our bodies the same as Jesus's body when He walked the face of the earth! Moses, Abraham, Ruth, Eve, Sarah—*all* the people in the Bible had the same number of body parts and organs we have! Nothing added, nothing taken away. Women of the Bible nursed their babies from breasts, which would look just like yours and mine in a mammogram x-ray. Yet we so often talk and think in terms of the Bible's relevance only to people back in "those days," not today. After all, these are modern times!

The Lord knew we would think this way, so He reminds us in Ecclesiastes 1:9–10, "What has been will be again, what has been done will be done again; there is nothing new under the sun. Is there anything of which one can say, 'Look! This is something new?' It was here already, long ago; it was here before our time." We may look different today, but what never changes is the basis for sustaining life by food, water, and oxygen. While we now extend life with artificial body parts, we still need certain vital organs to maintain life. Eyes are still required for seeing, noses for smelling, ears for hearing—from generation to generation and all that are to come.

Realizing this timeless truth helps us recognize the relevancy of all the Bible all the time. From cover to cover, from year to year, His words give direction, wisdom, comfort, and guidance for living our lives, regardless of the century. That is why I included so many scriptures in this book. I know and believe that there is no other self-help book more applicable to all circumstances in our lives than *the* Book . . . the Holy Bible. Throughout *Dear God, They Say It's Cancer,* you have read various Bible translations using current language and vocabulary, but it is all still God's Word . . . "God-breathed," as 2 Timothy 3:16 says.

Many of the women who shared their stories with you in this book referred to a scripture or scriptures that sustained them through the journey. Amazingly, none of them chose the same scripture! Why is that? Because scriptures are personal and address each of us differently at various times in our lives, just as we don't say the exact same things to every one of our children. We adapt our conversation to their ages, personalities, maturity level, and our knowledge of their personal uniqueness. Our heavenly Father does the same with us, His children. So a scripture that shouts out to me might not have the same relevance to you, and that's OK. Let the Bible speak to you in whatever way the Lord chooses. Here are scriptures that several of the breast cancer sisters found comforting:

- Kay Warren—Job 23:10: "But he knows the way that I take; when he has tested me, I will come forth as gold."

- Liz—Isaiah 43:1–2: "But now, this is what the LORD says—he who created you, O Jacob, he who formed you, O Israel: 'Fear not, for I have redeemed you; I have summoned you by name; you are mine. When you pass through the waters, I will be with you; and when you pass through the rivers, they will not sweep over you. When you walk through the fire, you will not be burned; the flames will not set you ablaze.'"

- Saddleback Church Breast Cancer Support Group—2 Corinthians 1:3–4: "Praise be to the God and Father of our Lord Jesus Christ, the Father of compassion and the God of all comfort, who comforts us in all our troubles, so that we can comfort those in any trouble with the comfort we ourselves have received from God."

- Shirley Neal—Philippians 4:4–8: "Rejoice in the Lord always. I will say it again: Rejoice! Let your gentleness be evident to all. The Lord is near. Do not be anxious about anything, but in everything, by prayer and petition, with thanksgiving, present your requests to God. And the peace of God, which transcends all understanding, will guard your hearts and your minds in Christ Jesus. Finally, brothers and sisters, whatever is true, whatever is noble, whatever is right, whatever is pure, whatever is lovely, whatever is admirable—if anything is excellent or praiseworthy—think about such things."

- Linda Taylor—Deuteronomy 31:8: "The LORD himself goes before you and will be with you; he will never leave you nor forsake you. Do not be afraid; do not be discouraged."

- Nancy Tuttle had many verses, including Psalm 18:2: "The LORD is my rock and my fortress and my deliverer; my God, my strength, in whom I will trust; my shield and the horn of my salvation, my stronghold." (NKJV)

- Lisha—James 1:2–4: "Consider it all joy, my brethren, when you encounter various trials, knowing that the testing of your faith produces endurance. And let endurance have its perfect result, so that you may be perfect and complete, lacking in nothing." (NASB)

- Gloria—Joshua 1:9: "Do not tremble or be dismayed, for the LORD your God is with you wherever you go." (NASB)

- Cheryl—Isaiah 26:3: "Thou wilt keep him in perfect peace whose mind is stayed on Thee, because he trusts in thee." (NBV)

- Sue—1 Corinthians 13:12–13: "For now we see in a mirror dimly, but then face to face; now I know in part, but then I will know fully just as I also have been fully known. But now faith, hope, love, abide these three; but the greatest of these is love." (NASB)

- Edna had three verses—Psalm 73:26: "My flesh and my heart may fail; but God is the strength of my heart and my portion forever"; Isaiah 41:10: "Do not fear, for I am with you. Do not be dismayed, for I am your God. I will strengthen you and help you. I will uphold you with my victorious right hand"; and Romans 12:12: "Be joyful in hope, patient in affliction, faithful in prayer."

- Grace Marestaing—Matthew 6:8: "Your Father knows exactly what you need even before you ask him!" (NLT)

Throughout this book in the "Let's Pray" sections, you and I personalized scriptures by simply inserting your name (and sometimes my name) and adding personal pronouns. I hope it has become a practice to use in your daily prayers. King David wrote many of his psalms during a very distressful and painful time of his life, so they are quite applicable to our crises. David and the other psalmists also wrote very uplifting praise songs and poems. Someone once suggested to me to read the book of Psalms during difficult situations. That practice has brought comfort many times, and it might to you too. If possible, read a modern-day translation or whatever Bible you enjoy. God's Word is God's Word, and He is the ultimate Author.

God's Love Letter to You

Dear_____, (fill in your name)
   You have been taught the holy Scriptures from childhood, and they

have given you the wisdom to receive the salvation that comes by trusting in my Son, Christ Jesus. All Scripture is inspired by me, God, and is useful to teach you what is true and to make you realize what is wrong in your life. It straightens you out and teaches you to do what is right. It is my way of preparing you in every way, fully equipped for every good thing I want you to do (2 Timothy 3:15–17 NLT paraphrased).

The Living, Breathing Word, God

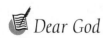 Let's Pray

Prayerfully personalize with me a psalm of David, Psalm 20:1–2, 4–5 NLT.

Father God, we pray Your precious Word back to You, just as David did . . .

In times of trouble, may the LORD respond to our, _____'s and Janet's, cry. May the God of Israel keep us, _____ and Janet, safe from all harm. May You send us help from Your sanctuary and strengthen us from Jerusalem. You grant our hearts' desires and fulfill all our plans. May we, _____ and Janet, shout for joy when we hear of our victory, flying banners to honor our, _____'s and Janet's, God. May the LORD answer all our prayers. Amen.

Pray for Your Doctors

Whoever has been praying can consider some prayers answered. My oncologist who is usually so stone faced, was nice and friendly today, and he actually smiled as he said, "Today is your last chemo treatment." —Linda M.

My work regularly brings me in close proximity to death. Like every doctor, I have learned how to compartmentalize the fear and anxiety it naturally provokes in order to function effectively at the bedside. —Dr Jerome Groopman[1]

GOD LOOKS AFTER US ALL, MAKES US ROBUST WITH LIFE—LUCKY TO BE IN THE LAND, WE'RE FREE FROM ENEMY WORRIES. WHENEVER WE'RE SICK AND IN BED, GOD BECOMES OUR NURSE, NURSES US BACK TO HEALTH. —PSALM 41:2–3 MSG

Dear God

Dear God,

I am only as good as my next doctor appointment or mammogram or some other "gram" or scan. Breast cancer always will look over my shoulder, and I in turn will look over the tech's and doctor's shoulders as they read test reports or look at films or computer screens. I'll hold my breath, searching their faces, eyes, tone of voice, touch to my shoulder, or big sigh for a revealing sign of impending bad news. Or, gratefully, let out my breath as they smilingly assure me, "Things look good for now. See you for your next checkup."

Just yesterday, going for a biannual mammogram on the recovering breast was like déjà vu as the radiologist thought she saw calcifications. Again I was in the radiologist's dark room, looking at white spots with a magnifying glass on the same computer screen, with a different radiologist's voice explaining what she saw. Trying to listen, my mind was screaming, *This can't be happening again so soon. I had radiation! I am taking Tamoxifen! This cannot be possible.* Still she talked on. Then suddenly in the darkness of the room, she gently took my hand and said, "You are going to be all right. I think these are 'fat necrosis' left from the surgery and radiation. They are scattered, not clustered, and we will just watch them." My legs felt weak as I mumbled how she had scared me.

My life is in the hands of You and my doctors and technicians who devote their careers to saving lives . . . including my life. You gifted them, and I am eternally grateful they use their gifts to help humanity. Please protect them. Watch over their own health from the stress of daily dealings with illness. Keep their hearts soft and kind as they work with each patient. Lord, give them clarity of thought, mind, and vision. Keep them accurate and precise. Bless their lives abundantly as they bless others.

Most importantly, I fervently pray each one will draw closer to You because I was their patient. Let me always be an example of Your undying love and grace, and at the end of my visit let them say, "I saw Jesus in Janet." Maybe they won't know it was You, because all my doctors and techs do not know You personally. But if You can use me in some way to change that, I willingly put myself at your disposal and pray You will give me courage for each new assignment.

Ready for Mission Possible, Janet

A Sister Shares

You'd be amazed at the kind of treatment you get when you get such a serious disease. Everyone's bedside manner improves. People can't seem to take care of you enough. Doctors, nurses, and technicians act like I'm their best friend and part of their families. And I've heard it only gets better. So there are some pluses to cancer. The word doesn't sound nearly as ugly and scary as it did a month ago. —Linda M.

☕ *Mentoring Moment*

In the midst of my scary mammogram experience, the mammography technician shared there are weeks where three mammograms turn out positive each day. She begins feeling guilty, and irrational thoughts go through her head like, *Am I spreading this from one woman to the next? Is it my fault? I don't want to touch another patient . . . I might be causing these positive results.* They are under terrific pressure, and some may mask their caring behind stoic exteriors.

Naturally, the foremost thought on our minds when first diagnosed is asking for prayers of healing, grace, and mercy for *ourselves*. However, it is so important also to ask for prayers for our devoted doctors, technicians, nurses, and physicians' assistants. Don't forget the receptionist answering the phones, the lab technician drawing our blood, the poor nurse trying to start an IV in our dehydrated veins, the skilled and capable surgeons who hold a steady hand with the scalpel over our bodies, and yes, even the office manager sending us a bill. Ask for abundant prayers and blessings on them all. They had career choices in their lives and willingly chose healthcare. Because of them we are not destitute when diagnosed. There is somewhere to go for help.

Of course, the *first* place we should go for help is the Lord. As we ask for His wisdom, guidance, and help, here are some practical ways to assure we don't forget to pray the same for our healthcare team. For each member of your healthcare team:

- Put them on your church prayer chain.

- Ask friends and family to include them in daily prayers.

- Pray with them at your appointments.

- Ask how you can pray for them . . . what are their prayer requests?

- Always let your surgeons, nurses, and technicians know others are praying for them, whether or not they are Christian. I have never heard of anyone turning down prayers.

- Pray for them yourself in a way only you can because you have a personal relationship.

- Pray for them personally and not just for your own benefit. It's easy to pray they will be skilled in our treatment, but how about praying for their marriages, families, health, salvation, and relationships?

- Look for positive changes in their lives. Maybe a softening heart or interaction with you. Things might begin to go more smoothly with the office staff. Trust me, you will see the results of your prayers.

📖 *God's Love Letter to You*

Dear_____, (fill in your name)
      As the mountains surround Jerusalem, so I, the LORD, *surround my people both now and forevermore (Psalm 125:2 paraphrased).*
Lovingly surrounding you and your healthcare team, God

🐰 *Let's Pray*

Lord, You gifted each healthcare professional. You know where they need prayer in their professional and personal lives, and so we petition Your intervention in enhancing and encouraging them. Daily they see sad and serious circumstances and face their inadequacy at stopping the inevitable end of earthly time for some of their patients. Comfort them in loss by drawing them closer to You as their source of strength and endurance so they can offer spiritual as well as physical hope to their patients. We praise You for their lives and ask that You reward them some day beyond their wildest expectations. We give our lives and hearts to You for Your ultimate care. Amen.

Pray for Everyone Touched by Your Breast Cancer

That is great news about your mammogram. Watching you go through this has been a very good learning experience for me, so I am sure you are influencing countless others even before the book comes out. —Lorna

The Big Fellow Upstairs never forgets those that remember Him. —President Ronald Reagan

PRAISE THE LORD! PRAISE THE LORD, I TELL MYSELF. I WILL PRAISE THE LORD AS LONG AS I LIVE. I WILL SING PRAISES TO MY GOD EVEN WITH MY DYING BREATH. —PSALM 146:1–2 NLT

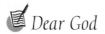 *Dear God*

Dear God,

The tentacles of breast cancer spread much further than just in my body. They wind and wrap, entwining the bodies of people You put in my path . . . affecting everyone who watches my story unfold. I am sure many observe from afar. There is certainly an abundance of close friends and family walking every step with me . . . continuously praying . . . still ready to help whenever needed. It is quite staggering to think so many eyes are on me when often I am just trying to make it from one day to the next.

Lord, I pray I have set a good example of truly living my talk . . . that others see I put my trust in You and in prayer . . . I press on, using each new day You give me. For those who do not know You, I pray my breast cancer experience has drawn them closer to the decision-making point; and when and if they encounter hardships, I pray they have seen a godly model of endurance that works.

I pray especially for my younger sister, Christie, and my daughter, Kim, that You spare them this affliction. Please don't let it be genetic but exclusive to me. Please also protect my other daughters, daughter-in-law, and granddaughters. I pray for my husband, Dave, who only yesterday so lovingly told me if ever a test or medical report revealed the final battle call, he would immediately quit his job and spend every moment with me! What love and reassurance that I am truly the love of his life. I am sure he lives with that thought every time I go for another mammogram or blood test, so I pray for comfort and peace in his soul.

Lord, You have blessed Woman to Woman Mentoring, and it continues expanding far beyond our church and me. As a result, thousands of women around the world have learned of my breast cancer, and I pray they see that ministry doesn't stop or slow down when the leader is stricken. A firm foundation and a continuous passing of the torch of responsibility keeps God's work humming right along.

Lord, I have no idea the neighbors, casual acquaintances, or the many people I talk to while going about my day who will perhaps be drawn to You because, in spite of my affliction, I still boldly proclaim that my Lord reigns. For any who came across me on a bad day when worry or pain got the best of me, please don't let them slip by . . . bring someone else into their lives to be a better example than I was. Help me always remember it is not about me but about You reaching others through me.

When I see You face to face, we won't talk about the details of my breast cancer journey. What we'll talk about is how many people will call heaven their permanent home because I, Janet, was in their lives. How many am I bringing with me? My constant prayer is for it to be more than I can count . . . more than I even know. You keep track of the numbers Lord, and I will continue on . . .

About His Work, Janet

♡ A Sister Shares

If I had a magic wand, I would ask each individual in my realm of friends and their friends that were so kind and helpful to me to step forward, taking a much deserved bow and accepting a rosebud from me for their every deed and thought. Words of encouragement and love were so abundant and seemed to come just when needed most. I have such a bounty of good memories that will keep me in loving debt for years to come. This was one battle in life's big war. The wound is healed, some pain is still around, and I'm sure more pain in other situations are in my future—but what a trail we took and met so many wonderful folks along the way. There are so many silent partners that were of much comfort to me . . . so many, I could never name them all . . . My needs were so great, that each administered so well, surly as we live, God gave the rewarding blessings in my behalf. God's love is sufficient. —Martha[2]

Mentoring Moment

If only we alone bore the scars of breast cancer. But many lives are touched by what happens to us. God planned for it to be that way; He calls it "community." It takes a village to take care of those who are sick. Whether our village is small, quaint, and intimate or very large and expansive, others surrounded us in our time of need, and their lives were touched as well. Women going through breast cancer alone usually have a community of volunteers or neighbors who step into the gap, and they always have their doctors, nurses, and God in their lives.

Even Dr. Jerri Nielsen, who discovered her breast cancer while working in a remote part of the South Pole where she was the only medical professional, had people assisting her long distance and rooting for her. Susan Sarandon, who played Dr. Nielsen in the TV movie *Ice Bound*, said in an interview that she hopes *Ice Bound* not only raises awareness about breast cancer detection but also makes "a statement about people's interdependence and the fact that we have to be there for each other. I think that's the bigger statement that involves men and women—education and empowerment, but also to in some way reach out to each other and be there for each other."[3]

Our lives affect others. We must give thanks for their help in our time of need and pray for God's plan and protection in their lives. Don't forget people like the taxi driver who drove you back and forth to the hospital, or the delivery boy who brought your medications, groceries, or pizza to the door—they matter to God, and so they should matter to us. We must not let this experience be wasted. Pray daily for each one as God brings them to mind.

God's Love Letter to You

Dear_____, *(fill in your name)*

My dear sisters, if anyone among you wanders away from the truth and is brought back again, you can be sure that the one who brings that person back will save that sinner from death and bring about the forgiveness of many sins (James 5:19–20 NLT paraphrased).
I love you all, God

Let's Pray

Our precious Lord and Savior, when we are having a tough time, it seems the world should stop and care for us . . . and for a while it did. But some of those whose lives touched ours during the cancer journey were also hurting physically, spiritually, and emotionally. No meeting was by chance. Father, bless their lives, heal their hurts, and restore or develop their right relationships with You. If we hurt any person along the way with a quick-tempered comment or were unkind, forgive us, and bring to mind any we should ask forgiveness of in person. Shine in us as godly role models of going through tough times. Help us remember others are more important than we are! This does not come easy, and we can't do it without You, but with You all things are possible. Amen.

Pray for All Your Breast Cancer Sisters

HEAR, O LORD, MY RIGHTEOUS PLEA; LISTEN TO MY CRY. GIVE EAR TO MY PRAYER.
—PSALM 17:1

THE LORD ANNOUNCES VICTORY, AND THRONGS OF WOMEN SHOUT THE HAPPY NEWS.
—PSALM 68:11 NLT

Dear God

Dear God,

Oh Lord, I pour out my heart to You . . . Please have mercy on each woman reading this book, journaling her journey, and facing her fears. I love each one, even though I may never know her name. But You love her even more than I do, and You do know her name.

Some will experience years of restored health, others will endure a constant battle until the end, and some have passed away. Let me never forget them, Lord. You might grant me the opportunity to meet some and hear how You touched and held them as they read Your "Love Letters" to them. But whether we meet personally, through e-mail, by phone, or never have the privilege until we meet in heaven, I lift them up to You now. I pray You open the eyes of those who do not know You yet, restore the faith of those that do, and keep them all cradled in Your righteous right hand.

Beseechingly Yours, Janet

A Sister Shares

Dear Janet,
Now I know why God has laid you heavy on my heart the last few days! I have sent blessings your way and prayed to our Father to strengthen you! You are such a *blessing* to me! God loves you bunches, and so do I. —Zephaniah 3:17, Linda Taylor

Mentoring Moment

You may recall I mentioned earlier that Linda Taylor and I met at a Woman to Woman Mentoring training I was leading. She was a participant and introduced herself as a breast cancer sister after I shared about my breast cancer. I met her only *once* for that brief moment and asked if she would like to send her story for inclusion in this book. She did and I thanked her. That was the extent of our communication. Later, when I needed her to sign a permission form, the above "Sister Shares" came as part of a handwritten letter she sent with the form. It sounds as if she's a good friend and we've known each other for years, doesn't it? But as you read, God put me on her heart to pray for, and it turned out she was praying right when I was in a stressful time. She loves me "bunches," and I am a "blessing" to her, even though we barely know each other!

I traced down Brenda Nardolillo after reading an article she had written in the newspaper about her breast cancer and noticed she also was the owner of the company we had used for our kitchen remodel!

I e-mailed her asking permission to use parts of her story and letting her know I was a satisfied customer. A relationship birthed as soon as she discovered I was another Christian breast cancer sister. We had never met, yet she offered to read the entire manuscript and sent encouraging "you can make it" e-mails as I persevered toward the goal of finishing this book.

How could this be? In today's busy world, two women who barely know me willing to give sacrificially of their prayers and time? The answer: we are *sisters*—connected by breast cancer and God. That was all it took to make two new praying friends!

I would like to share with you a poem that appears in the oncology ward of a local hospital and was lying on the checkout desk my first day at the oncologist's office. It has no author, but I think you will agree either a cancer patient or a family member must have written it. Hold on to these truths. Carry them in your mind at all times. You will be victorious. Cancer will not win. God always prevails.

> *What Cancer CANNOT Do*
> *Cancer is so limited . . .*
> *It cannot cripple love*
> *It cannot shatter hope*
> *It cannot corrode faith*
> *It cannot destroy peace*
> *It cannot kill friendship*
> *It cannot suppress memories*
> *It cannot silence courage*
> *It cannot invade the soul*
> *It cannot steal eternal life*
> *It cannot quench the Spirit*
> *It cannot lessen the power of the resurrection.*
> —ANONYMOUS

God's Love Letter to You

Dear_____, (fill in your name)
Hear, O my daughters, and I will speak, . . . I am God, your God. Sacrifice thank offerings to me, fulfill your vows to the Most High and call upon me in the day of trouble; I will deliver you, and you will honor me (Psalm 50:7, 14–15 paraphrased).
Your Most High Father, God

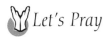 *Let's Pray*

All-seeing, all-knowing Father, we come to You as sisters in breast cancer and sisters in the Lord with the same heavenly Father—*You*! We know You do not want a single one lost, and Your eye is on each of us. We pray for all the women of the world who have breast cancer. You know their names . . . nationalities . . . diagnoses . . . prognoses, and where they need prayer this very moment. Please bring friends to comfort and support, family to love and provide, doctors to heal and ease pain, but most important, let them feel Your loving hope and blessed assurance like a loving arm around their shoulders or a warm hand caressing theirs. Thank You that all we have to do is call on Your name. Amen.

 Your Letter to God

Have you discovered comforting scriptures during your breast cancer journey? Isn't it a precious thought to think of praying for all those people God used to help you through this battle and those who are yet to come into your life? Take a moment to pray for the breast cancer sisters God brings to mind, as well as their families, who need a holy hug.

Dear God,   *Date:*

CHAPTER TWENTY-TWO

Ending at the Beginning

HE WILL REMOVE ALL OF THEIR SORROWS, AND THERE WILL BE NO MORE DEATH OR SORROW OR CRYING OR PAIN. FOR THE OLD WORLD AND ITS EVILS ARE GONE FOREVER. AND THE ONE SITTING ON THE THRONE SAID, "LOOK, I AM MAKING ALL THINGS NEW!" AND THEN HE SAID TO ME, "WRITE THIS DOWN, FOR WHAT I TELL YOU IS TRUSTWORTHY AND TRUE." AND HE ALSO SAID, "IT IS FINISHED! I AM THE ALPHA AND THE OMEGA—THE BEGINNING AND THE END. TO ALL WHO ARE THIRSTY I WILL GIVE THE SPRINGS OF THE WATER OF LIFE WITHOUT CHARGE!"

—Revelation 21:4–6 NLT

Preparing for the Inevitable

NO MAN KNOWS WHEN HIS HOUR WILL COME. —ECCLESIASTES 9:12

Death is a transition from life to life—that is, from creation life to resurrection life. —Anne Ortland¹

FOR WE ARE NOT OUR OWN MASTERS WHEN WE LIVE OR WHEN WE DIE. WHILE WE LIVE, WE LIVE TO PLEASE THE LORD. AND WHEN WE DIE, WE GO TO BE WITH THE LORD. SO IN LIFE AND IN DEATH, WE BELONG TO THE LORD. CHRIST DIED AND ROSE AGAIN FOR THIS VERY PURPOSE, SO THAT HE MIGHT BE LORD OF THOSE WHO ARE ALIVE AND OF THOSE WHO HAVE DIED. —ROMANS 14:7–9 NLT

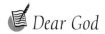 ## Dear God

Dear God,

I remember a conversation with a doctor who told me he noticed people with faith did better in treatment. You prompted me to say, "Doctor, your passion is to prolong a quality life, but one day we're all going to die. We can agree on that statistic. One hundred percent mortality rate. Right?" He nodded his head in agreement. I went on, "Thank you for prolonging my life and making it better for a few more years; however, one day, you and I will both die. Agreed?" Again, he nodded yes. "Doctor, my passion and mission is to help people understand that death does not have to be permanent. There is life after death for those of us who believe in the One, Jesus Christ, who conquered death by dying and resurrecting back to life. To those who believe in Jesus, death is not final."

Lord, I pray those words made a difference. Let the doctor think on them, and perhaps another patient will come along to reinforce eternal life in his heart and mind. Help me not fear death but accept it as the ultimate test of my faith. Death, where is your sting? There is no sting for those who believe in Your Son, Jesus Christ. I do believe, Lord. I find solace and comfort in the promise of eternal life.

Eternally Yours, Janet

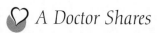 ## A Doctor Shares

Barbara was sixty-seven, a retired history teacher, active in her church, and the leader of its Sunday-school classes. . . . Barbara had found a lump in her left breast that was shown to be cancer. She had a lumpectomy and six months of chemotherapy. Now the cancer was found to be growing in her bones and liver. . . . As I reviewed the results of the biopsy and scans, there was no sign of distress or fear on her face. . . . She showed no fear, no anxiety, despite the prospects we were contemplating. Could someone really transcend the deep fear of death that seems to mark us all?

[Several months later, as Barbara was dying] For months Barbara had sustained a determined spirit. Now that she knew the grim reality of her condition, I had expected to see a change. But she seemed undeterred. I wondered if it would prove to be a façade that would ultimately crack. Or was it actually possible to subsume fear and face death with such apparent equanimity? "Are you afraid?" I asked. Her months of candor had encouraged mine. "You know, not really, not as much as I thought I might be." . . . "Why do you think that is?" "I'm not entirely sure. I have strange comforting thoughts. . . . When fear starts to creep up on me, I conjure the idea that millions and millions of people have passed away before me, and millions more will pass away after I do. Then I think, *My parents each died. I guess if they all did it, so can I.*" She paused. "As Ecclesiastes says, everything has its season—a time to be born and a time to die. As a Christian, I believe in a hereafter, that we can return to God. What form that takes no one can really say." Barbara grinned. "It's not like I'm expecting to get on the Up escalator and be delivered to paradise. Or find angels there playing harps . . ."

"I want to believe in an afterlife, but sometimes it's hard to imagine," I said. Barbara's tone turned grave. "Of course, I also have doubts. Everyone who believes has doubts if they're honest with themselves. I suppose it could all be an illusion. But deep inside it doesn't feel that way at all." For a while we shared silence. —Dr. Jerome Groopman[2]

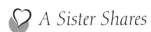 A Sister Shares

My stage-four cancer has *no* cure. I will always have it. However, my prayers have been answered, as I always planned, or at least figured, that I would be around long enough to watch Emily grow up. She will be an adult in three years. The doctor said I would be around for that long. He has stage-four breast cancer patients that are on seven to eight years of treatment now. It's rare to go beyond that point, *but not impossible.* Although it's hard to hear that, I simply can't dwell on it for too long. My treatments won't allow me to. I need to be most positive about this. I am not telling Emily about the how longs; she needs to focus on me just being Mom. —Linda M.

Mentoring Moment

I believe with all my heart that Jesus conquered death at the cross in order to grant us eternal life. Earthly death ushers in eternal life for those who accept Jesus as their personal Savior. Still, this earthly life is all we know; the unknown is a bit scary. Even as women of faith we often struggle with the paradox of knowing that the final, great reward is to be with Christ, where our bodies again will be whole, healthy, and pain free; yet we still hold on tightly to the only thing we have ever known—our earthly life. Our *mind* tells us this life is just a blink of an eye, but our *heart* still wants to stay. Peace comes when both our mind and heart accept that the real victory is when we enter heaven to spend eternal life with Christ.

"Faith is being sure of what we hope for and certain of what we do not see" (Hebrews 11:1). A certain element of surprise is always a thrill. The finality of life as we know it brings a sense of adventure and anticipation, laced with fear and sorrow. Fear of the unknown and sorrow for those we leave behind. They will be so sad. They will miss us desperately. There are so many things in life still to do, to see and experience—our children living a full life—grandchildren growing up. We even hoped for great-grandchildren! Yet the Bible tells us only God knows our last days. We can pray for longer days, and God might or might not grant them.

Perhaps, like me, you escaped death from your current bout with breast cancer. We sigh with relief and gratefulness at receiving more earthly days. Others of you are facing the inevitable truth that death comes to us all. A harsh, stark reality—one we seldom talk about because it is too painful. During my illness people looked at me with fear in their eyes—fear of my mortality, which reminded them of their own. It was a look I had never seen before but grew to dread. I am sure that is what keeps some people away when you need them most. They don't want reminders that the end of the story for all of us someday is death. Strange, we shy away from a universal occurrence. We seldom live each day as if it could be our last.

In eulogizing her dad, former president Ronald Reagan, Patty Reagan Davis said that when she was a little girl, her father taught her that new life always comes out of death. She remembered he never feared death or saw it as an ending. Once, taking her to property that had been burned by fire, he knelt down and showed her the new green growth already starting. When her goldfish died and they buried him, her dad explained that now the goldfish was free without the confines of the aquarium. When she suggested they kill all her other goldfish so they also could be free, Reagan explained to his daughter, "God's timing is always right and wise."

If you have a relationship with Jesus Christ, my prayer is that you are ready to go at any time. You are savoring the remaining earthly days, no matter how many or few, carrying in your heart the hope of someday being with Jesus. If your future is uncertain because you do not know Jesus as your personal Savior, I beg you to not leave any stone unturned in seeking out the truth about Jesus. Read the Bible in a modern-day translation. Talk to pastors or

Christian friends or relatives. Seek answers while you still can. Being a Christian is not about a *religion*, it is about a *relationship* with Jesus Christ, God's Son. You will find the hope, comfort, and peace you long for—that we all long for. It's the God-shaped hole in our hearts that only Jesus Christ can fill. Once we have a relationship with Christ that fills that hole in our hearts, we are complete; then we are ready to truly say, "Where, O death, is your sting?" (1 Corinthians 15:55).

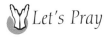 *God's Love Letter to You*

Dear_____, (fill in your name)

Every human being has an earthly body, but your heavenly bodies will be just like Christ's. . . . What I am saying, dear sisters, is that flesh and blood cannot inherit the Kingdom of God. Your perishable bodies are not able to live forever. But let me, God, tell you something wonderful. Not all of you will die, but will be transformed. It will happen in a moment, in the blinking of an eye, when the last trumpet is blown and the Christians who have died will be raised with transformed bodies. And then you who are living will have your earthly bodies transformed into heavenly bodies that never die. When this happens— . . . then at last my Scriptures will come true:

> *"Death is swallowed up in victory.*
> *O death, where is your victory?*
> *O death, where is your sting?"*

You should thank me, because I gave you victory over sin and death through my Son, Jesus Christ! So, my dear breast cancer sisters, be strong and steady, always enthusiastic about my work, for you know that nothing you do for me is ever useless (1 Corinthians 15:48–58 NLT paraphrased).
Waiting for you, God

Let's Pray

Prayerfully personalize Psalm 23 NLT.

O, God, I do know that . . .

The LORD is my, _____'s, shepherd; I, _____, have everything I need. He lets me rest in green meadows; he leads me

Death Is Only a Horizon

The saddest contradiction to the Christian life is all too often the average Christian funeral. While bereavement is a necessary part of any loved one's passing, the Christian has cause for rejoicing when a brother or sister in Christ is finally "absent from the body, and . . . present with the Lord" (2 Corinthians 5:8). There is hope and comfort in those words that the world knows nothing about.

The one sermon you can be sure everyone important to you will hear is the one preached over your casket. Have you given any thought to the words you want spoken on that occasion? Will those in attendance . . . find out why you could face death fearlessly, knowing it would bring you face to face with your Lord?

Jesus Christ turned every funeral He ever attended into a cause for celebration. The morbid wailing of the mourners would be cut short by the miraculous life-giving touch of the Savior, and the dead would live again. What plans are you making today to ensure that your funeral speaks as eloquently as your life that "for me to live is Christ, and to die is gain" (Philippians 1:21)?[3]

beside peaceful streams. He renews my strength. He guides me along right paths, bringing honor to his name. Even when I, _____, walk through the dark valley of death, I, _____, will not be afraid, for you are close beside me. Your rod and your staff protect and comfort me. You prepare a feast for me in the presence of my enemies. You welcome me as a guest, anointing my head with oil. My, _____'s, cup overflows with blessings. Surely your goodness and unfailing love will pursue me all the days of my life, and I, _____, will live in the house of the LORD forever. Amen.

We've Only Just Begun!

My cousin Eli is going to Jerusalem this month, and he offered to put a prayer for Leslie in the Western Wall. I mailed him a small slip of folded paper on which I requested that Leslie be granted a full recovery or, if that is not possible, a quick release from her suffering. —Bernard Wolfson[4]

REMEMBER THE FORMER THINGS, THOSE OF LONG AGO; I AM GOD, AND THERE IS NO OTHER;
I AM GOD, AND THERE IS NONE LIKE ME. I MAKE KNOWN THE END FROM THE BEGINNING,
FROM ANCIENT TIMES, WHAT IS STILL TO COME. I SAY:
MY PURPOSE WILL STAND, AND I WILL DO ALL THAT I PLEASE. —ISAIAH 46:9–10

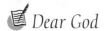 Dear God

Dear God,

I have come to the end of the book, and yet I feel like it is only the beginning of something new and spectacular. One thing I have come to grips with—finally—is that this journey is never over . . . each step is a new beginning. My breast cancer journey may never end, but it will add a new dimension to my life. Thank You for allowing me to journal my thoughts, feelings, regrets, joys, pains, gratitude . . . my heart and my soul poured out here before You in a thank offering. Use it how You plan; use me how You will; use this book to draw others closer to You and their eternal resting place.

It seems sad to write the last words, and yet in my heart You tell me it is only the beginning . . . after all, the first will be last; the last will be first. The great reversal! You are both the Alpha and Omega, residing in the beginning as well as the end. The end of each day is only the beginning of the next. As I watch the sunset over my backyard, I eagerly await the next sunrise in my front yard. The end of this life ushers in the beginning of a better one. So I go forward now with the promise in my heart that, indeed, I have survived for Your purpose, and I've only just begun.

Purposefully living for Christ, Janet

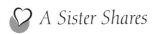 ## A Sister Shares

Dear God,

It's the beginning of a new year. What will 1998 hold for me?

Pain and blessings, life and death, spiritual growth unbounded, love of others and for others, strength to endure, courage to face trials, enthusiasm about the future, and a renewed faith.

What do you want me to do with the rest of my life?

Wait on the Lord. Be of good courage, and I will strengthen your heart. Mount up with wings like eagles, run and not be weary, walk and not faint. Learn to number your days, that you may apply your heart unto wisdom. God makes everything beautiful in its time.

Thank You for being there, for caring, and for Your mercy and grace.

Love, Nancy[5]

 ## Mentoring Moment

You, too, have come to the end of the book, but certainly not the end of the journey. You have chronicled the events, journaled your thoughts, poured out your heart to God, and, I trust, grown closer to Him. For some of you, that meant accepting Jesus as your personal Savior or rededicating your life. The old life shed, the new life ahead. As David wrote in Psalm 32:1–2, "Count yourself lucky, how happy you must be—you get a fresh start, your slate's wiped clean. Count yourself lucky—GOD holds nothing against you and you're holding nothing back from him" (MSG). *End* of a purposeless life before Jesus entered, *beginning* of a new life full of purpose, hope, and a future.

If you are still teetering on that decision—don't, even if you still have questions. What if Christians are right? Don't let another day pass. What would you have to lose? Nothing. But without Christ you lose everything—so why take the chance? At the end of this chapter, there is a simple salvation prayer you can pray to start your relationship with Jesus Christ.

Please don't let this be the end of your journaling and praying to God either. I hope it is the beginning of a new spiritual habit. One that brings you joy and peace as you draw close to God's ear each day, pouring out your praises and pleas to Him, and then listening for His reply. Buy another journal and keep going. Put this one in a treasured spot, and let it be a reminder of how much God loves you and a legacy that you leave for generations to come.

Your end and new beginning also might be . . .

- The end of all your treatments, beginning of a maintaining phase—Hallelujah!

- The end of one treatment or medication and the beginning of another—Praise God for more options.

- The end of cancer and the beginning of complete remission—Enjoy the days ahead.

- The end of life before cancer and the beginning of an era that will always have cancer treatments—Pray for endurance and blessings.

- The end of earthly life and the beginning of your eternal life with Christ—It can't get any better than that!

Nancy Tuttle lost the battle with breast cancer but won the war over death. Her passing was the end of life as we know it and the beginning of her eternal life with Christ. Lean over the shoulder of her son, Randall Niles, as he softly whispers in his mom's ear the releasing words she needed to hear to start her new beginning:

> "Everything here is done. It's OK to let your spirit go now."
>
> Within seconds she peacefully started to slow down her breathing. . . . And then, with a slight smile on her face, she drifted away and entered the loving arms of Jesus. He was so merciful; He was so faithful—there was no pain, only peace. We grieved, but we also embraced the joy of Mom entering into eternity with our Lord. At the moment her spirit departed, we could almost hear Jesus say, "Well done my good and faithful servant." What a precious and glorious memory for all of us. You couldn't have been in the hospital room and not left a believer . . . a believer in the presence, power, love and grace of our Lord and Savior, Jesus Christ.[6]

Wherever you are on your earthly journey, like any trip, it has a beginning and an end—the end signifies arrival at the destination, but another beginning starts with the adventure that awaits there. If you don't know your final destination, ask God to help you find the path leading to ultimate fulfillment in eternal life. If you are on that path and you know it, ask the Lord for comfort from His truth. Pray for help to make every moment left on earth count for something.

📖 God's Love Letter to You

Dear_____, (fill in your name)

My dear friends, I'm not writing anything new here. This is the oldest commandment in my book, and you've known it from day one. It's always been implicit in the Message you've heard from me. On the other hand, perhaps it is new, freshly minted as it is in both Christ and you—the darkness on its way out and the True Light already blazing! (1 John 2:7–8 MSG paraphrased).

I AM the Alpha and the Omega, the Beginning and the End, the New Beginning, God

🐰 Let's Pray

Please pray our closing prayer with me.

Lord, we, _____ and Janet, will miss our daily chats *together* with You, even though we, _____ and Janet, each commit to praying on our own. You also tell us that a chord of three strands, You, _____, and Janet, is not easily broken. Therefore, we look forward to our eternal reunion with each other and You on that glorious day we come together as sisters in Christ with a shared history of breast cancer. For now it is the time for us to do something spectacular with all that You have given us in whatever time we each have left. Lord, even if it is to reach out to a caregiver in our last hours or as powerful as a prodigal child accepting Jesus, we want You to use us till the *very end*—and each *new beginning*—and all the times in-between. Life has been dear, and we, _____ and Janet, cherish it. The future is unknown, but this we do know . . . all things are possible with Christ in our lives, and so we go forward ready for a *new beginning* with a faint memory of the past. It is in the name of your precious holy Son, Jesus Christ, that we, _____ and Janet, pray together. Amen.

✒️ Your Letter to God

You have written an entire book of letters to God. How does that feel? How has it helped you through this intricately wound maze of breast cancer? Where will it lead you? What will you do now? As you bring closure to your journal, think about what waits ahead for you. Each one of your *endings* will be so special and personal and the *beginning* of the rest of your life . . .

Dear God,   *Date:*

Step by Step
by Grace Marestaing

All of us walk a path—
Sometimes the way is gentle and smooth,
Our being hardly registering the forward movement.
We walk in the balmy, lulling warmth
and gentle breeze.
At times we walk out of habit,
unengaged and complacent,
as if we've seen it all before.
Fellow sojourners, we walk—step by step.
Sometimes the way turns rocky and hard,
and the path is steep and difficult.
The storm comes and we duck our head into the
freezing wind and stinging rain.
To stop the forward motion is to give up,
so we walk on—because we must.
Taking the leading edge of the storm head on,
we suddenly feel alone
and desperately look for a place of refuge—
for cover of answered questions,
for provision of looming needs,
for the stilling of fears and anxious thoughts.
The places of safety are there if we lift our head
just the slightest bit and look—
The crevices that would give us shelter,
the markers that point to hope are there—
if we'll just look.
They say we are courageous, the supporters
and observers of our progress.
Oh, if they only knew that God and they
are the source of light in the storm.
They speak the prayers we cannot voice.
They pull us forward, help us fight.
They keep us moving—step by step.
So we walk on.
©GMM, 2003

My New Beginning Prayer

I, _____, am scared to do this, Lord, because I _____ am not sure what it all means. But I do know that I couldn't be any more frightened than I am right now, not knowing where I will go when I die. I, _____, want to believe in you, God, and that You sent Your Son, Jesus, to wipe away my sins and give me eternal life with You. I don't understand everything about being a Christian, and I still have some questions; but I, _____, do know that I, _____, want to accept Jesus Christ today into my heart, and I am willing to learn more about what that means. Thank You for doing this for me . . . I feel strange and unworthy, but everything I have read in the Bible tells me that I, _____, am worthy and acceptable to You. Thank You for offering me this free gift of salvation. In Jesus's name, I, _____, pray. Amen!

Congratulations! You did it! You accepted Jesus into your heart as your personal Savior. Perhaps God's sole purpose in your breast cancer was to offer you eternal life. God wanted you to find Him, through this book or some other way, and give your life to Him. He forgave your sins and wiped the slate clean. God granted you a fresh start and eternal life in heaven. Nothing can take that away from you—absolutely nothing! Cancer can't, and neither can death. Isn't that good news in light of all the bad news you've received lately? Hang on tightly to the promise of God: "Be strong and courageous. Do not be afraid or terrified because of the enemy cancer, for I, the LORD your God, go with you; I will never leave you nor forsake you" (Deuteronomy 31:6 paraphrased).

You might want to go back through this book and reread "God's Love Letters to You" and *really* pray those prayers we prayed together under "Let's Pray." They will have so much more meaning and significance to you now.

If you are up to it, go to church this Sunday. If not, many church services are available on the Web. If you don't have a Bible and don't feel like going out to get one, order one online. Maybe you have enjoyed one of the translations I used in this book. I recommend any of them. Just remember that *The Message* is a paraphrase and not the actual translation. The *New Living Translation* would probably be a good Bible to start with. If your church has a breast cancer support group, it would be a great place to find other believers going through the same thing you are.

Above all, pray and talk to God about everything.

Appendix A

Remembering When

Trust the Lord
and his mighty power.
Worship him always.
Remember his miracles
and all his wonders
and his fair decisions.
You belong to the family.

—*1 Chronicles 16:11–13 CEV*

Dates That Changed Your Life

HOUR BY HOUR I PLACE MY DAYS IN YOUR HAND. —PSALM 31:15 MSG

Throughout the book most of the story contributors included specific dates as they related the events of their breast cancer. Did you notice that? Those dates are so important to them and imprinted in their memories just like birthdays and anniversaries. When one year rolled around for me, I knew exactly the anniversaries of all the initial appointments, biopsy day, diagnosis day, surgery day, start and completion of radiation dates. These are milestones etched in your and my histories. It is important we remember them to schedule annual checkups and know how long we have been on medications, but we also have a new way to mark time. "It was the month after my surgery" or "the year before I had breast cancer" or "the night before my mastectomy." We talk in terms also of years cancer-free or years since prognosis time.

As I was pondering whether these dates would be important to you, the Lord spoke clearly to me that those dates were like dates of battles fought and won in history, and I needed to give them the same reverence, honor, and respect. So I made sure they were included. Here is a place for you to keep track of all those significant dates, both for your personal use and as a medical reference. Remember, they are also anniversaries to celebrate and thank God for another year . . . day . . . moment of life.

Date   *Occurrence*

_____

_____

_____

_____

_____

_____

_____

_____

_____

_____

_____

Date *Occurrence*

ℛ_____

ℛ_____

ℛ_____

ℛ_____

ℛ_____

ℛ_____

ℛ_____

ℛ_____

ℛ_____

ℛ_____

ℛ_____

ℛ_____

ℛ_____

ℛ_____

ℛ_____

ℛ_____

ℛ_____

ℛ_____

ℛ_____

ℛ_____

ℛ_____

ℛ_____

Date   Occurrence

Memory Notes

Here is a page for you to write whatever you need to remember: grocery lists, names, instructions, directions, and so forth. Whether it's "chemo brain," "radiation brain," "Tamoxifen brain," or "early-middles brain," we all forget things, so write them down. Of course, if you're like me, you might forget you wrote them here!

Picture Me . . .

REMEMBER THIS MONTH AS A TIME WHEN OUR SORROW WAS TURNED TO JOY, AND CELEBRATION TOOK THE PLACE OF CRYING. CELEBRATE BY HAVING PARTIES AND BY GIVING TO THE POOR AND BY SHARING GIFTS OF FOOD WITH EACH OTHER. —ESTHER 9:22 CEV

I did finally lose most of my hair, and I have a beautiful head. John [her husband] is still taking a progression of pictures, and I will then post them to a Web site for all you interested baldy fans. —Linda M.

My friend Jane had her camera in the pre-surgery prep area, but my other friends would not let her take pictures of me and my doctors. I later regretted that. So when I started my radiation treatment, Jane brought her camera and literally did a documentary starting with the yellow radiation sign and going right through their prepping me for the treatment. I had her hand me the camera while I was lying down, and I took a picture of the cross cut in the ceiling that I told you about. She took pictures of Mary Ann, the radiation therapist, and we even have one of Jane with the physicist. Of course, there are pictures of Liz and Grace also. We compiled this into a PowerPoint presentation that I use when speaking.

We have pictures of me holding brand-new baby Micah the day before surgery and then having fun with all the grandkids who were home for the holidays during my recuperation. Shirley, who had the hat party, sent me fun collages of herself wearing all her hats and wigs and pictures from bald to stubble as well as pictures of her with her sister-in-law, who also was going through breast cancer chemotherapy. Shirley used this collage for her Christmas card. She said she wanted her family back in England to know she was alive and well. Shirley also mentioned putting all her pictures, e-mails, and cards in a "big C" scrapbook. Darlene Gee said she didn't take pictures, but now she wished she had. She knows of one woman whose daughter gave her a Creative Memories book when she started her treatments. They took pictures all through her journey, and she had her mom journal next to the pictures as they went along. When it was all over, she had a completed pictorial and written record in her own words, just as you have been writing in this book.

When you finish radiation and chemo, they often give you a certificate of completion. Admittedly, on my last day of radiation I was just glad to be done, but it did bring a smile as I came across it the other day. You might want to slip that in here too.

Perhaps you will want to put a smiling picture of your family or a friend to look at while you sit through those long waits or chemo treatments. This is your book, so do whatever feels right; use these next few pages in whatever way pleases you.

Appendix B
Sanity Tools

At the end of that time, I, Nebuchadnezzar, raised my eyes toward heaven, and my sanity was restored. Then I praised the Most High; I honored and glorified him who lives forever. . . . At the same time that my sanity was restored, my honor and splendor were returned to me for the glory of my kingdom.

—*Daniel 4:34, 36*

NOTE: In this section I've offered tools that would have been so helpful to me when I was going through my breast cancer journey. You might find it helpful to use a set of Post-its—they come in all colors!—to mark the pages you want to find quickly. You may also want to make extra copies of some of the forms before you write on them.

Doing Research

After the initial shock of learning I had cancer came the overwhelming task of choosing doctors and treatment options. I got lots of advice about alternative treatments from friends as well as medical advice from doctors. The more research I did, the more overwhelmed I felt. There are hundreds of cancer "cures" out there, in addition to the surgery, radiation, and chemotherapy offered by the medical profession. —Nancy Tuttle[1]

With cancer there is a fine line between educating yourself and inundating yourself with facts, statistics, and survival rates that are never going to apply to you. —Darlene Gee

Doing research is valuable, and there are many sources available—books, brochures, Web sites, calling the National Breast Cancer organizations, or talking to other breast cancer women. One of the sanity tools is a "National Contacts" list (page 345). Check with your doctors for handouts, publications, organizations, and Web sites they recommend for your particular type of breast cancer and treatment. My breast care center has a complete library with computers set up for our use. If you don't have access to a computer, they are available at most libraries. There may also be local cancer organizations in your area. You have read some of Heather's story in this book. She established a local organization to assist women going through breast cancer treatment who had no help or means of financial support. I read about another voluntary group that does something similar. If you have the energy, don't leave any stone unturned in finding financial aid and assistance. If you don't have the energy, enlist your friends and family to help.

Another sanity tool is a "Books Janet Found Helpful" list (page 346). By no means is this an exhaustive list. I could only absorb so much at a time and actually didn't even own some of these books until I started doing research for this book. Don't feel you need to read them all—they cover many of the same issues. When you begin to see confirming statements and are moving toward a decision, you probably have read enough. I found several personal-testimony books helpful. Even when they were not exactly about my type of cancer, the emotions expressed were the same, and it helped to validate my own feelings. However, one or two of these was sufficient, and then it was time to get on with my own story. You will want to do the same, I am sure.

When conducting research, it helps to have a central place to take notes. This prepares you for making peace-filled decisions as you work through the "Peacekeeping Worksheet."

Use these next few pages to jot down information, but here is a good benchmark—don't feel you have to fill them all. When and if they are full, you probably are ready to move to the decision phase. Warning: don't let yourself get into information overload—that can be overwhelming and paralyzing.

Research Notes

Source: _____

Area of Treatment: _____

Notes: _____

_____

Source: _____

Area of Treatment: _____

Notes: _____

_____

Source: _____

Area of Treatment: _____

Notes: _____

_____

Source: _____

Area of Treatment: _____

Notes: _____

_____

Source: _____

Area of Treatment: _____

Notes: _____

_____

Source: _____

Area of Treatment: _____

Notes: _____

_____

Research Notes

Source: _____

Area of Treatment: _____

Notes: _____

_____

Source: _____

Area of Treatment: _____

Notes: _____

_____

Source: _____

Area of Treatment: _____

Notes: _____

_____

Source: _____

Area of Treatment: _____

Notes: _____

_____

Source: _____

Area of Treatment: _____

Notes: _____

_____

Source: _____

Area of Treatment: _____

Notes: _____

_____

Source: _____

Area of Treatment: _____

Notes: _____

_____

Source: _____

Area of Treatment: _____

Notes: _____

_____

National Contacts

American Cancer Society
- www.cancer.org
- 1-800-ACS-2345 (1-800-227-2345)
- An extensive source of information on virtually every aspect of breast cancer and living with it

Susan G. Komen Breast Cancer Foundation
- www.komen.org OR www.breastcancerinfo.com
- helpline: 1-800-I'M-AWARE (1-800-462-9273)
- A comprehensive source for information on screening and treatment, news, public events, and survivor stories

Cancer News on the Net
- www.cancernews.com

Breast Cancer.Net (BCN)
- www.breastcancer.net

The National Cancer Institute
- www.cancer.gov OR www.nci.nih.gov OR www.cancernet.nci.nih.gov
- 1-800-4-CANCER (1-800-422-6237)
- Offers a huge volume of information from national statistics to the latest in detection, treatment, and clinical trials

Cancer Care, Inc
- www.cancercare.org
- 1-800-813-HOPE (1-800-813-4673)

Cancerlinks Building Opportunities for Self-Sufficiency (BOSS)
- www.cancerlinks.org

National Coalition for Cancer Survivorship (NCCS)
- www.canceradvocacy.org
- 1-877-622-7937 or 1-877-NCCS-YES or 1-888-650-9127

Susan Love, MD, Web site for Women
- www.susanlovemd.com

"Look Good . . . Feel Better" Program
- www.lookgoodfeelbetter.org
- 1-800-395-LOOK (1-800-395-5665) or call your local American Cancer Society office, or the American Cancer Society

The National Lymphedema Network
- www.lymphnet.org

Pink Ribbon.com
- www.pinkribbon.com
- A breast cancer resource center

Y-ME National Breast Cancer Organization
- www.y-me.org
- 1-800-221-2141 (English) or 1-800-986-9505 (Spanish)
- They provide a twenty-four-hour hotline with breast cancer survivors operating the phones, as well as affordable prosthesis information

Headcovers Unlimited
- www.headcovers.com
- Hats, turbans, and wigs for hair loss

Kids Konnected
- www.kidskonnected.org
- An online community for children whose parents are battling any type of cancer, it also has books and other links recommended on the Susan G. Komen Breast Cancer Foundation Web site (see above)

Gilda's Club
- www.gildasclub.org
- 1-888-Gilda-4-U (1-800-445-3248)
- A special place where the focus is on *living* with cancer and where men, women, and children with any kind of cancer and their family members and friends can plan and build life-changing emotional and social support

Books Janet Found Helpful

Spiritual Books
The Holy Bible

A Spiritual Journey through Breast Cancer: Strength for Today, Hope for Tomorrow, Judy Asti (Chicago: Northfield, 2002)

Disciplines of the Heart: Tuning Your Inner Life to God, Anne Ortland (Nashville: W Publishing, 1989)

The Cancer Survival Guide: Practical Help, Spiritual Hope, Kay Marshall Strom (New York: Beacon Hill, 2002)

The Purpose Driven Life, Rick Warren (Grand Rapids: Zondervan, 2002)

Medical Books

Tamoxifen and Breast Cancer—What Everyone Should Know about the Treatment of Breast Cancer, second edition, Michael W. DeGregorio and Valerie J. Wiebe. (New Haven, Conn.: Yale University Press, 1999)

The Breast Cancer Survival Manual: A Step-by-Step Guide for the Woman with Newly Diagnosed Breast Cancer, third edition, John Link, MD, et al (New York: Owl Books, 2003)

Dr. Susan Love's Breast Book, fourth edition, Susan M. Love, MD, and Karen Lindsey (Cambridge, Mass.: Da Capo Lifelong Books, 2005)

Living beyond Breast Cancer: A Survivor's Guide for When Treatment Ends and the Rest of Your Life Begins, Marisa C. Weiss, MD, and Ellen Weiss (New York: Three Rivers Press, 1998)

Nutritional Books

The Breast Cancer Prevention Diet, Dr. Robert Arnot (New York: Little, Brown and Company, 1999)

RawSome Recipes: Whole Foods for Vital Nutrition, third edition, Robyn Boyd (Life Sciences Press, 2005)

Tell Me What to Eat to Help Prevent Breast Cancer, Elaine Magee, MPH, RD (Franklin Lakes, N.J.: Career Press, 2000)

The Breast Cancer Prevention and Recovery Diet, Suzannah Olivier (Orem, Utah: Woodland, 2001)

The Maker's Diet: The 40 Day Health Experience That Will Change Your Life Forever, Jordan S. Rubin, MD, PhD (Lake Mary, Fla.: Siloam, 2004)

Testimonial Books

Getting Better, Not Bitter: A Spiritual Prescription for Breast Cancer, Brenda Ladun (Birmingham, Ala.: New Hope Publishers, 2002)

Fiction Books

After Anne, Roxanne Henke (Eugene, Ore.: Harvest House, 2002)

Decisions, Decisions, Decisions

Perhaps, as a result of continuous research in breast cancer, or the awareness brought by women and the media, the "old days" of the doctor deciding everything and the patient just following instructions are mostly in the past. The resulting interactions in the process following a positive diagnosis are ultimately good for all concerned but do have some challenges. Becoming a co–decision maker with the doctors is an immediate challenge to one's own lack of knowledge. I found myself having to absorb a lot of information and educate myself very quickly in order to make an informed decision. Of course, I put a great deal of trust in my doctors, and they were great in helping me sort through the information, but there were at least a couple of options for treatment and each would take me down a different path. My decision to have bilateral mastectomies was the result of my recent experiences with my mother's breast cancer, the process of decision making with my doctors, and much prayer. —Grace Marestaing

The needle biopsy was my first step after the suspicious mammogram, but yours might be another diagnostic procedure. Or maybe your first biopsy was benign, but a later one was positive. Perhaps you took the first option the radiologist gave me and decided just to have the area taken out without the cost or pain of the biopsy. Others of you had treatment to reduce the tumor before surgery. Each of us, in our own way and with the expertise of our medical teams, makes the decisions we feel are best for us. There are so many: Who are the right doctors? Should we get a second opinion? What course of treatment to select? Do we stay close to home or see a specialist farther away? Who should we tell? Who will watch the children? Should we try to continue working? To reconstruct or not?

When faced with the many overwhelming decisions, I found it helpful to:

- Write down what the doctors said.

- Do some research.

- Consult my family.

- Ask others to pray specifically for the decision.

- Pray about all of the above.

- Arrive at a decision that gave me peace.

I thought it might be helpful for you, also, to have a place to go through this "peacekeeping exercise," so I am including the following form for you to process decisions and then arrive at the conclusion that provides you the most peace. You might be thinking at this point, *What does she mean, "peace"? This is a chaotic, terrible time in my life. How can I feel peace about anything?* For sure, on our own, we can't. However, I discovered that seeking the Lord for answers and direction and enlisting the prayers of everyone I knew resulted in peaceful decisions.

It is exciting to see God confirm His presence throughout the cancer experience, as He did with the newspaper article about my surgeon and radiologist. There were more signs to come. Doctors are very educated and gifted humans. Our family and friends love us, but I found only the Lord could grant me perfect peace. Jesus says in John 16:33, "I have told you these things, so that in me you may have peace. In this world you will have trouble. But take heart! I have overcome the world." Paul wrote in Philippians 4:5–7, "The Lord is near. Do not be anxious about anything, but in everything, by prayer and petition, with thanksgiving, present your requests to God. And the peace of God, which transcends all understanding, will guard your hearts and your minds in Christ Jesus."

Then I began to pray, and it was as if I heard the Lord say, "I will take care of this." I immediately had a peace that continues through today. —Cheryl

Peacekeeping Worksheet for Decisions about . . .

_____

Facts from Doctors _____

_____

_____

_____

Facts from Research _____

_____

_____

_____

Facts from Consultations _____

_____

_____

Doctors' Opinions and Suggestions _____

_____

_____

_____

Input from Family/Friends _____

_____

_____

Time with God in Prayer _____

_____

_____

My Peace-Filled Decision Is: _____

_____

_____

Peacekeeping Worksheet for Decisions about . . .

_____

Facts from Doctors_____

_____

_____

_____

Facts from Research _____

_____

_____

_____

Facts from Consultations _____

_____

_____

_____

Doctors' Opinions and Suggestions _____

_____

_____

_____

Input from Family/Friends_____

_____

_____

Time with God in Prayer _____

_____

_____

My Peace-Filled Decision Is:_____

_____

_____

Appointments, Appointments, Appointments

On appointment day my little faithful was right here to go with me. Sue and I went a little early to fill in all forms and turn in my report. He [the doctor] gave my upper quadrant a thorough examination. Sue took a few notes as I was answering his questions. —Martha[2]

Medical studies indicate most people suffer a 68 percent hearing loss when naked. —United Health Foundation

The last quote above was the title in an advertisement run in magazines and newspapers encouraging people to get the most out of their doctor appointments. Another United Health Foundation ad is titled "There Are 126 Schools in the Country That Teach You How to Be a Physician, but Not One for How to Be a Patient." Here were some of their suggestions:

- Take a friend for support, someone who will help you remember important information.

- Educate yourself. Gather trustworthy information on your condition.

- Have key information with you, including your medical history and medication history.

- Be up-front. Tell your doctors everything, or they might miss something important.

- You have to ask in order to receive. If you want answers, you have to ask questions. Write them out ahead of time.

It is very important to keep good records of all your appointments:

- The plan and purpose for each appointment

- Questions you want to ask

- The outcome, instructions, and action to take after each appointment

- Phone conversations you have with the doctors and medical facilities between appointments

- Copies of all your medical records

I found myself writing all this down on scraps of paper and numerous Realtor notepads. Even if you are a Day-Timer or notebook-type person, the rest of your life is also written in that Day-Timer. It takes time and energy to search for medical-appointment notes intermingled with other aspects of your life. I longed for *one* place to keep everything relevant to my breast cancer. Things happened so fast, I never found a dedicated place. I designed this book to be that for you. Following are some recordkeeping pages.

Questions will continuously run through your mind at odd times of the day and night. Keep this book handy to jot them down on the appointment space for the appropriate doctor or technician. Then you are well prepared during appointments or phone calls from doctors and their offices or when you call them. When the phone rings, grab your book. If you forget, excuse yourself for one moment and go get it *before* they start giving you information. Frequently there are new terms or procedures explained, or maybe shocking news. If I did not write down everything they said as they were talking, I couldn't remember half of it when I hung up.

Same thing at the doctor's office—write down *everything* they say. Even better, take someone with you to take notes into your book. Some have found it helpful to take a tape recorder and tape conversations with the doctor so you can replay them later and accurately fill in the blanks of your memory. Be sure you explain to your doctors the reason for the tape recorder so they will not feel intimidated by it. If you don't understand something or they talk too fast, ask them to slow down and repeat.

You are entitled to copies of all your medical records. They will be helpful in the future and for a family history. I waited until the end of my treatment and requested them from the radiation oncologist, who gladly had his office staff copy my medical folder. Since he was the last doctor in that series of treatments, he had everything in one place. Your cancer oncologist, whom you continue with for follow-up treatment, should also have a culmination of all your records. Always ask for a copy of the results of any blood work, x-ray reports, and mammogram reports—essentially anything you have done. I have provided you a form to keep track of any reports or information given to you verbally.

Then put all of this information in a safe place. If you have a file cabinet, dedicate a portion of it to your cancer care. I find it helpful to have a folder for each doctor. When I come across an article about new drugs or treatment, I slip it in the appropriate doctor's folder. Before an appointment I review that doctor's folder and prepare questions to ask. When they give me copies of reports or blood work, it all goes in these folders.

I know this sounds terribly organized when you are just trying to get through this battle. This, again, could be something you ask someone to help you set up and maintain. It saves so much stress and worry when you are trying to find that important article in a magazine and you only have five minutes to get to the doctor. Another factor—we trust our doctors, but they are only human; it is important to double-check test results and reports. I was the one who pointed out to my first gynecologist that I might be going through menopause and that was why my Pap smears constantly came back irregular. Guess what, I was right! I also changed my gynecologist, and the new doctor turned out to be the one whom God used to discover my breast cancer.

Do you remember my saying earlier that I had a folder titled Menopause? I started it long before menopause was in my realm of reality, but that file was invaluable for going through "the change" and having relevant, accessible breast cancer information. Be a student of yourself. Keep your eyes open. Cut things out when you see them, or write down when you hear them, and tuck it all in folders for future reference. Maybe you are actually saving some of these things to help someone else too!

Appointment Notes

Appointment with:_____ Date:_____ Time:_____ Place:_____

Purpose of Appointment:_____

- Question to ask: _____

  Answer: _____

  _____

- Question to ask: _____

  Answer: _____

  _____

  _____

- Question to ask: _____

  Answer: _____

  _____

  _____

Doctor's information and instructions: _____

_____

_____

_____

_____

_____

_____

_____

Appointment Notes

Appointment with:_____ Date:_____ Time:_____ Place:_____

Purpose of Appointment:_____

- Question to ask: _____

  Answer: _____

  _____

- Question to ask: _____

  Answer: _____

  _____

  _____

- Question to ask: _____

  Answer: _____

  _____

  _____

Doctor's information and instructions:_____

_____

_____

_____

_____

_____

_____

_____

_____

_____

_____

Appointment Notes

Appointment with:_____ Date:_____ Time:_____ Place:_____

Purpose of Appointment:_____

- Question to ask: _____

  Answer: _____

  _____

- Question to ask: _____

  Answer: _____

  _____

  _____

- Question to ask: _____

  Answer: _____

  _____

  _____

Doctor's information and instructions:_____

_____

_____

_____

_____

_____

_____

_____

_____

_____

_____

_____

_____

Appointment Notes

Appointment with:_____ Date:_____ Time:_____ Place:_____

Purpose of Appointment:_____

- Question to ask: _____

  Answer: _____

  _____

- Question to ask: _____

  Answer: _____

  _____

  _____

- Question to ask: _____

  Answer: _____

  _____

  _____

Doctor's information and instructions:_____

_____

_____

_____

_____

_____

_____

_____

_____

_____

_____

Oh No! I Just Remembered . . .

Often questions arise right after your appointments. You are driving home or wake up the next morning and can't believe you forgot to ask a really important question. Or during the day questions just pop into your head, and you don't want to forget them. Doctors and technicians encourage you to call, even if it is not urgent. They do not want you worrying or fretting. Here are a couple of pages to jot down those questions so you can be equipped when the time comes to ask them. I spent a lot of time fumbling through my purse for the scrap of paper I wrote something on, or the grocery list or envelope I had in my hand when the question came to mind. If I was fortunate enough to find it, I wrote the answer there too. Then, oh my, now where did it go?

Questions -and-Answers Note Page

Question: _____

Person to Ask: _____

Answer: _____

What to Do Next: _____

Question: _____

Person to Ask: _____

Answer: _____

What to Do Next: _____

Question: _____

Person to Ask: _____

Answer: _____

What to Do Next: _____

Question: _____

Person to Ask: _____

Answer: _____

What to Do Next: _____

Question: _____

Person to Ask: _____

Answer: _____

What to Do Next: _____

Question: _____

Person to Ask: _____

Answer: _____

What to Do Next: _____

Question: _____

Person to Ask: _____

Answer: _____

What to Do Next: _____

Question: _____

Person to Ask: _____

Answer: _____

What to Do Next: _____

Question: _____

Person to Ask: _____

Answer: _____

What to Do Next: _____

Question: _____

Person to Ask: _____

Answer: _____

What to Do Next: _____

There's the Phone Again

Your phone will ring frequently. Don't answer it if you don't feel up to talking. Let the answering machine or someone else pick it up. There were so many times when I had no energy for phone conversation but now would love a record of all the people who called. Of course, when one of your medical team calls, you want to answer and write down everything they say. Here is a spot for taking phone notes.

Phone Notes

Date: _____ Time: _____ Who called: _____

Message: _____

My response to the call: _____

_____

Date: _____ Time: _____ Who called: _____

Message: _____

My response to the call: _____

_____

Date: _____ Time: _____ Who called: _____

Message: _____

My response to the call: _____

_____

Date: _____ Time: _____ Who called: _____

Message: _____

My response to the call: _____

_____

Date: _____ Time: _____ Who called: _____

Message: _____

My response to the call: _____

_____

Date: _____ Time: _____ Who called: _____

Message: _____

My response to the call: _____

_____

Date: _____ Time: _____ Who called: _____

Message: _____

My response to the call: _____

_____

Date: _____ Time: _____ Who called: _____

Message: _____

My response to the call: _____

_____

Date: _____ Time: _____ Who called: _____

Message: _____

My response to the call: _____

_____

Date: _____ Time: _____ Who called: _____

Message: _____

My response to the call: _____

_____

We Are in This Together

As treatment progresses, you will meet many fellow patients in waiting rooms, during chemo treatments, at support groups, and so on. A common bond develops among strangers fighting the same battle. Some of us exchanged business cards, but, frankly, my focus was on getting through the ordeal. I didn't feel much like making contact with other cancer patients, except when our paths crossed. Now I would love to know how they are doing. Here is a place to write down their information. And don't forget to slip in their business cards or contact information in the pocket of this book, and you can keep some of your own ready to hand out.

New Friend's Name _____ Where Met _____
Telephone_____ Cell Phone_____ E-mail _____
Address_____
_____

New Friend's Name _____ Where Met _____
Telephone_____ Cell Phone_____ E-mail _____
Address_____
_____

New Friend's Name _____ Where Met _____
Telephone_____ Cell Phone_____ E-mail _____
Address_____
_____

New Friend's Name _____ Where Met _____
Telephone_____ Cell Phone_____ E-mail _____
Address_____
_____

New Friend's Name _____ Where Met _____
Telephone_____ Cell Phone_____ E-mail _____
Address_____
_____

New Friend's Name _____ Where Met _____
Telephone_____ Cell Phone_____ E-mail _____
Address_____
_____

My Medical Team

Every professional taking part in your treatment will give you a business card, often doubling as your next appointment card. The pockets in the cover of this book are a place to put those cards, as well as other handouts they give you, until you can transcribe the information to the appropriate form in the "Sanity Tools." This information is a lifeline when you need it, but often, trying to find it means rummaging through your purse, pants pocket, the floor of the car, or a book. If I had allotted some organization time, or had this book, it would have made a hectic period so much less stressful. I actually am a very organized person, and you probably are, too, but don't you feel things are moving so rapidly, there is just no time to stop and clean out your purse or organize your desk? You are fighting for your life for goodness' sake! (Although you might actually get that urge to clean later—I did.)

You need a place to write down all the necessary contact information for your medical team in case you lose or misplace those valuable business cards. Do everything you can to eliminate stress and frustration. Here is a spot to help you with that.

Important Information about My Medical Team

Name _____

Role in my treatment _____

Phone_____ Fax_____ E-mail_____

Address_____

Nurse Contact _____ Phone/Ext. _____

Billing Office Contact _____ Phone/Ext. _____

Name _____

Role in my treatment _____

Phone_____ Fax_____ E-mail_____

Address_____

Nurse Contact _____ Phone/Ext. _____

Billing Office Contact _____ Phone/Ext. _____

Name _____

Role in my treatment _____

Phone_____ Fax_____ E-mail_____

Address_____

Nurse Contact _____ Phone/Ext. _____

Billing Office Contact _____ Phone/Ext. _____

Name _____

Role in my treatment _____

Phone_____ Fax_____ E-mail_____

Address_____

Nurse Contact _____ Phone/Ext. _____

Billing Office Contact _____ Phone/Ext. _____

Name _____

Role in my treatment _____

Phone_____ Fax_____ E-mail_____

Address_____

Nurse Contact _____ Phone/Ext. _____

Billing Office Contact _____ Phone/Ext. _____

Name _____

Role in my treatment _____

Phone_____ Fax_____ E-mail_____

Address_____

Nurse Contact _____ Phone/Ext. _____

Billing Office Contact _____ Phone/Ext. _____

Name _____

Role in my treatment _____

Phone_____ Fax_____ E-mail_____

Address_____

Nurse Contact _____ Phone/Ext. _____

Billing Office Contact _____ Phone/Ext. _____

Name _____

Role in my treatment _____

Phone_____ Fax_____ E-mail_____

Address_____

Nurse Contact _____ Phone/Ext. _____

Billing Office Contact _____ Phone/Ext. _____

Additional Numbers Others or I May Need

Hospital _____

Address_____

Phone_____ Billing Phone _____

Emergency Room Phone _____ Oncology Unit Phone_____

Emergency Phone Numbers

Fire Department_____ Police _____

Ambulance_____ Paramedics _____

Pharmacy _____ Pharmacist _____

Address_____

Phone_____ After-Hours Phone _____

Delivery Available_____

Mammogram Center _____

Address_____

Phone_____ Billing Phone _____

Contact Person_____ Ext._____

Counselor/Support Group/Social Services

Name of Agency_____

Address_____

Phone_____ Meeting Times _____

Services They Provide _____

Contact Person_____

Home Health/Hospice Services

Name of Agency_____

Address_____

Phone_____ Nurse Case Manager_____

Nursing Services They Provide:

- ❑ Physical Therapy
- ❑ Rehabilitation Services
- ❑ Medication Management
- ❑ Bath Aide

- ❑ Occupational Therapy
- ❑ Side-Effect Management
- ❑ Chore Services
- ❑ Other_____

Insurance Company _____

Address_____

Phone_____ Policy Number _____

Group # _____ Subscriber Number _____

Medicare Number _____ Public Assistance # _____

Case Manager_____

Nutritional Assistance

Registered Dietitian _____ Phone _____

Address_____

Meals-on-Wheels Contact Person _____ Phone _____

Restaurants that Deliver

Restaurant _____ Phone _____

Restaurant _____ Phone _____

Restaurant _____ Phone _____

Restaurant _____ Phone _____

Restaurant _____ Phone _____

Personal-Assistance Contacts

Prosthesis and Bra Fitting_____ Phone _____

Wig Fitting_____ Phone _____

Breast Cancer Massage Therapist _____ Phone _____

Prosthesis and Bra Fitting_____ Phone _____

Prosthesis and Bra Fitting_____ Phone _____

Transportation Services

Taxi _____ Phone _____

Shuttle Services _____ Phone _____

Private Ride Services_____ Phone _____

Transportation Ministries_____ Phone _____

Church_____

Pastor_____ Phone_____ After Hours _____

Prayer Chain Number _____ Meals Ministry _____

Support Group Contact _____ Phone _____

Family and Friends

Name_____ Phone_____

Name_____ Phone_____

Name_____ Phone_____

Name_____ Phone_____

Name_____ Phone_____

Name_____ Phone_____

Name_____ Phone_____

Name_____ Phone_____

Name_____ Phone_____

People I Can Talk to Any Time of Day or Night

Name_____ Phone_____

Name_____ Phone_____

Name_____ Phone_____

Name_____ Phone_____

Name_____ Phone_____

Name_____ Phone_____

Name_____ Phone_____

Name_____ Phone_____

Name_____ Phone_____

Keeping Good Records

My blood-cell count had recovered well. I did not know I was supposed to ask and keep track of what my count is. It took another cancer patient (my mother-in-law) to tell me I should know that information. She has a little book where they record the count for her. —Linda M.

THEY LOOKED HIGH AND LOW FOR THEIR FAMILY RECORDS BUT COULDN'T FIND THEM.
—NEHEMIAH 7:64 MSG

I cannot stress enough the importance of keeping all your breast cancer information in one place. Utilizing the following sanity-tool forms can help you do that and stay sane at the same time. You are entitled to copies of all tests and blood work, and you should ask for them. Doctor offices are busy—there is always the possibility for something to go unnoticed or be misplaced. Nancy Tuttle found out too late that her file mistakenly ended up in a doctor's office drawer, and she never received a phone call to retest an elevated CEA cancer marker. The oversight went undiscovered until she changed doctors, but by then the cancer had spread through her lymph system to her spine. The lessons she said she learned include:

- Ask for copies of all blood tests.

- Ask a lot more questions.

- Take a more active role in my health care.

The following chart is a place where you can keep track of all your test results.

Test Results

Date	Test Name	Results	Retest Date

Test Results

Date	Test Name	Results	Retest Date

Taking My Meds

I helped my friend Cheryl when she had knee-replacement surgery. Cheryl had quite a regime of medications. Her husband wrote down what we gave her and the time so we would not have to remember if she took her medications or not. I soon realized the need for something very similar myself. I don't know if it's age, menopause, radiation, or Tamoxifen, but I no longer have a photographic memory. Are you tracking with me? It was shocking not to remember taking my vitamins or Tamoxifen! I tried setting them out so if they were gone, it meant I took them, but then I questioned whether they were set out that day!

This was a real struggle until I came across a pillbox to use for traveling, which now gets daily use. It contains a pop-out row for every day of the week. Each pop-out has four compartments, labeled with the day of the week and Breakfast, Lunch, Dinner, and one for afternoon or evening. Monday mornings I get out all medications and vitamins and fill the boxes for the entire week. Now each day I just take out that day's compartment (knowing they were filled on Monday) and take my meds. Hope that makes sense. It was less than ten dollars at the pharmacy. See if you can find something similar. It is one less thing to think or stress about.

Following is a medication-record form to use during those times when you don't have the energy to fill up little boxes but need to keep track of your medications. It is also a good record of what medications and dosages you are taking, which is often requested information on doctors' forms.

Medication Record

Drug	Dose/Freq	Date/Time	Reason	"X" When Taken

Medication Record

Drug	Dose/Freq	Date/Time	Reason	"X" When Taken

My Breast Cancer Journey Map

Are you the kind of person who likes to chart your course? This next page is for you. On the "Milestone" lines write in your treatment plan and the projected dates. Then you can check off or highlight them as you pass one milestone and move on to the next. You'll begin to feel a sense of accomplishment and be encouraged as you move down the page and more and more is behind you. It also gives you an overview in one glance of the journey you are traveling.

Breast Cancer Journey Map

Milestone

Date

GIVE ME YOUR LANTERN AND COMPASS, GIVE ME A MAP, SO I CAN FIND MY WAY TO THE SACRED MOUNTAIN, TO THE PLACE OF YOUR PRESENCE, TO ENTER THE PLACE OF WORSHIP, MEET MY EXUBERANT GOD, SING MY THANKS WITH A HARP, MAGNIFICENT GOD, MY GOD.

—PSALM 43:3–4 MSG

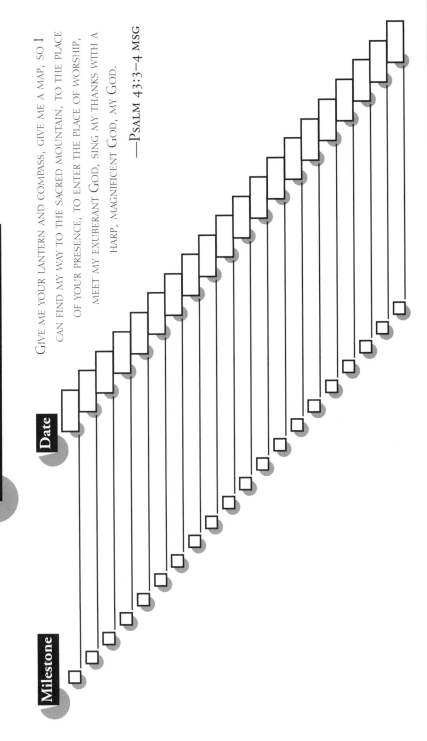

My Support and Help Team

You will need help in the upcoming weeks. It is humbling to acknowledge this, but when you do, it frees you to begin enlisting the services of close friends, relatives, coworkers, neighbors, and your church. Sit down right now and make a list of people you can count on. Don't be surprised if people you don't have on your list also come forward offering assistance. It is important to have the contact information of your support team close at hand.

Name _____ Home Phone _____

Work Phone _____ Cell Phone _____

Address _____ E-mail _____

How Could This Person Help Me? _____

What Did They Offer to Do? _____

Name _____ Home Phone _____

Work Phone _____ Cell Phone _____

Address _____ E-mail _____

How Could This Person Help Me? _____

What Did They Offer to Do? _____

Name _____ Home Phone _____

Work Phone _____ Cell Phone _____

Address _____ E-mail _____

How Could This Person Help Me? _____

What Did They Offer to Do? _____

Name _____ Home Phone _____

Work Phone _____ Cell Phone _____

Address _____ E-mail _____

How Could This Person Help Me? _____

What Did They Offer to Do? _____

Name _____ Home Phone _____

Work Phone _____ Cell Phone _____

Address _____ E-mail _____

How Could This Person Help Me? _____

What Did They Offer to Do? _____

Minding the Doctor

Do not think people can "read" your mind. If you want or need someone to do something for you, let them know! —Linda Taylor

Listen carefully when the doctors explain your limitations, possible reactions, complications, restrictions on activity, and so on. Don't panic. You just made a list of people you can call on. This is not the time to play the tough role. You need to do what the doctor says and focus on getting well. Rest is a big part of the body's healing process. However, problems arise when we do not know how to receive help, and others don't know how to offer it. I found myself staring blankly when people said things like, "Just call me if you need anything," "Where do you need help?" "What can I do?" My mind raced through a never-ending list. I wanted to say, "I need everything!" but usually no response came out. I didn't know what they were willing to do. Did they mean clean my house? Give me a ride? Fix a meal? I didn't want to put them on the spot, and I wasn't sure how much of themselves they were expecting to give.

To avoid those awkward moments when you don't know how to respond to an offer of assistance, make a list of all the areas where you need help. When someone asks where he or she can help, say something like, "Oh, thank you so much for your kind offer. I really do need help in these areas. Is there one that might fit your schedule?" Then hand them your list, or the one on the following page, and let them choose. As people make selections, mark those off the list. You don't want everyone bringing you a meal and then you don't have a ride to a treatment or doctor appointment. This takes the pressure off you and gives them a chance to gracefully say where they are comfortable helping. *Then take their help!* No one expects you to be superwoman or thinks less of you for needing help. It is easier to give than to receive—that is true. Nevertheless, it is a gift to allow people to serve. The Woman to Woman Mentoring Ministry calls it "an opportunity to serve."

In *Today's Christian Woman* magazine, S. K. Whang wrote an article titled "The Joy of Being Served" during her battle with breast cancer. A line that jumped out at me was, "Through this experience, God taught me that letting others serve me can be as much an act of faith as reaching out to others in need."[3]

More than one woman has said she frantically had to think of things for her friends to do because they all wanted to help. They were actually offended if she couldn't think of anything. For many of your friends and family, helping you is their way of showing how much they love you and want to be a part of your healing and recovery. Receive it gracefully, knowing that it does not make you any less a homemaker or wife or mother. When you are well, return the favors you received by being there for someone needing assistance. You can be sure God will put those people in your path. However, for right now, that needy person is *you*. I will start the list, and then you personalize and add to it. Be sure to tuck the list in your purse to have handy when someone says, "How can I help?"

Bless You! Here's Where I Need Help

- ❏ Rides:
  - ❏ When
  - ❏ Where
  - ❏ How long it will take

- ❏ Meals:
  - ❏ Breakfast
  - ❏ Lunch
  - ❏ Dinner

- ❏ Shopping:
  - ❏ Groceries
  - ❏ Medications
  - ❏ Personal Items
  - ❏ Other

- ❏ Childcare:
  - ❏ What days?
  - ❏ What hours?
  - ❏ Your home
  - ❏ My home

- ❏ "Me" Care
  - ❏ What hours?
  - ❏ Your home
  - ❏ My home

- ❏ Rides for the kids
  (Specify days and times)
  - ❏ School
  - ❏ Sports
  - ❏ Church
  - ❏ Activities
  - ❏ Other

- ❏ Prayer Partners

- ❏ Someone to call when I'm down

- ❏ Someone to call when I'm up

- ❏ Housecleaning

- ❏ Laundry

- ❏ Answering e-mails

- ❏ Sending thank-you notes

- ❏ Running errands

- ❏ Paying bills and assisting with financial obligations

- ❏ Checking with my insurance plan to see what's covered, including:
  - ❏ Wigs
  - ❏ Prosthesis
  - ❏ Reconstruction
  - ❏ Surgery on the "well" breast for symmetry
  - ❏ Home care

- ❏ Taking over some commitments I have at church or on a committee

- ❏ Filling in for me at work

- ❏ Doing yard work

- ❏ Helping with my car:
  - ❏ Fill with gas
  - ❏ Wash
  - ❏ Maintenance

☐ Doing maintenance around the house

☐ Accompany me to doctor appointments and treatments

☐ Accompany me to my first support group

☐ Go shopping with me to buy:
    ☐ Wig
    ☐ Prosthesis
    ☐ First bra after surgery

☐ _____
☐ _____
☐ _____

When I Need Comfort or Someone to Talk To

This is an emotional time of life. You are probably saying, "That is an understatement! Without a doubt, this tops anything I have ever experienced emotionally. I am all over the board with my feelings." Some describe it as a "roller coaster of emotions."

You know yourself and how you react to life situations. Where are you going to need moral support? We usually have different people in our lives we go to for various kinds of support. Take a moment now to list feelings you already have experienced or feel you might in the future. Who could you call or ask to come over when you are feeling this way? Again, I will give you a few ideas to start with, and then you add to it or cross off ones that don't apply to you. With something as personal as breast cancer, most women find they need to talk to another woman. As much as the men in our lives love us, they cannot readily identify with some of the feelings we have, and chances are, they have their own struggles to work through.

Who Will I Call or Where Will I Go When I Am Feeling . . .

☐ In need of prayer _____

☐ Sad _____

☐ Happy_____

❑ Bad in general _____

❑ Discouraged _____

❑ Depressed _____

❑ Encouraged_____

❑ Scared _____

❑ Like I want to cry _____

❑ Like I need to laugh _____

❑ Physically ill _____

❑ Lonely_____

❑ Overwhelmed _____

❑ At peace and want to share it_____

❑ Other Areas_____

Where Can My Husband and Family Go for Comfort?

It's all about you right now. Everyone tells you that and, honestly, you feel that way. Husbands, fiancés, boyfriends, children, immediate family, and extended family can sometimes get lost in the shuffle and may not even realize they are not dealing with the new you. Brainstorm ideas to suggest to them for support or an outlet. If they are reticent, consider making a few calls yourself, and ask dear and trusted friends to make themselves available for a golf game or dinner or a play date with the kids—anything that can bring a sense of normalcy back into their lives.

Support System for My Family and Friends

• Who will this most affect?

• What areas will be hard for them?

• Who could help?

• What would help?

My Breast Cancer Purpose and Plan

Use this space to take notes as the Lord reveals to you in the unfolding months the plan and purpose He will fulfill through your breast cancer journey.

BECAUSE OF THE SACRIFICE OF THE MESSIAH . . . WE'RE A FREE PEOPLE—FREE OF PENALTIES AND PUNISHMENTS CHALKED UP BY ALL OUR MISDEEDS. AND NOT JUST BARELY FREE, EITHER. ABUNDANTLY FREE! HE THOUGHT OF EVERYTHING, PROVIDED FOR EVERYTHING WE COULD POSSIBLY NEED, LETTING US IN ON THE PLANS HE TOOK SUCH DELIGHT IN MAKING. HE SET IT ALL OUT BEFORE US IN CHRIST, A LONG-RANGE PLAN IN WHICH EVERYTHING WOULD BE BROUGHT TOGETHER AND SUMMED UP IN HIM, EVERYTHING IN DEEPEST HEAVEN, EVERYTHING ON PLANET EARTH. IT'S IN CHRIST THAT WE FIND OUT WHO WE ARE AND WHAT WE ARE LIVING FOR. LONG BEFORE WE FIRST HEARD OF CHRIST AND GOT OUR HOPES UP, HE HAD HIS EYE ON US, HAD DESIGNS ON US FOR GLORIOUS LIVING, PART OF THE OVERALL PURPOSE HE IS WORKING OUT IN EVERYTHING AND EVERYONE. —EPHESIANS 1:7–12 MSG

Prayer-and-Praise Journal

The best sanity tool I can think of is a place to write specific prayer requests and then record the answers. These pages give you that opportunity. After you have written your requests to God, be sure to come back and make a notation of the day and way He answered. When you are having a low day, read these pages and see God in action. Revisit your journal on really good days, too, so you remember from where your joy comes.

<table>
<tr><td>

I YELL OUT TO MY GOD,
I YELL WITH ALL MY MIGHT,
I YELL AT THE TOP OF MY LUNGS.
HE LISTENS.
—PSALM 77:1 MSG

</td><td>

ONCE AGAIN I'LL GO OVER WHAT GOD HAS DONE, LAY OUT ON THE TABLE THE ANCIENT WONDERS; I'LL PONDER ALL THE THINGS YOU'VE ACCOMPLISHED, AND GIVE A LONG, LOVING LOOK AT YOUR ACTS.
—PSALM 77:11–12 MSG

</td></tr>
</table>

Prayer Request	Praise

Prayer Request	Praise

Express Yourself!

This page is for you to let loose all your feelings and do whatever you want. You might want to draw, scribble, dig your pen in and just go crazy, write a poem . . . feel free. It's all yours!

About the Author

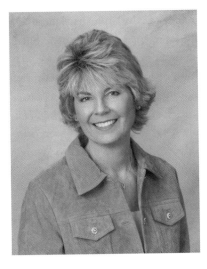

Janet Thompson became a Christian at age eleven, a year after the murder of her father, a highway patrolman shot on duty with his own gun. Janet's family learned how to deal with tragedy at an early age, as she was ten, her sister four, and her mom a young widow at thirty-two. They each had a different way of dealing with his death. For Janet, it was accepting Christ as her heavenly Father in place of "my dearly loved earthly father" whom she had just lost.

Janet was on fire for the Lord throughout her teens, even when crippling scoliosis kept her at home for two years in a plaster body cast. She stayed faithful to God during her college years. However, the day after graduating from college, Janet married without consulting the Lord. Sadly, that marriage only lasted six years, but God blessed her with a sweet baby girl, Kimberly Michele. The next seventeen years Janet was a single parent, moving up a successful worldly career ladder. They were times of great backsliding away from the Lord.

In 1992, Janet rededicated her life to Christ and met her future, godly husband, Dave. They married and became a blended family with Dave's three children, Michelle, Shannon, Sean, and Janet's Kim. Dave and Janet quickly accepted each other's children as their own.

The spring of 1995, Janet received a call from the Lord to "feed My sheep." Within months God revealed the "sheep" were women and the "feeding" was mentoring. So she quit a lucrative career in insurance to start the Woman to Woman Mentoring Ministry at her home church, Saddleback Church in Lake Forest, California. Three months later, Dave went through a layoff and was out of work for a year and a half. As friends and family asked if Janet was going back to work, Dave repeatedly answered, "She *is* working." When asked, "At what?" He replied, "She is about the Lord's work"—thus the name of Janet's writing and speaking ministry, *About His Work (AHW)* Ministries. *AHW* Ministries has now expanded to *AHW* Publishing and *Two about His Work*, a speaking ministry with Janet's best friend and coworker for Christ, Jane Crick. You can find out more about *AHW* Ministries at their Web site: www.womantowomanmentoring.com.

Dave and Janet live in Lake Forest, California, and have been members of Saddleback Church since 1987. All four of their children are married, and they have nine wonderful grandchildren—six boys and three girls! Janet and Dave are enjoying the empty-nest season of life Janet refers to as "parents time to rest"—although they often comment it seems busier being about the Lord's work than any time in their lives.

About His Work Ministries

About His Work Ministries is Janet Thompson's writing and speaking ministry. Janet has a passion for today's women to live significant lives regardless of their circumstances. She is about His work helping women realize the importance and value of relationships and God's call in Titus 2:3–5 to teach and train the next generation of women through mentoring and loving them. Janet leads the Woman to Woman Mentoring Ministry, which she started in 1996 at Saddleback Church. Through her resources, *Woman to Woman Mentoring: How to Start, Grow, and Maintain a Mentoring Ministry,* and a Bible study series, Mentoring God's Way, she has helped numerous churches around the world start Woman to Woman Mentoring.

For More Information and to Contact Janet

Two about His Work

Janet and her best friend, Jane Crick, have a speaking ministry called *Two about His Work.* To contact them about speaking availability:

> Tom Crick—*Two about His Work* Ministries
> Phone/Fax 949-380-0690
> Tom@2ahw.com

Woman to Woman Mentoring

For information about *Woman to Woman Mentoring: How to Start, Grow, and Maintain a Mentoring Ministry:*

> www.lifeway.com
> Call LifeWay at 1-800-458-2772
> Visit your nearest LifeWay Bookstore

Mentoring God's Way Bible Study

For information about the Mentoring God's Way Bible Study series:

> E-mail: ahwpublishing@sbcglobal.net
> Call *AHW* Publishing at 559-713-0421

To Contact Janet Thompson and *About His Work* Ministries

> Janet would love to hear now this book has impacted you or someone else's life:
> Phone/Fax: 949-837-0614
> E-mail: ahw@sbcglobal.net
> www.womantowomanmentoring.com

NOTES

Introduction: Sharing Sister to Sister

1. Nancy Tuttle, *Purpose in Trial: Finding Joy and Meaning in the Midst of Cancer* (Mission Viejo, Calif: Kenosis, 2002).

2. Nancy Tuttle with Randall Niles, *The Prodigal Prayer* (Mission Viejo, Calif.: Kenosis, 2002), v–vi.

Chapter One: Making the Annual Appointments

1. Bonnie Davidson, www.pinkribbon.com/my_story.htm. Accessed 04/12/04.

2. American Cancer Society, "How Is Breast Cancer Found?" http://www.cancer.org/docroot/CRI/content/CRI_2_2_3X_How_is_breast_cancer_found_5.asp?sitearea= (Accessed May 11, 2006)

3. Martha Ramsey, *To Cry or Not to Cry: Coping and Winning the Battle after Mastectomy* (Lufkin, Tex.: Pineywoods Printing, 1995), 12.

4. Ramsey, *To Cry or Not to Cry*, 16–17.

Chapter Two: Facing the Dreaded Diagnosis

1. Jennifer Leclaire, "To the Max: Margaret Kelly's Post-Cancer Lessons on Living Life to the Fullest," *Better Nutrition*, June 2003, 37.

2. Martha Ramsey, *To Cry or Not to Cry: Coping and Winning the Battle after Mastectomy* (Lufkin, Tex.: Pineywoods, 1995), 10.

3. Ramsey, *To Cry or Not to Cry*, 9.

4. Mayrav Saar, "Race Unites Generations," *Orange County Register,* September 29, 2003, 5.

Chapter Three: Paralyzing Shock

1. Bonnie Davidson, www.pinkribbon.com/my_story.htm (accessed 04/12/04).

2. Tuttle, *Purpose in Trial*.

3. Dr. Jerome Groopman, "The Patient I Will Never Forget," *Parade,* December 21,

2003, 4. Reprinted with permission from *Parade*, copyright © 2003.

    4. Leslie Furth, "In Her Own Words," *Orange County Register*, January 18, 2004, 5.

    5. S. K. Whang, "The Joy of Being Served," *Today's Christian Woman*, March/April 2004, 29.

    6. Martha Ramsey, *To Cry or Not to Cry: Coping and Winning the Battle after Mastectomy* (Lufkin, Tex.: Pineywoods, 1995), 4, 14.

Chapter Four: Asking What If? What About? Why?

    1. Tuttle, *Purpose in Trial*

    2. Bernard Wolfson, "A Turning Point," *Orange County Register*, June 6, 2004, 3.

    3. Bonnie Davidson, www.pinkribbon.com/my_story.htm. Accessed 04/12/04.

    4. Rick Warren, e-mail message to Saddleback Chruch, December 19, 2003. Used by permission.

    5. Davidson, www.pinkribbon.com/my_story.htm.

    6. Tuttle, *Purpose in Trial*.

Chapter Five: Dealing with People's Reactions

    1. Terri Green, *Simple Acts of Kindness: Practical Ways to Help People in Need* (Grand Rapids, Mich.: Revell, 2004).

    2. Nancy Tuttle with Randall Niles, *The Prodigal Prayer* (Mission Viejo, Calif.: Kenosis, 2002).

Chapter Six: Preparing for What Comes Next

    1. Martha Ramsey, *To Cry or Not to Cry: Coping and Winning the Battle after Mastectomy* (Lufkin, Tex.: Pineywoods, 1995), 14–15.

Chapter Seven: Starting Treatment

    1. Dianne Hales, "Why Prayer Could Be Good Medicine, *Parade*, March 23, 2003, 4–5. Reprinted with permission from *Parade*, copyright © 2003.

    2. Bernard Wolfson, "A New Kind of Normal," *Orange County Register*, March 21, 2004, 3.

    3. Brenda Ladun, *Getting Better, Not Bitter: A Spiritual Prescription for Breast Cancer* (Birmingham, Ala.: New Hope, 2002), 96–97.

    4. Janet Gornick, "Surrounded by Love," *Orange County Register*, March 14, 2004, 3.

    5. Leslie Furth, "Light Amid Shadows," *Orange County Register*, February 1, 2004, 3.

    6. Furth, "Light Amid Shadows," 1, 3.

    7. Furth, "Light Amid Shadows," 1, 3.

Chapter Eight: Enjoying the Good Days

    1. Martha Ramsey, *To Cry or Not to Cry: Coping and Winning the Battle after Mastectomy* (Lufkin, Tex.: Pineywoods, 1995), 84.

    2. Roxanne Sayler Henke, *After Anne* (Eugene, Ore.: Harvest House, 2002), 260.

    3. Leslie Furth, "Light Amid Shadows," *Orange County Register*, February 1, 2004, 3.

    4. Camerin Courtney, "The Real Facts—and Fun!—of Life," *Today's Christian Woman*, May/June, 2004, 40.

    5. Ramsey, *To Cry or Not to Cry*, 85.

    6. Ramsey, *To Cry or Not to Cry*, 41.

    7. Leslie Furth, "New Beginning," *Orange County Register*, September 13, 2002, 12.

    8. Furth, "Light Amid Shadows," 3.

    9. Bernard Wolfson, "Rest and Reflection," *Orange County Register*, April 4, 2004, 3.

    10. Janet Gornick, "Surrounded by Love," *Orange County Register*, March 14, 2004, 3.

    11. Nancy Tuttle, *Correspondence with God: The Heart of Prayer Captured in Letters to Our Lord* (Mission Viejo, Calif.: Kenosis, 2002).

Chapter Nine: *Making It through the Bad Days*

1. Nancy Tuttle, *Correspondence with God: The Heart of Prayer Captured in Letters to Our Lord* (Mission Viejo, Calif.: Kenosis, 2002).

2. Brenda Ladun, *Getting Better, Not Bitter: A Spiritual Prescription for Breast Cancer* (Birmingham, Ala.: New Hope, 2002), 51–52.

3. Martha Ramsey, *To Cry or Not to Cry: Coping and Winning the Battle after Mastectomy* (Lufkin, Tex.: Pineywoods, 1995), 22.

4. Ramsey, *To Cry or Not to Cry*, 111.

5. Ramsey, *To Cry or Not to Cry*, 102.

6. Tuttle, *Correspondence with God.*

7. Ramsey, *To Cry or Not to Cry*, 46.

8. Bonnie Davidson, www.pinkribbon.com/my_story.htm.

9. Ramsey, *To Cry or Not to Cry*, 21.

Chapter Ten: *Getting Needed Support*

1. Jane Glenn Haas, "The Second Cancer," *Orange County Register,* September 17, 2003, 8.

2. Brenda Ladun, *Getting Better, Not Bitter: A Spiritual Prescription for Breast Cancer* (Birmingham, Ala.: New Hope, 2002), 153.

3. Nancy Tuttle, *Purpose in Trial: Finding Joy and Meaning in the Midst of Cancer* (Mission Viejo, Calif: Kenosis, 2002).

4. Tuttle, *Purpose in Trial.*

5. Bernard Wolfson, "A New Kind of Normal," *Orange County Register,* March 21, 2004, 3.

6. Wolfson, "A New Kind of Normal."

7. Bernard Wolfson, "One Step at a Time," *Orange County Register,* January 25, 2004, 3.

8. Jennifer Leclaire, "To the Max: Margaret Kelly's Post-Cancer Lessons on Living Life to the Fullest," *Better Nutrition,* June 2003, 39.

Chapter Eleven: *Knowing Who Is in Control*

1. Nancy Tuttle, *Purpose in Trial: Finding Joy and Meaning in the Midst of Cancer* (Mission Viejo, Calif: Kenosis, 2002).

2. Brenda Ladun, *Getting Better, Not Bitter: A Spiritual Prescription for Breast Cancer* (Birmingham, Ala.: New Hope, 2002), 56–57.

3. Leslie Furth, "New Beginning," *Orange County Register,* September 13, 2002, 13.

4. Martha Ramsey, *To Cry or Not to Cry: Coping and Winning the Battle after Mastectomy* (Lufkin, Tex.: Pineywoods, 1995), 55.

5. Tuttle, *Purpose in Trial.*

Chapter Twelve: *Adjusting to a New Normal*

1. Tuttle, *Purpose in Trial.*

2. Bernard Wolfson, "A New Kind of Normal," *Orange County Register,* March 21, 2004), 3.

3. Tuttle, *Purpose in Trial.*

4. Leslie Furth, "New Beginning," *Orange County Register,* September 13, 2002, 3, 12.

5. John Link, MD, *The Breast Cancer Survival Manual* (New York: Henry Holt, 2000), 95.

6. Marisa C. Weiss, MD, and Ellen Weiss, *Living Beyond Breast Cancer* (New York: Three Rivers Press, 1998), 268.

7. Link, *Breast Cancer Survival Manual,* 94–95.

8. Weiss and Weiss, *Living Beyond Breast Cancer,* 268–69.

9. Tuttle, *Purpose in Trial.*

10. Tuttle, *Purpose in Trial.*

Chapter Thirteen: Adapting to Body Changes

1. Nancy Tuttle, *Correspondence with God: The Heart of Prayer Captured in Letters to Our Lord* (Mission Viejo, Calif.: Kenosis , 2002).
2. Bernard Wolfson, "Comfort and Care," *Orange County Register,* March 7, 2004, 3.
3. Elyse Fitzpatrick, and Carol Cornish, *Women Helping Women* (Eugene, Ore.: Harvest House, 1997), 519.
4. Lisa Liddane, "Choices Comfort of Prostheses Rise," *Orange County Register,* September 13, 2002), 9.
5. Ibid.
6. Ibid.
7. Lisa Liddane, "Restoring the Breast and the Hope," *Orange County Register,* September 13, 2002, 8.

Chapter Fourteen: Coping with the Private Issues

1. Nancy Tuttle, *Purpose in Trial: Finding Joy and Meaning in the Midst of Cancer* (Mission Viejo, Calif: Kenosis, 2002).
2. Brenda Ladun, *Getting Better, Not Bitter: A Spiritual Prescription for Breast Cancer* (Birmingham, Ala.: New Hope, 2002), 46.
3. Jane Glenn Haas, "The Second Cancer," *Orange County Register,* September 17, 2003, 8.

Chapter 15—Grieving the Losses

1. Martha Ramsey, *To Cry or Not to Cry: Coping and Winning the Battle after Mastectomy* (Lufkin, Tex.: Pineywoods, 1995), 97.
2. Brenda Ladun, *Getting Better, Not Bitter: A Spiritual Prescription for Breast Cancer* (Birmingham, Ala.: New Hope, 2002), 99–100.
3. Margaret Blackstone, "Living Well with a Chronic Illness," *Parade,* October 12, 2003, 5. Reprinted with permission from *Parade,* copyright © 2003.
4. Ladun, *Getting Better, Not Bitter,* 152–53.
5. Nancy Tuttle, *Purpose in Trial: Finding Joy and Meaning in the Midst of Cancer* (Mission Viejo, Calif: Kenosis, 2002).
6. Anne Ortlund, *The Gentle Ways of the Beautiful Woman* (New York: Inspirational Press, 1998), 47.

Chapter Sixteen: Restoring the Joy!

1. Martha Ramsey, *To Cry or Not to Cry: Coping and Winning the Battle after Mastectomy* (Lufkin, Tex.: Pineywoods, 1995), 115–16.
2. Nancy Tuttle, *Purpose in Trial: Finding Joy and Meaning in the Midst of Cancer* (Mission Viejo, Calif: Kenosis, 2002).
3. Tuttle, *Purpose in Trial.*

Chapter 17—Discovering a New Focus and Purpose

1. Nancy Tuttle, *Correspondence with God: The Heart of Prayer Captured in Letters to Our Lord* (Mission Viejo, Calif.: Kenosis, 2002).
2. Jennifer Leclaire, "To the Max: Margaret Kelly's Post-Cancer Lessons on Living Life to the Fullest," *Better Nutrition,* June 2003, 39.
3. Rick Warren, *The Purpose Driven Life* (Grand Rapids, Mich.: Zondervan, 2002), 35.
4. Kay Marshall Strom, *The Cancer Survival Guide* (Kansas City, Mo.: Beacon Hill, 2002), 86.
5. Warren, *Purpose Driven Life,* 17–18.
6. Warren, *Purpose Driven Life,* 27–33.

7. Nancy Tuttle, *Purpose in Trial: Finding Joy and Meaning in the Midst of Cancer* (Mission Viejo, Calif: Kenosis, 2002).

8. Michele Koidin, "News Anchor's Cancer Battle Goes on the Air," *Orange County Register,* April 29, 2001, 14.

9. Brenda Ladun, *Getting Better, Not Bitter: A Spiritual Prescription for Breast Cancer* (Birmingham, Ala.: New Hope, 2002), 49–50, 52.

10. Robert J. Morgan, comp., *Nelson's Complete Book of Stories, Illustrations, and Quotes* (Nashville: Thomas Nelson, 2000), 779.

Chapter Eighteen: Living with Breast Cancer

1. Bonnie Davidson, www.pinkribbon.com/my_story.htm. Accessed 04/12/04.

2. Sharon Overton, "Healing Baking," *Better Homes and Gardens,* April 2004, 30.

3. Jennifer Leclaire, "To the Max: Margaret Kelly's Post-Cancer Lessons on Living Life to the Fullest," *Better Nutrition,* June 2003, 39.

4. Nancy Tuttle, *Correspondence with God: The Heart of Prayer Captured in Letters to Our Lord* (Mission Viejo, Calif.: Kenosis, 2002).

5. Nancy Tuttle, *Purpose in Trial: Finding Joy and Meaning in the Midst of Cancer* (Mission Viejo, Calif: Kenosis, 2002).

Chapter Nineteen: Relying on God

1. Gordon Dillow, "Prayers Heard, Not Always Answered," *Orange County Register,* March 9, 2004, 1.

2. Frank S. Mead, *12,000 Religious Quotations* (Grand Rapids, Mich.: Baker, 1989), 236.

3. Robert J. Morgan, comp., *Nelson's Complete Book of Stories, Illustrations, and Quotes* (Nashville: Thomas Nelson, 2000), 448.

4. Nancy Tuttle, *Purpose in Trial: Finding Joy and Meaning in the Midst of Cancer* (Mission Viejo, Calif: Kenosis, 2002).

Chapter Twenty: Making a Difference

1. Jane Glenn Haas, "The Second Cancer," *Orange County Register,* September 17, 2003, 8.

2. Brenda Ladun, *Getting Better, Not Bitter: A Spiritual Prescription for Breast Cancer* (Birmingham, Ala.: New Hope, 2002), 153.

3. "The Power of Caring Inspired by Their Mother, the Arquettes Fight Cancer," Cigna Special Advertising Feature, copyright ©2002, Time Inc.

4. Diane Hales, "The Quiet Heroes," *Parade,* March 21, 2004, 4. Reprinted with permission from *Parade,* copyright © 2004.

5. "The Power of Caring Inspired by Their Mother, the Arquettes Fight Cancer."

6. Hales, "The Quiet Heroes."

Chapter Twenty-One: Praying Expectantly

1. Dr. Jerome Groopman, "The Patient I Will Never Forget," *Parade,* December 21, 2003, 6. Reprinted with permission from *Parade,* copyright © 2003.

2. Martha Ramsey, *To Cry or Not to Cry: Coping and Winning the Battle after Mastectomy* (Lufkin, Tex.: Pineywoods, 1995), 135–37.

3. Valerie Kuklenski, "'Ice Bound' Is about People, Not Disease," *Orange County Register,* April 20, 2003, 9.

Chapter Twenty-Two: Ending at the Beginning

1. Anne Ortlund, *The Gentle Ways of the Beautiful Woman* (New York: Inspirational Press, 1998), 212.

2. Dr. Jerome Groopman, "The Patient I Will Never Forget," *Parade,* December 21, 2003, 4–5. Reprinted with permission from *Parade,* copyright © 2003.

3. *Daily Walk,* "David's Kingdom Passed on to Solomon," April 20, 2004, 25. Used by permission.

4. Bernard Wolfson, "Worn and Weary," *Orange County Register,* May 23, 2004, 3.

5. Nancy Tuttle, *Correspondence with God: The Heart of Prayer Captured in Letters to Our Lord* (Mission Viejo, Calif.: Kenosis , 2002).

6. Tuttle, *Correspondence with God.*

Appendix B: Sanity Tools

1. Nancy Tuttle, *Purpose in Trial* (Mission Viejo, Calif: Kenosis, 2002).

2. Martha Ramsey, *To Cry or Not to Cry: Coping and Winning the Battle after Mastectomy* (Lufkin, Tex.: Pineywoods, 1995), 91.

3. S. K. Whang, "The Joy of Being Served," *Today's Christian Woman,* March/April 2004, 29.